Nurses: A Political Force

D0760674

NURSES:
A POLITICAL FORCE

Sarah Ellen Archer
UNIVERSITY OF CALIFORNIA, San Francisco

Patricia A. Goehner
GARFIELD NURSING HOME, Oakland, California

WADSWORTH HEALTH SCIENCES DIVISION
Monterey, California

TO OUR FAMILIES
  Helen, Ross, and Beth Archer
  Gene, Lynn, and Gina Goehner

Sponsoring Editor: Edward F. Murphy
Production: Brian Williams, San Francisco
Manuscript Editor: Carolyn Miller
Interior Design: Wendy Calmenson
Cover Design: Al Burkhardt
Illustrations: Carl Brown
Typesetting: Graphic Typesetting Service, Los Angeles
Production Services Coordinator: Stacey C. Sawyer
Coordinating Designer: Jamie Sue Brooks

WADSWORTH HEALTH SCIENCES DIVISION
A Division of Wadsworth, Inc.

© 1982 by Wadsworth, Inc., Belmont, California 94002. All rights reserved. No
part of this book may be reproduced, stored in a retrieval system, or transcribed,
in any form or by any means—electronic, mechanical, photocopying, recording,
or otherwise—without the prior written permission of the publisher, Wadsworth
Health Sciences Division, Monterey, California 93940, a division of Wadsworth,
Inc.

Printed in the United States of America

10   9   8   7   6   5   4   3   2   1

Library of Congress Cataloging in Publication Data:

Archer, Sarah Ellen.
  Nurses, a political force.

  Bibliography: p.
  Includes index.
    1. Nursing—Political aspects—United States.
  2. Nurses—United States—Political activities.
  3. United States—Politics and government.
  I. Goehner, Patricia A.   II. Title.
  RT86.5.A73   322'.2   81-16206
  ISBN 0-8185-0513-3   AACR2

Foreword

Margretta M. Styles, EdD

Dean, School of Nursing; University of California, San Francisco

FOR THOSE NURSES who view politics as contemptible, irrelevant, mysterious, too big to tackle, or fine for other nurses to be involved in . . .

For those who consider political activity to be a less critical aspect of the nursing role than the management of patient problems or the management of health care units . . .

For those who are convinced of their rightful role as political activists but don't quite know how to go about filling it . . .

For those who want to teach and learn about political activism . . .

For all of the above—whether teachers, students, or practicing nurses—*Nurses: A Political Force* is the book to read. It motivates; it explains; it informs; it illustrates. This volume includes contributions from nurses who are activists themselves, with diverse backgrounds: faculty member, administrator, professional-organization lobbyist, state assemblyperson, congressional committee staff member, local appointive officeholder. The range of subjects included is correspondingly broad and complete: history, theory, conceptual framework, definitions, a typology of political participation, and a catalog of resources. All those subjects are discussed here to stimulate and prepare us for success in fulfilling our political responsibilities as nurses. Why? As stated by the authors, so that we can be "shaped into a cohesive community that can have a considerable impact on the decisions and policies that affect health care in the United States." For us to do less is to fail our mission to society.

The authors found, in a survey among nurse leaders, that the major reason given for low participation in political affairs is lack of know-how. This finding supports the need to include content of this nature in basic and advanced curricula in nursing. You hold in your hand an exceedingly valuable resource for such courses.

We should all read on, and then act with political awareness, acumen, and vigor.

Acknowledgments

WE WISH TO thank the following people for their invaluable support and assistance in making this book possible:

To several generations of graduate students in our "Legislative Processes and Strategies" course, who have urged us on by clamoring for a text. They were our incentive to begin this work, they have sustained our enthusiasm for it, and they will be our severest and most welcome critics.

To Ruth Fleshman, whose critiques and editing, especially of Sarah's spelling, vastly improved our work.

To Hanna Regev, Gina Goehner, and Tess Jones, whose "magic fingers" typed and typed and typed . . .

To Joanne Rabinowe, Kit Kerwick and Nancy Snyder, who saw us through the whole thing.

Sarah Ellen Archer
Patricia A. Goehner

The Contributors

Sarah Ellen Archer, RN, DrPH,
FAPHA, FAAN, CNAA
Associate Professor
Community Health Nursing and
Administration
Department of Mental Health and
Community Nursing
School of Nursing
University of California, San
Francisco
Trustee and Secretary, Nursing
Dynamics Corporation
Mill Valley, CA

Cheryl Beversdorf, RN, MScHy
Legislative Assistant
New York State Office of Federal
Affairs
Washington, DC
Formerly: Member of Senator Alan
Cranston's Staff
Veterans' Affairs Committee
United States Senate

Dona Wilcox Cutting, RN, MS
Administrative Aide
Congressman Ronald Dellums
Lafayette, CA

Ruth P. Fleshman, RN, PhD
President
Nursing Dynamics Corporation
Mill Valley, CA

Patricia A. Goehner, RN, MS
Director of Nursing Services
Garfield Nursing Home
Oakland, CA
Trustee, Nursing Dynamics
Corporation
Mill Valley, CA

Claire Mailhot, RN, MS
Clinical Coordinator
Stanford–Palo Alto Medical Center
Palo Alto, CA

Jean M. Moorhead, RN, MS
Assemblywoman
5th District
California State Legislature
Sacramento, CA

Contents

Nurses: A Political Force

Part I

WHETHER USED in formal courses or independently, this book is designed to help nurses become more politically effective. The contributors have been chosen, therefore, because they are role models of nurse-activism. In Chapter 1, we set the stage by briefly reviewing pertinent literature on nursing and politics. We then offer definitions of politics and a typology of political participation, followed by an overview of the book.

Chapter 2, "The Women's Movement: How We Got Where We Are," by Claire Mailhot and Sarah Ellen Archer, traces the development of the women's movement in the United States from Colonial times to ERA. The purpose of this chapter is to raise female nurses' consciousness regarding the limitations that their socialization as women and as nurses places on them. Political activism, particularly collective activism, offers opportunities for nurses to bring about changes not only in their own status but also in health care provision and the kinds of services their clients receive.

In Chapter 3, Sarah Ellen Archer discusses some fundamental political concepts for nurse-activists. She begins with a detailed presentation of systems theory from a political perspective and presents a political-systems model. The typology of power describes a number of kinds of power including legitimate, expert, corruptive, referrent, associative, lower-participant, nutrient, rational, charismatic, and sexually based. Each kind of power is discussed as it applies to the political arena. Other concepts dealt with in the chapter are decision making, conflict, and change.

In Chapter 4, Sarah Ellen Archer begins her discussion of political

Theoretical Background

strategies with a section on assertiveness, an essential skill for nurses who want to be politically effective. Role models, mentors, and networking are much-needed tools in the nurse's political kit. Role models and mentors show the way and run interference. Networking draws together people of like minds and similar interests for professional, political, and personal support. Archer then presents some guidelines for getting involved in campaigns for candidates and for ballot initiatives before turning to a brief discussion of some ways to influence policy. Since many nurses are public employees, she includes a brief discussion of what kinds of political activities the Hatch Act does and does not prohibit. Finally, political parties and political action committees are considered because they are both vehicles nurses can use to become more politically active.

In Chapter 5, Patricia A. Goehner looks at legislatures, legislators, and the processes a bill goes through in each state and on the national level on the way to becoming a law. A large part of nursing practice is governed by legislation, and Goehner describes how nurses can be active participants in this lawmaking process. As nurses read this chapter, they will become aware of the steps a bill progresses through before becoming a law, and where they can provide input during this process so as to become influential and active participants. In learning how to use the legislative process, nurses will become known, heard, and recognized. Such effective recognition will enable nurses to determine the future of their profession as well as the future of much of the health care system. Thus nurses will become indispensible in health care decision making.

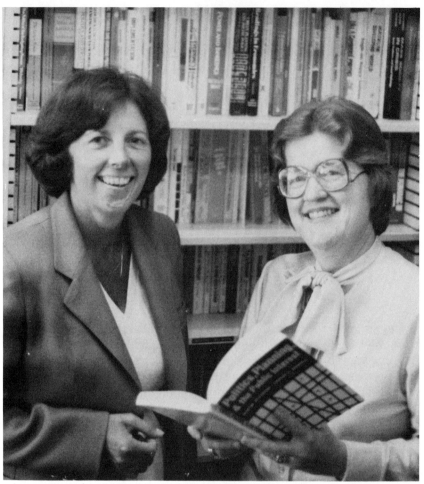

Patricia A. Goehner (left) and Sarah Ellen Archer. *(Photo by Katherine McInerney)*

CHAPTER 1

Introduction and Overview

Sarah Ellen Archer and Patricia A. Goehner

IN SPITE of the concern about dropouts, nurses are still the largest group of licensed health care providers in the United States. The 1977 National Sample of Registered Nurses shows that, of the 1,401,633 RNs with current licenses, 70 percent were employed in nursing (Moses & Roth, 1979). This figure means that approximately 981,000 nurses are in some kind of active practice. By sheer force of numbers we should and could have much more say than we do on health care provision, health care policy, cost containment, and reimbursement. Effective participation in any and all of these arenas requires an understanding of the politics involved. One of the reasons why nurses do not have significant influence in these areas is that we are neither as united nor as well financed in political activities as are other special-interest groups such as the American Medical Association and the American Hospital Association (Diers 1978; Grissum & Spengler, 1976 Holt, 1976; Moorhead, 1979; Mullane, 1979; see also Chapter 4).

Other reasons for nurses' lack of participation, as determined in our own study of nurse-administrators across the country, include lack of preparation for participation, apathy, lack of awareness of issues, and failure to realize the importance of participation (Archer & Goehner,

SARAH ELLEN ARCHER, RN, DrPH, FAPHA, FAAN, CNAA, FRSH, is associate professor, community health nursing and administration, in the Department of Mental Health and Community Nursing, School of Nursing, University of California at San Francisco. She is also trustee and secretary, Nursing Dynamics Corporation, in Mill Valley, California.
PATRICIA A. GOEHNER, RN, MS, is director of nursing services, Garfield Nursing Home, in Oakland, and trustee, Nursing Dynamics Corporation.

forthcoming). Kalish (1978), Lawrence (1976), and Matejski (1979) state that the greatest threat to the nursing profession is nurses' apathy about social and health care issues. Still more reasons nurses do not have influence in politics relate to our socialization as nurses and our failure to realize our potential political clout. Deloughery and Gebbie state that nurses' involvement in political activities is societally based (1975). Holt (1976) more specifically states that female nurses are politically naïve because of their socialization into the woman's role and the service role (see Chapter 2). We feel that all of these reasons for nurses' low political participation are related to an overriding deficit: nurses are generally not taught or encouraged to become politically active. Levinson expresses concern over nurses' lack of legislative education (1977). Kalish and Kalish state that nurses need to overcome our political apathy and adopt positive attitudes toward political activity (1976). They feel that this conversion process should begin in nursing education with a class on the politics of nursing. Indeed, the broadening of nurses' knowledge of the political process will enable us to identify and speak to the unmet needs of the profession and the unmet health needs of Americans (Anderson, Leonard, & Yates, 1974; Matejski, 1979).

Nurses must be better prepared for political participation and be rewarded for those activities. The role of nurse-activist in a variety of political arenas must be further developed and perfected. Many of us already play such roles and have not only learned how to do so but also have experienced the euphoria of success as well as the depression of failure. Having learned much from both kinds of experiences, we are ready to move on to the next issue, the next contest. Nurses have clout and must learn to use it. The contributors to this book have all learned their lessons well and, by sharing their experiences with you, seek to motivate you to become nurse-activists also.

In this chapter we discuss the purposes of the book and offer some definitions by way of setting the semantic stage for what will follow. The bulk of the definitions section is devoted to a presentation of the typology of political participation that we developed and used in our study of nurse-leaders' political participation (Archer & Goehner, forthcoming). We then provide an overview of the contents of the book.

Most of what we and our contributors have written about focuses on political arenas outside of single agencies or organizations. This is because we believe that most of us are more familiar with and more adept at working in and around internal organizational political situations than we are in the external arena. Of course, many of the strategies presented are equally as applicable to internal organizational politics as they are to politics on local, state, and national levels. We feel that political preparation for nurses at this time must focus on these larger arenas.

We have assiduously avoided making this a civics book, since there are many excellent books that address political science in general and the particular history and development of political institutions and practices in the United States (Easton, 1979; Nie, Verba, & Petrocik, 1976; Redman, 1973; Sabine & Thorson, 1973). We have included a number of these in the annotated bibliography at the end of the book for your further reading. Also, because this is a book about political participation in the United States, its content is not applicable to other countries or political systems. Of course, some of the strategies presented are transferable, but even then caution must be used. We have chosen to concentrate on providing United States nurses with workable and practical preparation so that our participation will be more effective in whatever political arena or arenas we elect to become nurse-activists.

PURPOSES OF THE BOOK

As noted, the overriding goal of this book is to help to prepare nurses to be more politically effective. To do this we and our contributors address some specific objectives:

1. *To assist faculty in all levels of nursing curricula, continuing education, and in-service education to devise and teach courses or parts of courses to prepare their students to be nurse-activists.* One of our motivations for writing this book was that we could not find a dynamic text for our own political-strategies course. Elsewhere we have provided a guide for faculty who want to develop a course in political participation for nurses. We have discussed objectives, requirements, content to be included in the course itself, content that can be drawn from other nursing courses and cognates, and suggestions for field experience and projects (Archer & Goehner, 1981). Chapters 3, 4, and 5 are theoretical and strategic bases for political participation. The Yellow Pages, Chapter 10, provides information on many political organizations across the United States, about which nurses who become political activists may wish to know more. Chapters 6 through 9 are case studies of nurse-activists' participation. Chapter 2 provides background on the women's movement.
2. *To provide students enrolled in all levels of nursing education with a basic reference with which to increase their preparation for political activity. It can be used either in formal courses or as an independent study vehicle if no formal courses are available.* We and our contributors have focused on providing concrete

examples of a variety of nurse-activist preparations that we hope will help others to pursue similar kinds of roles.

3. *To provide the individual practicing nurse with an independent study opportunity to increase her or his understanding of how to become more involved in political activities.* We hope to reach our colleagues already in practice, in order to stimulate their interest, augment their expertise, and intensify their political participation.

4. *To provide role models of a variety of nurse-activists.* All of the contributors to this book are politically active women and nurses. We have described many of our own political activities because they are what we know best. Our intent is to serve as examples for others who want to increase their involvement as nurse-activists.

SOME DEFINITIONS

Before we go any further in this discussion of what the book is about, we need to define some critical terms so that our readers will understand the sense in which we use them.

Politics

There are probably as many definitions of politics as there are people thinking about it. The following definitions are all useful in describing what we mean when we talk about politics.

> Politics is the art of creating actions by entire communities. Politics is shaping many disparate social elements into societal, not private action. It is the art of directing societies (Novack 1973:9).

This definition reinforces our conviction that nurses can be shaped into a cohesive community that can have a considerable impact on the decisions and policies that affect health care in the United States. Nursing is not now a cohesive community. If we were to recognize the potential clout that we have, if we were more unified, then we might be willing to settle some of our internal differences and present a more united front.

Aristotle, in one of the earliest known writings on politics, points out that politics has to do with power, and with authority relationships between people and among institutions. Much of the political process, therefore, is focused on deciding who the supreme authority will be and what decisions will be under the purview of that individual or small group (1952). Weber describes political action in terms of the enforcement of an order within a given territorial or geographic area; the enforcement is predicated on the threat of physical force by those in authority to ensure that their wishes are carried out (1947). (We shall hear much more of power and Weber in Chapter 3.) Political decisions are translated into laws and regulations that increasingly affect everything we do in both our personal and professional lives. Failing to be actively involved in concerted efforts to influence and shape such decisions, is to resign ourselves to passive participation in our society, and sets the stage for us to be reactors to what others decide for us rather than actors on our own behalf.

Leininger defines politics as "the art of influencing another's thoughts and actions for individual self-interests, group needs, and/or societal goals" (1978:2). This process of influencing others either for one's own interests or on behalf of another group involves decision making, community organization, interest articulation, coalition formation, lobbying, and monitoring functions, all of which we shall hear more about later in this book.

The common themes that run through these and other definitions of politics involve power, influence, and authority in interpersonal and intergroup relationships within a defined jurisdiction or territory. For example, the United States Congress passes laws that can directly affect what every man, woman, and child in our country may or may not do. Failure to follow these laws can lead to sanctions, because the government has the power to enforce what it believes is in the best interests of the society, even if an individual may not be enthusiastic about complying.

The element of conflict is implicit in all of these definitions. Conflict arises the minute more than one demand is made on scarce resources. As long as everyone can have all that he or she wants, then there is little reason for conflict to arise; however, this happy state of affairs rarely exists, and so competing claims for finite resources result. To avoid violence, competing parties must have the opportunity to meet, negotiate, compromise, and reach at least temporary agreement. Conflict management and resolution are essential components of political activities. Many of these concepts are dealt with at length in Chapter 3.

Political Participation

We use the term *political participation* in an extremely broad sense to encompass many kinds of activities. The typology of political participation developed from our initial study of nurse-leaders is shown in

Table 1.1. (Archer & Goehner, forthcoming). We have divided our typology into three sections on the basis of whether the activities are active or passive and involve commitment of long- or short-term time and effort.

TABLE 1.1
Typology of Political Participation

Active Long-Term Political Participation

Organize local groups to work on health-related problems

Serve as a working member of local boards or commissions such as health-systems agencies, League of Women Voters, the Agency on Aging

Serve as a working member of state boards or commissions such as a state Board of Health, gubernatorial commissions, task forces, advisory commissions

Serve as a working member of national-level commissions or task forces such as presidential advisory councils

Run for and hold elective office at any level of government

Participating on political parties' committees such as platform committees

Participate on nursing organizations' political committees such as N-CAP, state N-PAC

Participate in general political activities of ANA, NLN, or one of the nursing specialty organizations

Participate in politically oriented organizations such as the League of Women Voters, the National Women's Political Caucus, the Health Action Coalition.

Active Short-Term Political Participation

Work for the election of local, state, or national candidates known to support health care and nursing issues

Work to qualify issues as ballot initiatives or referenda

Give testimony on health- or nursing-related issues before legislative committees' or regulatory bodies' hearings at the local level

Give testimony on health- or nursing-related issues before legislative committees' or regulatory bodies' hearings at the state level

Give testimony on health- or nursing-related issues before legislative committees' or regulatory bodies' hearings at the national level

Visit policy makers to lobby for specific issues

Write or telephone policy makers to lobby for specific issues

Passive Political Participation

Contribute money to candidates and/or initiative campaigns

Contribute money to political parties or political action committees

Vote

Active Long-Term Participation. The activities in this classification require an on-going commitment by participants and often a great deal of time and work. Most of them involve organization building and maintenance. The most time-consuming ones, in our experience, are the organizing of local groups and being an active member of boards or commissions at local, state, and national levels. Participation in organizations such as the American Nurses' Association, N-CAP, the League of Women Voters, and the National Women's Political Caucus as elected officers or committee chairpeople also requires considerable time, often approaching a full-time job. Although many of these positions are strictly voluntary, they provide considerable work experience and responsibility, especially in the areas of administration and public relations. Remember this fact when you are making up a résumé, and include those positions in it. Clearly, the activities listed in this section of the typology have a life much greater than the duration of a single election.

Running for and holding elective office, activities we did not include in our study because of the population to whom it was addressed, are perhaps the ultimate in active long-term participation. More nurses are seeking and winning elective office; we need to do all that we can to foster this encouraging trend.

Active Short-Term Participation. The activities listed here require considerable effort but for a relatively short period of time, generally one election. Many are limited to the duration of one campaign or to the occasion of providing testimony at hearings of legislative or regulatory bodies. Again the major criterion separating them from active long-term participation activities is the time, effort, and commitment they require.

Passive Participation. Contributing money and voting are the activities that fall into this classification of political activities. Such participation involves neither significant time nor effort. This fact is not meant to demean their importance by any means, but rather to point out that they are qualitatively and quantitatively different from both active long- and short-term participation, activities in which nurse-activists are sorely needed.

Our typology includes many of the political activities that Milbraith describes (1965, 1968). He categorized political activities as follows: (1) "spectator activities," which involve voting, proselytizing, and wearing a campaign button; (2) "transitional activities," such as giving money and attending meetings; and (3) "gladiator activities," which include working in a campaign, joining a club, and other activities that we have defined as active long-term participation (1965).

We did not include such activities as street demonstrations and riots because we felt they are not applicable to the populations we studied. Although on-site and informational picketing are highly political activities, we did not include them, either, because the population we studied consisted of administrators. The typology of political participation presented here is more extensive than the one developed by Verba and Nie (1972), although many of the activities we have listed are similar to theirs.

OVERVIEW OF THE BOOK

Part I: "Theoretical Background." This first part includes this chapter on introduction and definitions, a discussion of the women's movement, two chapters on fundamental concepts and strategies for political participation, and a chapter on the processes in the several states and territories through which an idea goes to become a law.

Chapter 2: "The Women's Movement: How We Got Where We Are," as the title suggests, focuses on the development of women's political activism in the United States from Colonial times until the present. Since this is a book by women about political participation by members of a profession that is more than 90 percent women, talking about women's issues is appropriate. Although men in nursing may find themselves having to deal with many of the kinds of discrimination women face, women are generally socialized to avoid risks, to shun conflict, to acquiesce to authority, and generally to keep a lower profile than are men. Such behaviors are antithetical to effective political participation and women must unlearn them. The point of Chapter 2 is to provide a brief consciousness-raising experience for readers not already familiar with women's history in the United States.

Chapter 3: "Selected Concepts Fundamental to Nurses' Political Activism" presents a basic conceptual framework for political participation. Systems theory applied to political processes sets the stage. A political-systems model (Figure 5.1) shows the interdependencies and intradependencies of the political system and its internal and external environments. A typology of power is developed and discussed as a means of illustrating the many faces power can and does wear in political arenas. The crux of public policy is the decision-making process. As long as there are fewer claimants than there are resources, decision making is relatively easy and conflicts are minimal. When there are more claimants than resources, decision making becomes a political process. A decision matrix is presented as an aid to policy makers in their deliberations. Conflict is seen as an unavoidable and indeed often beneficial element in politics and change. Types of conflict and strategies for dealing with conflict are discussed. Finally, three types of change strategies are considered.

Chapter 4: "Political Strategies for Nurses' Involvement" includes selected techniques for political participation. We begin with assertiveness, a key to being effective in any situation. A short values-clarification exercise precedes the discussion of assertiveness, aggressiveness, and avoidance/acquiescence behaviors as they vary in terms of personal characteristics such as leadership style, the ability to take risks, and perceptions of conflict. Role models, mentors, and networking are presented as ideas whose time have come for women in general and female nurses in particular. Some strategies for working in political campaigns for individuals and issues as well as techniques for influencing policy makers are briefly presented. Since many nurses are public employees, a listing is given of the areas the Hatch Act does and does not cover in prohibiting public employee involvement in partisan politics. Finally, political parties and political action committees, both vehicles for political involvement, are also discussed.

Chapter 5: "Legislatures and Legislation" is a basic "how to" presentation of how ideas become bills, become laws, and become regulations. The roles of Congress, state legislatures, and local legislative bodies are discussed. There are some surprising differences in procedures from state to state. Each of us must know the exact process in our own state in order to intervene effectively in the procedure.

Part II: "Nurses' Roles in Political Processes." This part contains in-depth descriptions by nurses of their experience in local, state, and national political arenas: lobbying, running for office, organizing grassroots political activities, and serving as a staff member of a congressional committee.

Chapter 6: "The Nurse as Lobbyist" focuses on the processes nurses can use to actively influence policy makers. Starting with a historical perspective on the development of lobbying, the right to peacefully petition government, this chapter contains detailed information about lobbying strategies. Information on the regulation of lobbyists and other campaign regulations is included. Nurses and nursing organizations increasingly recognize that using individual and collective clout to intervene early and effectively in political processes is vital to the quality of health care available to the American public as well as to the practice of nursing. Activities of nurses' organizations are discussed as positive and effective steps toward making nurses' clout felt. Political decisions are much too vital to health care, nurses, and nursing to be left in the hands of politicians. Nurses must learn to be more effective lobbyists, and this chapter provides some valuable guidelines on doing just that.

Chapter 7: "Running for Office" provides another insight into one way nurses can influence policy making—by becoming policy makers. The more nurses we have on the inside of legislative and regulatory bodies, the better we will be able to develop and implement policies that affect health care and nursing. This very human description of the joys and frustrations of being a candidate is a realistic picture of what those who decide to run for office can expect. The author was a lobbyist on the California Nurses' Association's Governmental Relations staff before she made her successful bid for the state Assembly. She learned a tremendous amount about the workings of the legislature, campaigning, and politics in general before she ever undertook her own election race. She has stated publicly that she believes her preparation and practice as a community health nurse is the best background she could have had for her job as assemblywoman. We would concur! We hope that more nurses will follow the lead of nurse-legislators and run for offices at all levels of government.

Chapter 8: "Nurses in Local Political Organizations" is another real-life description of nurses working in community organizing activities. Particular emphasis is given to nurses' roles as advocates, documentors, and organizers for consumer and provider coalitions to improve the quality, quantity, and accessibility of health care services on a local level. The author makes a convincing case for her belief that the local arena, in her case a county, is a place where nurse's political participation is needed and can be highly effective.

Chapter 9: "The Nurse as a Congressional Committee Staff Member" provides insight into the author's role as the only health professional on the Senate Veterans' Affairs Committee in Washington. Using her experience as an example, she offers some hints about how other nurses can prepare for and obtain similar positions. She comes from a background in public health and community health nursing and has worked as a staff member for several professional organizations. She has made all these pieces fit together in attaining her goal of being a staff member on "the Hill."

Part III: "Resources." This final section includes a three-part listing of resources available to the nurse-activist, as well as an extensive reading list.

Chapter 10: "The Nurses' Political Yellow Pages" seeks to acquaint nurses with some of the vast variety of resources available to those nurses interested in various facets of politics. Section 1 presents brief descriptions of a number of national political and professional organizations and agencies. The American Nurses' Association, the National League for Nursing, and all of the current members of the Federation of Nursing Specialty Organizations and ANA are included. Section 2 lists political and professional organization resources on a state-by-state basis. This individual state listing will help nurses to make contacts and to begin networking within their own states. Those who do so will become aware of many more resources that are available on the local level. Nurses should develop their own Yellow Pages for specific locales and special areas of interest. We invite additional listings for our Yellow Pages so that we may update and expand them periodically. Such a resource can never be either complete or totally up-to-date. Section 3 contains a selected list of political publications, mostly periodicals, that can be highly valuable sources of much-needed information.

Chapter 11: "State-by-State Bill-to-Law Procedures" refers to the specific bill-to-law procedures of all of the states and territories in the United States.

The annotated bibliography at the end of the book is included for those who wish to undertake more extensive reading in political science and other aspects of nursing and politics.

REFERENCES

Anderson EM, Leonard BM, Yates J: Epigenesis of the nurse practitioner role. *American Journal of Nursing* 74: 1816, October 1974.

Archer SE, Goehner PA: Acquiring political clout: Guidelines for nurse administrators. *Journal of Nursing Administration.* Forthcoming.

Archer SE, Goehner PA: *Speaking Out: The Views of Nurse Leaders.* New York, National League for Nursing, Pub. No. 15-1847, 1981.

Aristotle: *Politics.* The Great Books Series, Vol. 9. Chicago, University of Chicago Press, 1952.

Deloughery GL, Gebbie KM: *Political Dynamics: Impact on Nurses and Nursing.* St. Louis, Mo, CV Mosby Co., 1975.

Diers D: A different kind of energy: Nurse power. *Nursing Outlook* 26: 51-55, January 1978.

Easton D: *A Systems Analysis of Political Life.* 1965. Reprint. Chicago, University of Chicago Press, 1979.

Glenn N, Grimes M: Aging, voting, and political interest. *American Sociological Review* 33:563-575, 1968.

Grissum Mr, Spengler C: *Women, Power, and Health Care.* Boston, Little, Brown & Co., 1976.

Holt JP: The struggles inside nursing's body politics. *Nursing Forum* 15:324-340, April 1976.

Kalish BJ: The promise of power. *Nursing Outlook* 26:42-46, January 1978.

————, Kalish PA: A discourse on the politics of nursing. *Journal of Nursing Administration* 6:29-33, March 1976.

Lawrence JC: Confronting nurses' political apathy. *Nursing Forum* 15:363, 1976.

Leininger M: Political nursing: Essential for health service and education systems for tomorrow. *Nursing Administration Quarterly* 2:1-16, Spring 1978.

Levinson R: Knowledge of professional nursing legislation. *Nursing Times* 73:674-676, 1977.

Matejski MS: Politics, the nurse, and the political process. *Nursing Leadership* 2:31-37, January 1979.

Milbraith, LW: *Political Participation*. Chicago, Rand McNally Co., 1965.

————: The nature of political beliefs and the relationship of the individual to the government. *American Behavioral Scientist* 12:31-32, November-December 1968.

Monsma SV: *American Politics: A Systems Approach*. New York, Holt, Rinehart, & Winston, 1969.

Moorhead JM: Community health nurses' involvement in legislative activities, in Archer SE, Fleshman RP (eds): *Community Health Nursing: Patterns and Practice*, ed 2. North Scituate, Mass, Duxbury Press, 1979, pp 566-591.

Moses E, Roth A: Nurse Power. *American Journal of Nursing* 79:1745-1756, October 1979.

Mullane MK: Nursing care and the political arena. *Nursing Outlook* 23:699-701, November 1975.

Nie NH, Verba S, Petrocik JR: *The Changing American Voter*. Cambridge, Mass, Harvard University Press, 1976.

Novak M: Politics as drama. *The Center Magazine* 3:9, Summer 1969.

Redman E: *The Dance of Legislation*. New York, Simon & Schuster, 1973.

Sabine GH, Thorson TL: *A History of Political Thought*, ed 4. Hinsdale, Ill, Dryden Press, 1973.

Verba S, Nie NH: *Participation in America: Political Democracy and Social Equity*. New York, Harper & Row, 1972.

Weber M: *The Theory of Social and Economic Organization*, Parsons T (trans). New York, Oxford University Press, 1947.

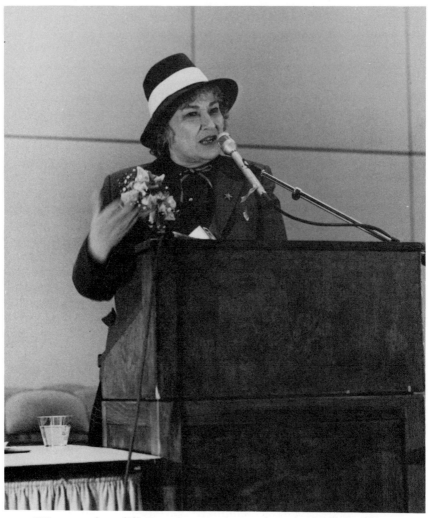

"We can make a difference," women's movement leader Bella Abzug
tells the California Nurses' Association 1981 Convention. *(Photo
courtesy California Nurses' Association)*

CHAPTER 2

The Women's Movement: How We Got Where We Are

Claire Mailhot and Sarah Ellen Archer

IF WE AS women are to understand how we have reached our present state of affairs in our search for equal rights, autonomy, and self-esteem, we need at least a brief introduction to the history of women in the United States and the quest for equality. Fascinating though the topic is, the scope of this book limits the depth to which we can plumb the history of the women's movement. We have discussed some of the major highlights of the movement and have included a fairly extensive bibliography for those of you who want more. We have talked a little about some of the changes nursing has been and is going through, and we raise some questions about why nurses are not more visible in the women's movement. Appendixes A and B of the book relate to this chapter; the first appendix presents selected laws and executive orders affecting women's rights. The second appendix contains a brief presentation of survey data from 88 community nurse-practitioners who were asked what impact the women's movement was having on nursing and on them as individuals.

THE FIRST WOMEN'S MOVEMENT IN THE UNITED STATES

Early History

European settlers coming to the New World brought with them their religious, social, and political customs. These customs included a long-held belief in the basic inferiority of women to men, particularly in

CLAIRE MAILHOT, R.N., M.S., is clinical coordinator at Stanford–Palo Alto Medical Center, Palo Alto, California.

political and economic affairs outside of the home. Thus, with few exceptions, the lot of the white woman was little different from that of the Black people who were brought into the new country as slaves for the southern plantations. All were socially, economically, and politically under the direct control of white men—husbands or owners. This basic social pattern was institutionalized in the state constitutions, which permitted only free men who owned property to vote and thus to participate in political affairs. Universal white male suffrage evolved gradually within the states and at the federal level, but Black men were not permitted to vote until the ratification of the 25th Amendment to the US Constitution in March 1870, and no woman was permitted to vote until the ratification of the 29th Amendment in August 1920.

In Colonial America, therefore, white women and Blacks had no voice in public matters. Certainly women had considerable say in the management and organization of their families. Life in Colonial America was rigorous, to say the least, and division of labor within the household was essential for the family's survival. Because of the vital role they played in this struggle for survival, wives attained a good deal of influence, even controlling household matters. With few exceptions, this sphere of influence seldom extended beyond the edge of the family's property.

One of the most notable of these exceptions was attorney Mistress Margaret Brent of Maryland, who owned and managed her own estate and participated in political and legal activities connected with her own and her family's affairs. She also served as administrator for many Colonists' estates. In 1647 she was named executrix of the will of Maryland's governor, Leonard Calvert. As such for a period of time she managed not only his estates, but also administered the affairs of Maryland. She clearly demonstrated by her deeds, as well as by her words, that women could have a place and a voice in government. Many in Maryland believed that she should be elected governor of the colony in her own right, but that was not to be (Hymowitz & Weissman, 1978). That event, the election of a woman as governor of a state in her own right rather than as a successor to her husband, did not occur until 1974, when Ella Grasso became governor of Connecticut.

The influence that wives have had on their husband's political aspirations and activities is apparent from the earliest moments in our history. Abigail Adams managed the Adams family's farms and accounts throughout the time that John was away working on the Declaration of Independence, the Revolution, the Constitution, and the country's relations with European allies. Her correspondence, in addition to day-to-day details of family and business affairs, shows her keen interest in and grasp of the issues of the day, and documents the pleas for recognition of women's political rights—not always welcome—that she directed to John (Adams, 1972; Butterfield, 1963). Although their letters have been lost, there is considerable evidence that Martha Jefferson exerted a deep and lasting influence on her husband, Thomas Jefferson (Brodie, 1974). Eleanor Roosevelt, more recently, was for Franklin Roosevelt a vital extension into a world in which he could not easily travel (Lash, 1971). Eleanor was also a staunch supporter of women's rights (Roosevelt, 1933).

Colonial women were of necessity partners with their men. They often took over farm or business when something happened to their men-folk. Such relationships of relative equality and interdependence persisted among the settlers who moved West, but for their sisters in settled areas of the country, changes began to occur. A new personality theory gradually developed that stressed "man's sphere" and "woman's sphere" and the great differences and separations between the two. This development accompanied the emergence of the middle class as a result of increased urbanization and the growth of commerce, particularly in the Northeastern states. Urbanization made families less dependent on their women to produce their clothing, to raise and preserve their food, and to be the sole providers of other essential goods and services. Increasingly men worked outside of the home in trade and manufacturing. Their salaries were used to buy those goods the urban family's women no longer produced. Work became associated with money, and so women, who earned no money, became increasingly dependent on their husbands. The results of these factors were the rise of the middle class, the loss of the balance of division of labor between men and women within families, and the doctrine that a woman's "sphere" was in the home where she was to labor in isolation and without pay at her traditional tasks of child rearing and homemaking (Hymowitz & Weissman, 1978). These societal changes increased the social, economic, and political gaps between men and women. The prevailing attitude was that "nice women" were those who stayed at home, took care of their husbands and children, and left the workings of the real world beyond their front gate to men, who were much better suited for such activities.

The spread of the Industrial Revolution, with its shift from home production of goods to large-scale centralized manufacturing, joined with these events to reshape women's roles still further and to make the struggle for equal rights even more difficult. In the 1800s the belief in women's inferiority continued, although with some changes. Two definite classes of women were becoming more apparent in urban American society: middle- and upper-class women and working-class women. The wealthy were made so because of the rapid growth of industrialization, which their men dominated. The working class provided the labor on which this wealth was built (Ehrenreich & English, 1973). Much of the cheap labor needed for factories and mills in communities such as Lowell, Massachusetts, and other industry towns, was provided by lower-class women and their children, often under deplorable conditions.

Women's social roles in these two classes were polar opposites. Affluent women were expected to live leisurely and quietly and not to indulge in any physical work or mental strain because of their innate frailties. Working-class women were expected to do back-breaking work, to manage their homes, and to raise their children. These two views of women's abilities were obviously in direct conflict. Women could not be seen as frail yet strong enough to work in factories. Therefore, biomedical thought justified these two fundamentally contradictory roles of women with the theory that there were two different species of women. Affluent women were inherently sick, and too weak and delicate for anything but the mildest pastimes, while working-class women, having come from different stock, were inherently strong and robust. In reality, the opposite was true. The affluent woman, because of her more sheltered environment, was much less disease prone although more physically frail than the working-class woman, who put in long hours, got little rest, was poorly nourished, and lived in unsanitary conditions. Doctors gradually realized that the soft life of upper-class women contributed to their frailty. Many capitalized on this fact because well-to-do women were the only ones who could afford doctors. Some physicians encouraged long periods of convalescence, requiring continuous medical supervision. Since, at that time, all unacceptable behavior on women's part was considered an illness, any woman attempting to become active in a social cause was quickly put to bed and led to believe that she was ill. Frequently husbands called in physicians when their wives became opinionated, sought greater sexual activity, or demanded more recognition. Thus men continued to define women's roles.

Doctors realized that lower-class women did not faint or develop "female problems" as frequently because of their active life-styles. But their environment increased their risk of typhoid, cholera, and venereal diseases. The doctors did not often intervene with medical care for these women. Someone had to carry out chores in the homes of affluent women, and lower-class women were also needed in the labor force. After all, lower-class women could not pay a physician or afford the luxury of leisure time prescribed for healing. Underlying all this conflict in women's roles were two sexist ideologies: contempt for women who were weak and frail, and a fear of any other kind of woman as dangerous and polluting (Ehrenreich & English, 1973).

Many women began to see and to resent the attitude that they were inferior and should be subject to their husband's and other men's decisions about all aspects of their lives. This awakening of women's desires for identities of their own, the development of political concerns for individual rights and freedom, and the prevailing societal attitudes of women's inferiority and weakness set the stage for women's struggles for equal rights for themselves as well as for men who were deprived of their "natural rights." The battle is far from over.

Women Reformers

Great is the temptation to turn this chapter into an in-depth study of the leaders of the first women's movement, but that is beyond the scope and purpose of this book. Their stories are fascinating and those of you who are interested in pursuing the study of the roots of feminism will find at least a beginning point in the bibliography. A few of our forebears must be mentioned all too briefly.

In 1792, Mary Wollstonecraft, a British woman, wrote *A Vindication of the Rights of Women*, a book that was to become the handbook of the feminist movement (Wollstonecraft, 1973). In this work, Wollstonecraft spoke out in favor of "natural rights" and against all kinds of enslavement, including that of women by men, even as the American and French revolutions were overthrowing governments that sought to enslave their citizens. The doctrine of "natural rights" is clearly present in our own Declaration of Independence: ". . . that they are endowed by their Creator with certain inalienable rights; that among these are life, liberty, and the pursuit of happiness." Little did the authors of these words realize how soon they would come back to haunt them. For these words formed part of the platform on which the reform movements of the 1800s were built.

Religion was, and often remains, largely the concern of women, because of their role as child rearers. In the 1800s religion played a large and vital role in the socialization of children. Thus it was "all right" for women to engage in religious activities, even if these pursuits soon became inextricably involved with politics. Feminist leaders Lucretia Mott, Sarah and Angelina Grimke, Lucy Stone, and Elizabeth Cady Stanton got their start in the anti-slavery movement; Susan B. Anthony made her debut in the reform movement as the organizer of Daughters of Temperance societies. All of these women soon realized that their rights as women were as sorely compromised as were those of the slaves they sought to set free. In fact, it was when Lucretia Mott and Elizabeth Cady Stanton, as well as all other women, were barred from participating in the World Anti-Slavery Convention in London in 1840, after they had crossed the Atlantic Ocean to do so, that they resolved to form a society for the advancement of women's rights when they returned home (Hymowitz & Weissman, 1978).

True to their vow, the Women's Rights Convention was held in Seneca Falls, New York, in July 1848, with more than 300 women in attendance. The convention adopted the Declaration of Sentiments, which chronicled women's subservient position in marriage, education, employment, politics, franchise, property ownership, guardianship of children, and moral standards. It also agreed upon 12 resolutions to overcome these inequities. Eleven moved through with little discussion; the 12th, introduced by Elizabeth Cady Stanton, to give women the right to vote, met with great resistance and nearly failed to pass. From that time forward, women's rights were real goals to be actively pursued. One member of the first convention, Charlotte Woorward, lived to see women get the vote—72 years later (Hymowitz & Weissman, 1978).

These women realized that they could not secure action on their 12 resolutions without help from men. They set out to gain this help. It was the belief of many women leaders during the 1800s that men did not want the power they held over women and could be persuaded to change unjust laws if women could overcome their timidity and begin to speak out for action. Women found however, that, despite their unity, large numbers, and assertive demand for justice, male support was difficult to obtain. So women turned to and found support from the abolitionists. This support was not surprising, since many of the early leaders of the women's rights movement were themselves abolitionists. It was only natural that women fighting for equality and justice for themselves on all levels should become strong advocates of Blacks in the fight against slavery.

Male abolitionists were far from united on the issue of whether or not women were equal to men. Some believed that women's "inferiority" was God's Will, whereas others supported women's rights activities, recognizing that white women based their demands for citizenship and equal rights on the same moral premises on which abolitionists based their antislavery beliefs. Many men recognized the invaluable contributions that women made to the abolition movement and felt it their duty, in return, to support women in their fight for recognition. A strong supportive link continued between both movements. Abolitionists such as William Lloyd Garrison discussed women's issues and supported their cause when addressing groups throughout the country in his fight against slavery.

Despite the general agreement that the fight for abolition and women's rights stemmed from essentially the same moral base, extremists of both groups continued to have some reservations about being linked too closely together. Unfortunately, conservative abolitionists feared that women's rights issues might hamper their fight against slavery. The issue of abolition was a much stronger cause and had more public attention, due to the brutality inflicted upon slaves in the South.

Not all white women were in agreement with Anthony and Stanton's views. Many were reluctant to ally themselves with the abolitionists. They feared that the free Black man would come to his own defense as a man before he would support women—Black or white.

Nonetheless, women's rights activities stopped for the duration of the Civil War, while reformers put their energies into pressing for emancipation and supporting the war effort. Toward the end of the war, Stanton, Anthony, and Anna Dickinson organized the National Woman's Loyal League, which gathered thousands of signatures in support of expanding the Emancipation Proclamation to abolish slavery in all the states and territories. The League also passed a resolution calling for equal rights for Blacks and women. The fruit of their work is the 13th Amendment to the US Constitution.

Strong debate as to whether or not women's rights should be supported until the question of slavery and equal rights for Blacks was settled continued. Women had fought hard and long for Black equality and felt that all issues of equality should be dealt with simultaneously. They were horrified to learn that the draft of the 14th Amendment explicitly limited its concern to Black male citizens. The proposed amendment not only failed to mention women, but also introduced the word "male" into the Constitution; so doing would institutionalize discrimination on the basis of sex. Up to this point the Constitution had not mentioned sex, and women had been excluded from suffrage under individual states' laws. Now they were to be excluded by the federal Constitution itself. Anthony, Stanton, and Lucy Stone Blackwell led the opposition to the 14th Amendment because of its exclusion of women. They organized a petition campaign to Congress requesting that the amendment prohibit disfranchising any United States citizens on account of sex, race, or color. This was the first time Congress had been directly petitioned, since in the past only state legislatures had been petitioned for women's rights. The Republican reconstructionists, who cared little about women's rights, much less their suffrage, prevailed. The 14th Amendment to the US Constitution, ratified in 1868, explicitly gives men the right to vote and excludes women. This action served to galvanize women into action on their own behalf.

The Popular Health Movement

One way to view the impact of the political process on the lives of individual women during the 19th century is to examine nursing, a profession that was dominated by women. In the early 1800s most health care was provided by women. Their focus was mainly health maintenance and disease prevention, as little scientific knowledge was available for the treatment of disease. They did, however, prepare herbs and potions, knew something of basic anatomy, and delivered babies. Health care at this time was considered an extension of home services: cleaning, bandaging, and caring for the dying.

A decade later several schools of medicine were founded in the United States. The greatest distinction between graduates of these schools and lay practitioners was that the formally trained physicians were male, usually middle class, and much more expensive. Their practice was primarily confined to those who could afford their services: the middle class and the wealthy. In terms of knowledge and skills, the physician had little more knowledge than did the lay practitioner. The greatest difference was that the physician believed in the "heroic" approach to cure, which entailed massive bleeding, huge doses of laxatives, and opium. Their "cures" were often fatal (Ehrenreich & English, 1973). The lay practitioners, who were mostly women, were much more conservative. They believed in herbal medications, dietary changes, and laying on of hands (as in our current belief in the power of touch). Their knowledge was no better than the physicians' but their treatments were definitely safer.

Tired of the quackery promoted by physicians, the popular health movement developed in the 1830s and 40s. Again, this movement was headed by women. They began teaching the public simple anatomy and personal hygiene. They emphasized preventive care instead of the life-threatening "cures" that physicians offered. The practices they supported included frequent bathing, loose-fitting clothing for women, nutrition, and birth control—all things that had previously been regarded as taboo.

The popular health movement was initiated by women and coincided with the first women's movement in the United States. The crusade for women's rights, its members were convinced, was inseparable from the need for women to have better, more humane health care, and for women to gain access to medical education to provide that care. Thus the popular health movement emerged as a new medical philosophy to challenge and compete with traditional male physicians. The movement opened its own medical schools, which focused on disease prevention and mild herbal treatments. These medical schools welcomed women as vigorously as traditional medical schools had excluded them (Ehrenreich & English, 1973).

Elizabeth Blackwell, sister-in-law of Lucy Stone Blackwell, was an exception to the rule of exclusion of women from traditional medical education. Blackwell was the first woman to receive an MD degree. She practiced medicine for a short period of time before turning her energies to hospital administration and then to public health and sanitation. She and her sister Emily, also a physician, founded the first infirmary for women and children in New York. The care was provided by women physicians, and they even established their own medical school for women at the infirmary (Rossi, 1973). The Drs. Blackwells' *Medicine as a Profession for Women* (1860) is a landmark in feminist literature and could well have been to their day what *Our Bodies, Ourselves* has become to ours (Boston Women's Health Collective, 1971).

At the height of the popular health movement in the 1830s and 40s, doctors became fearful of loosing control and power over the American people. Later, as the movement lost momentum in the mid 1800s, traditional doctors regrouped and developed their first national organization: the American Medical Association. Its main focus was reform. Women lay practitioners, along with women physicians, were the first to be persecuted. The arguments against women physicians were sexist and paternalistic: how could a respectable woman travel alone at night to a medical emergency (Ehrenreich & English, 1973)? Even if a woman managed to overcome the constant harassment from her peers and professors in medical school, in many instances she faced greater struggles after attaining her degree. Internship programs were generally closed to women, hospitals were reluctant to hire them, and if they managed to open a small private practice, traditional doctors would not refer patients to them.

Finally, in order to survive, women doctors who followed the new philosophy of the popular health movement had to join the ranks of traditional medicine. All this occurred at a time when traditional physicians still had little scientific knowledge on which to base their practice. Once again male dominance succeeded. Middle-class women of the new medical philosophy largely gave up their attack and accepted their prescribed role and the terms dictated by male doctors.

Medicine became recognized as a profession only after the discovery of the germ theory in the 1850s by French and German scientists and the extensive donation of funds by philanthropists for the purpose of educating American doctors. A reformist zeal filled the ranks of doctors as their knowledge base developed. Newly trained doctors set up the first American-German–style medical school, Johns Hopkins. The new curriculum included laboratory training in conjunction with clinical practice. Other reforms included the hiring of a full-time faculty, an emphasis on research, associating medical centers with universities, and a new pattern for medical training: four years of college followed by four years of medical school. The length and expense of this preparation limited its availability to families who could afford the costs. Since the enrollment to schools consisted mainly of upper-middle-class white males, physicians became elites.

NURSING IN THE 1800s

Women with an interest in science and a desire to become physicians were often discriminated against and thus likely to fail. The alternative many chose was nursing. Nursing in the early 19th century consisted primarily of caring for sick and aging family members. Employment was available in hospitals and to some extent in homes. Hospitals were at that time mainly refuge centers for the dying poor and degenerates. Token care was provided by disreputable women prone to drunkenness, prostitution, and thievery, personified by Sarah Gamp in the writing of Charles Dickens (1975). Conditions in hospitals were often scandalous.

Nursing was not an attractive field for women workers, but it intrigued and lured women reformers. The reformer believed that if nursing could attract women of good character, the hospital setting could become an acceptable health care facility and nursing could become an acceptable occupation for women from good families. As is often the case, war provided opportunities for women that peacetime does not afford. The Civil War brought thousands of women into nursing to care for the sick and wounded. If civilian hospital conditions were bad, military hospitals were almost intolerable. Little was known about treating injuries successfully, and even less was understood about the transmission of disease or of asepsis. But even in the face of incredible suffering, physicians preferred untrained male attendants to skilled female nurses. Thousands of women volunteers, as well as army nurses who flocked to the military hospitals, overcame their resistance by showing what they could do. Dr. Elizabeth Blackwell spearheaded training nurses for the Northern army and led to the creation of the Sanitary Commission to coordinate care, supplies, and staff. Dorothea Dix became a superintendent of nurses and took over responsibility for preparing nurses for service in military hospitals. Ms Dix went on to lead the reform of insane asylums, prisons, and almshouses. Confederate nurses were neither as well trained nor as well equipped as their Northern counterparts. Mary Bickerdyke traveled with General Sherman's army and conducted her own personal war on incompetent and derelict physicians. Clara Barton, another nurse, worked with soldiers on both sides of the conflict, and her beliefs that medical aid to the wounded should offer help to any and all who needed it led her to found the American and International Red Cross following the war. Although the Civil War ended in 1865, it was not until 1892 that the US Congress recognized the contribution that nurses had made to the care of the nation's military and passed a bill to provide a $12 per month pension for Civil War nurses (Hymowitz & Weissman, 1973). These nurses were of a new breed: sober, disciplined, well trained, many from the middle class; they proved their value to both physicians and hospitals.

Of course no discussion of this period and of the effects of war on nurses and nursing is possible without inclusion of the work of Florence Nightingale, that upper-class Victorian Englishwoman and nurse who took on the entire British military and civilian hospital systems and reformed them both. The Crimean War, 1853-1856, provided the proving ground for her ideas and practices. And prove them she and her colleagues did (Aynes, 1973).

After the wars, nursing schools began to appear in England and the United States. At the same time, the number of hospitals increased to keep pace with the increased needs of medical education. Medical students needed good hospitals to train in; good hospitals, as the physicians were learning, needed good nurses (Ehrenreich & English, 1973).

Nightingale and her colleagues attempted to attract aristocrats and upper-middle-class women to nursing schools. Their philosophy was that the nurse should be an ideal woman, transplanted from the home to the hospital. She should bring the wifely virtue of absolute obedience to the physician and the selfless devotion of a mother to the patients, To lower-level hospital workers she should provide the kindly, guiding discipline of a household manager accustomed to dealing with servants. Her entire training was to be focused on character, as opposed to skills (Ehrenreich & English, 1973).

Despite the more socially acceptable new image of the nurse, the work was heavy and workers poorly paid, and women coming into nursing were mostly of the working class or lower-middle class. The philosophy of nurses' training did not waver despite the lack of aristocrats in the field. Nurses were expected to be ladylike at all times, to follow orders, to be obedient helpers, and to do all the menial tasks involved in total patient care.

The feminist movement did not challenge nursing as an oppressive female role. In fact, by the late 19th century, feminists were supporting this newly recognized role of the nurse-mother. Women had found a secure and valued niche in the health care field. Although the nurses who helped bring this phenomenon about are not generally thought of as leaders of the women's movement, they were role models for other women by showing them what other women could and did accomplish. In the meantime, the leaders of the women's suffrage movement were far from idle.

THE WOMEN'S SUFFRAGE MOVEMENT

In 1869, one year after the ratification of the 14th Amendment, Stanton and Anthony completely broke with the abolitionists and formed the National Women's Suffrage Association (NWSA). Many, but not all, of their supporters followed them into the new organization. A group of Boston women, led by Lucy Stone and Julia Ward Howe, refused to break off their association with the Boston-based abolitionist movement and were excluded from NWSA. In 1870 this Boston group formed its own organization, the American Women's Suffrage Association (AWSA). This split the women's suffrage movement along ideological lines concerning its means and ends; the rift was to continue for 20 years and to weaken efforts towards attaining women's suffrage and other rights (Hymowitz & Weissman, 1978).

Settlement of the West had been accelerated by the Civil War as well as by the discovery of gold in California. On the frontier, women were again equal with men in settling the land and developing the new territories. Lawmakers realized that settling the West had to be made attractive to women as well as to men if the country was to move beyond the frontier stage. This realization is reflected in the Homestead Acts of 1860 and 1890, which gave men and women equal amounts of free land. Thus a single person, male or female, could claim 320 acres for homestead; a married couple could claim 640 acres. In the West, the wife could control the title to her own lands from the start, a right that had been won by the women of New York in 1860, only after a hard fight. With these attitudes and precedents it is little wonder that a western state, Wyoming, was the first to grant women the vote. The law was passed in 1869, the same year that the splintered women's suffrage movements were launched in the East.

During the last half of the 19th century, a reform movement was to galvanize women together in another crusade; this time the cause was temperance. "Demon Rum" was seen as an enemy of all women and children and, thereby, of the American family as well. The Women's Christian Temperance Union (WCTU), founded in 1874, became a formidable force in American life, and culminated in 1919 with the ratification of the 18th Amendment to the US Constitution prohibiting "the manufacture, sale, or transportation of intoxicating liquors." Frances Willard, the WCTU's leader for 20 years, fortunately was also an advocate of any reform that would benefit women and children. Thus her scope of concern included child labor laws, prison reform, laws to protect working women, and women's suffrage. She believed that women's rights were essential to insure women's position in home and family. Her rallying cry, "Do Everything," neatly encompassed all of these concerns. Many women were drawn to the temperance cause who would not have joined the women's rights movement; once in the WCTU they were exposed to these other causes and many joined in them as well. Willard's emphasis on the preservation of women's position in the home and family, however, while drawing many men and women to her movement, was antithetical to many of the positions feminists have taken before and since with regard to women's rights for equality and opportunities outside of the home (Smith, 1970). Willard, her ideas, and her WCTU organization helped to win the battle for women's suffrage, but caused problems in the battle for women's rights that still constrain us.

By 1878, Susan B. Anthony and Elizabeth Cady Stanton realized that many barriers had to be overcome if the rights of women were to be recognized in every state. They finally decided what would be most helpful and expedient would be an amendment to the United States Constitution. They petitioned and received help from Aaron Sargent of California. He was able to introduce the "Anthony Amendment" in the Senate. In essence, it stated that the right of citizens of the United States to vote should not be denied or abridged by the United States or by any state on account of sex. The amendment was defeated over and over again but each time by a smaller margin of votes. Doubtless this shrinking margin was caused in no small part by the activities of women reformers such as those in the WCTU, as well as by the examples of Wyoming and other western states that came into the Union having already given their women suffrage.

Other reform groups were also busily at work throughout the country. The Young Women's Christian Association (YWCA) and the General Federation of Women's Clubs (GFWC) were both on the rise. The GFWC provided an outlet for the reform desires of upper- and middle-class white native-born women; it also provided them with an escape from the boredom of their homes. Babysitters and household help were easily recruited from the ranks of the millions of immigrant women who came to the United States in the 19th and early 20th centuries. Thus freed from their household responsibilities, these American women were able to devote their time and talents, as well as their husbands' resources, to any number of causes. Unfortunately these causes often included all rights and needs except women's rights and needs for equality (Hymowitz & Weissman, 1978).

The early 1900s saw the rise of the settlement-house movement, largely brought about by the upper-class college-educated White native-born women who were determined to do something for society. Jane Addams, founder of Chicago's Hull House, which provided social services for the immigrant families with whom she and her colleagues chose to work, demonstrated once again that women could organize, manage, and lead as well as men (Addams, 1960). Addams was instrumental in the development of the Progressive Party's reform platform of 1912. Planks dealt with an eight-hour work day and a six-day work week, improved labor laws, the prohibition of child labor, old age assistance, and women's suffrage.

The unwillingness of the male world to accept women as equals was apparent in the work force. Many women went to work because their husband's salary was inadequate to supply family needs. Others worked to support themselves; many widows were the sole support of their children. There was no Social Security or welfare in the early years of the 20th century. Women workers were consistently given the least skilled jobs and the lowest pay. Even when men and women did the same job, women were paid one-third to one-half what men were (Smuts, 1971), a situation that still exists today in some places. For example, the median annual income for women in the craft and kindred workers category in 1977 was $6,742; for males in the same category it was $12,827 (*Current Population Reports*, Series P-60, no 118, 1979; Lawrence, 1978). Promotions went to men, and so women, regardless of their skills or experience, remained at the bottom of the employment ladder. Since no child care facilities were available either in the community or at the work place, women could either leave their children unattended, pay sitters out of their inadequate wages, or take their children into the often deplorable conditions in the work place. Part of the problem of child care often was "solved" by putting even very young children to work; the few cents a day that the children were paid augmented the family income.

During the 1800s, labor unions, which were then organizing in most industrializing countries, paid little attention to women workers. The unions used much the same rationale for this behavior that the employers did in refusing to pay women equal wages: either women were only temporary workers and would drop out soon, or they were only working for extra money. Overtones of this same attitude toward women in the work force continue today. In 1881 the Knights of Labor, a national labor union, offered support for working women. This organization advocated an eight-hour day, putting a stop to child and convict labor, improved health and safety regulations, and arbitration to take the place of strikes. The Knights of Labor led the way in demanding equal pay for women for equal work done. The Knights of Labor, as well as much of the labor movement involving unskilled workers, went into a decline in the late 1880s. Eugene Debs and the Socialist Party, organized in 1901, took up the role of advocate for unskilled men and women workers. This led to a rivalry between the Socialist Party and the American Federation of Labor, which championed the rights of skilled workers but largely ignored the needs of the unskilled.

One of the early women organizers in the Knights of Labor union was Mary Harris Jones, better known as Mother Jones. She referred to herself as a "hell raiser" (Noyes, 1978); others used this and other names for her during her 50 years as an organizer among the miners and mill workers. She was also instrumental in the founding of the Industrial Workers of the World in 1905 (Jones, 1972; see also *Mother Jones* magazine). Other women, including Kate Richards, Rose Pastor Stokes, Elizabeth Gurley Flynn and Rose Schneiderman, followed her example, and women's participation and inclusion in the labor movement increased. Strikes by the needle trades in New York around 1910, called the Great Uprising, turned the International Ladies Garment Workers' Union (ILGWU) into a trade union to be reckoned with (Levine, 1924). Women's voices could never again be ignored by either labor or management. Think about this the next time you see an ILGWU tag in an article of clothing.

All of these activites were making women more visible throughout American society. They were also making more and more men and women aware of the stupidity of the denial of women's rights to property, equal wages, and the vote. The women's suffrage movement had managed to reunite itself in 1890 with the warring New York-based National Women's Suffrage Association (NWSA) and the Boston-headquartered American Women's Suffrage Association, forming the NASWA, an organization that continued to center its efforts on getting women the vote. Western and southern women sought to gain the right to vote at the state level, as a "states rights" issue, meeting with considerable success in the West. They therefore saw little need to continue the push for an amendment to the federal Constitution giving them this right. Thus, following the 1894 NWSA convention, much of the members' efforts to obtain the vote took place at the state level. The old leaders, Stanton and Anthony, who held out for federal-level action, lost their power in the organization and the movement. The women who moved public opinion between 1890 and 1920, when the 19th Amendment to the Constitution of the United States was ratified, were those who pushed unconventional leaders and radical positions out of the movement and put their efforts into winning the support of middle-class women throughout the country (Hymowitz & Weissman, 1978). They were successful in their efforts. As we, in the early 1980s, approach the Equal Rights Amendment's final hours, we may well have to adopt precisely the same strategy.

The final push toward the 19th Amendment began in earnest in 1910, when Washington state passed its women's suffrage amendment, the first since 1896. California, Oregon, Arizona, Kansas, Montana, and Nevada rapidly followed suit. The militant suffragette movement in England was also underway, and many American women learned new and useful strategies from women such as the Pankhursts, who were dramatized in the United States in the mid 1970s PBS series "Shoulder to Shoulder" (Pankhurst, 1977; Strachey, 1978). Alice Paul, an American of Quaker birth, who had been involved in the Pankhurst demonstrations while a graduate student in England, and others with similar backgrounds exerted considerable influence on NWSA and on American women. Paul lost power in 1915 to Carrie Chapman Catt, who had followed Susan B. Anthony as president of NWSA between 1900 and

1904. Again the movement splintered, with Paul going off to form The Women's Party (TWP), a much more radical suffrage group than the NWSA. Many TWP members were jailed for demonstrations and picketing. Both NWSA and TWP campaigned hard against Woodrow Wilson because of his opposition to suffrage for women. The First World War intervened, and American women in general and particularly those involved in the NWSA supported the war effort; many TWP members were pacifists. By the end of the war, the question was no longer whether women would be allowed to vote, but when. The first woman elected to be a representative to Congress, Jeanette Rankin of Montana, introduced the measure that was to become the 19th Amendment to the US Constitution onto the floor of the House of Representatives on January 10, 1918. The amendment passed, receiving one more vote than the needed two-thirds majority. Tennessee, the 36th and last state needed for ratification, passed it on August 26, 1920. Women could vote (Hymowitz & Weissman, 1978).

FROM THE 19th TO THE EQUAL RIGHTS AMENDMENT

Following a time-honored tradition, instead of NWSA and TWP fading away after they had attained their goal of obtaining women's suffrage, they both lingered on. NWSA evolved into the League of Women Voters. TWP has continued the fight for equal rights, particularly when it became apparent that, although women had been granted the right to vote, not much else had changed for them. Dual standards of morality continued: men could have affairs and mistresses, but women who followed similar courses were socially ostracized. Women such as Emma Goldman believed that women's liberation depended on freedom of sexual expression and enjoyment. It was being said that the woman's role in marriage amounted to trading sexual favors for economic security; not a new theme. During the Roaring Twenties there was much talk about women's new-found freedom in terms of their own sexuality; one has the suspicion, however, that for most women there was much more talk than activity for many reasons, the fear of pregnancy and venereal disease being at least two.

In the first decade of the century, Margaret Sanger, a public health nurse, was in Europe, preparing to raise the American consciousness about birth control. Sanger had studied the use of the diaphragm in Holland and had seen that because it allowed for the spacing of pregnancies and required frequent medical examinations, it resulted in cutting maternal mortality in half. Prior to the development of the diaphragm, the major methods of contraception had been withdrawal and the condom, both of which placed the burden of effective use on the man. The diaphragm permitted women to take control of ensuring that unwanted pregnancies did not occur. When Sanger returned to the United States and opened her first birth-control clinic in New York in 1917, the dispensing of birth control devices was prohibited by the existing obscenity laws, except in situations where they were needed to prevent disease. Disease was interpreted to mean venereal disease, and thus legal contraception was limited to the condom. After several years, and a few stints in jail for Sanger, the laws' interpretation was liberalized, at least in New York, to permit contraception to be prescribed to prevent diseases that were complications of pregnancy. Sanger's New York clinic was the harbinger of the Planned Parenthood program, which has developed and spread throughout the country and the world (Sanger, 1971).

The Great Depression brought hardship to virtually everyone. Especially hard hit were poor, minority, and immigrant families whose incomes were marginal even before the Depression. In these families women, regardless of the ages of their children, were forced to seek whatever employment they could find to augment their husband's salary, if their husband was lucky enough to have a job at all. Many of these women, as well as single women and those who were heads of households, ran into tremendous discrimination in the work place and were admonished that they must not take jobs away from men. Twenty-six states had laws forbidding employment of married women during the Depression years, and from 1932 to 1937 the federal government prohibited more than one member of a family from holding a civil service job (Hymowitz & Weissman, 1978). Even when women were employed, they were paid less than men for the same work and were not eligible for hiring or promoting into better-paying upwardly mobile positions. Changes in the availability of jobs for women and the kinds of jobs they could hold did not occur until World War II. Rosie the Riveter is famous as a prototype of the American women who took over men's jobs while they were fighting in the war, did them well until the end of the war, and then were laid off and sent out of the work force and back into the home when the men returned.

Few women remained politically involved in the 1920s or in the Depression years. Hattie Caraway, in 1938, made a significant step as a woman in politics when she was elected to the US Senate. She had held the Senate seat since her husband had died in office, and she had been asked to take over his position. Her reelection broke an important barrier. Unfortunately she was not reelected in 1944. Traditionally women have been more successful in attaining and holding lower-ranking offices (see Chapter 3). In the 1940s and 1950s, thirty-four women were elected to the House of Representatives. Twenty-one of these women ran for election as bona fide candidates; the remaining 11 were the widows of Congressmen, who served out their husband's term. This ten-year period produced two great women leaders in the Congress: Frances Payne Bolton served in Congress until 1968 and rose to become ranking minority leader on the House Foreign Affairs Committee. Margaret Chase Smith from Maine ran for the Senate in 1948 without party endorsement and won. She served until 1972 and became the first woman to hold a party leadership post in the US Senate.

Despite the increased role of women in federal government, progress continues to be slow. Stereotypes of women, as well as the socialization to believe these stereotypes, have consistently been among the greatest barriers to equality (Rivers, Barnett, & Baruch, 1979). Men have considered the political arena as exclusively their domain. Many double standards exist. Women have not been taken seriously, and are not protected by the media or by the "old boys" concept, as are their male counterparts in politics. For example, it was acceptable in the 1960s for the opponent of Congresswoman Coya Knutson to extract a statement from her alcoholic husband saying, "Coya come home," and have it publicized (Papachristou, 1976). Many in Washington felt that this ploy strongly contributed to Knutson's political defeat. Much more tantalizing stories were available about some of the men running for political office at the time, yet the media and the candidates' political opponents would not have considered using the information as political weapons.

There was little organized women's movement activity from 1940 to 1960 to support the few women who were then breaking into the political arena. Among the reasons for this relative void were the elite class base from which many of the suffragists came, and the limited ideology of the women's suffrage movement. The League of Women Voters continued its nonpartisan educational activities, but its mailing list decreased from 2 million in 1940 to 106,000 in 1960. Organizations such as the YWCA, the Business and Professional Women clubs, and the American Association of University Women also survived, but membership was small and their primary interest lay in social or professional reform—not reforms related to women's liberation (Deckard, 1975).

The Women's Party, the sole survivor of the militant suffragists' groups, had a narrow perspective. They fought for equal rights but ignored the housewife's inferior position in the home, the special problems of minority women, and the exploitation of women workers. This lack of interest in major social, economic, and racial problems affecting women alienated militant women from the group. This dissension created a hostile atmosphere that also deterred moderate women from being attracted to the organization. Many members of this group were slow to see that although suffrage had been achieved, women were still far from equal in most phases of American life: educational, political, social, and economic.

The male-dominated system cannot be held totally responsible for the oppression of women. Many women, whether consciously or unconsciously, fought and continue to fight against achieving equal rights. Many participate fully in their own oppression. This is illustrated by the social role of women in the 1940s and 50s.

As World War II ended, the majority of middle-class women willingly left the factories and returned to their homes. Men were back from war and could once again take over their role of "provider." As the country prospered, salaries increased and one income became adequate to support a family. Most women were content to return to the home and the wife/mother roles they had been socialized to accept. They knew what church, state, and men expected and wanted from them. The return of middle-class women to the home was applauded by experts in all fields; psychologists with their Freudian sophistication, pediatricians, publishers of women's magazines, churches, educators, men, and women themselves. Women were recognized for their femininity, adjustment, and new maturity. Only unhappy women sought careers, higher education, political power, and the independence that the old-fashioned feminists had championed.

By the late 1940s, the ratio of women to men in college had dropped by 12 percent. Attending college was a high price to pay when the goal was finding a husband rather than pursuing an education for a career. By 1950, 60 percent of the women students were leaving college to marry or because they felt higher education would be a deterrent to marriage. The average marrying age for American women dropped from the 20s to the teens. By the end of the 1950s, the United States' birthrate was overtaking India's. The Baby Boom was in full tilt. Statisticians were astounded to find a phenomenal increase in the number of babies being born to women college graduates. Earlier, women in this group had had one or two children, now they had four, five, or six. Women who had once wanted careers now found a career in having babies (Friedan, 1963).

As women became more and more home-bound, a new marketing focus developed. Kitchens were no longer considered solely functional; mosaics and murals were included by interior designers. Windows were built over kitchen sinks, since women spent a large part of their days preparing food and doing dishes. Home sewing became extremely fashionable. Making clothes, curtains, and gifts occupied part of almost every housewife's day. Many women left their homes only to chauffeur their children back and forth from school, to do needed shopping, and to attend social functions with their husbands and children. As someone has correctly quipped, women deliver children once vaginally and then forever after by car. Identity conflicts ensued for middle-class women whose previous educational experience had led them to believe that there might be more to life than these activities, rewarding though many of them are.

By the late 1950s a sociological phenomenon had become apparent. One third of the female population was in the work force, but few were young. Most of these women were temporarily employed to help finance husbands or sons through college. Some were widows supporting families. Few were in professional careers. As a result there was a sharp decline in professions that women had generally dominated, such as teaching, nursing, and social work. These shortages caused crises in almost every American city. (Friedan, 1963).

That women's place was in the home was a belief that was well supported until the dawn of the space age. Then it suddenly occurred to scientists that half of the country's potential brain power was being underutilized. So, as in World Wars I and II, women were once again called out to contribute to the country. Scholarships became available for young women who demonstrated a high aptitude in the sciences. Many of these monies were refused by their potential recipients on the basis the scientific professions were unfeminine. Young women wanted the fulfilling life of the suburban housewife as described in women's magazines: live in a big white house, kiss your husband goodbye at the door, drive the children to school in the family station wagon, clean the house until it is spotless, take rug-hooking classes, and sew your own clothes. Their only dream was to be a perfect wife and mother, their highest ambition to have several children, and their only fight to keep their husbands (Friedan, 1963).

In 1960 the civil rights movement awakened the country to a full realization of the discriminiation and prejudice that penetrated the lives of many Americans. Spurred by labor and women's groups, President Kennedy established the Presidential Commission on the Status of Women. The committee was to examine any outmoded customs or prejudices that impinged on women's basic rights. It was then to make recommendations in the areas of employment practice, tax laws, and labor laws, and to assess services needed by women, such as child care (Papachristou, 1976).

Months after these recommendations were made, an executive order was issued from the commission to further reiterate them. It did not, however, recommend an enforcement procedure. Therefore the main value of the committee was in its recognition of women's inequality and the publicity that it provided. It was the first official body to make a thorough study of the status of women in the United States (Hale & Levine, 1971).

But others were making studies of the situations of American women. In 1963 Betty Friedan published her landmark book, *The Feminine Mystique*. Although the work had little to offer working-class and poor women or minorities, it did address the problems and needs of middle-class women. It helped them give names to the vague insights they were having about their situations, and, most important of all, it told them that their problems were not unique but were shared by thousands of other women like themselves. Once this realization was made, what Hymowitz and Weissman define as the most important insight of modern feminism—that "the personal is political"—was not far behind (1978:350). In this climate the seeds of the second women's movement took root.

Reform was in the air not only for women but also for minorities and the poor. During the Depression the United States had been preoccupied by problems such as economic unrest and foreign wars and, in 1945, its awesome rise to world power and prosperity (Papachristou, 1976). After its resolution of these problems, the country looked at its internal organization and began further reform. It recognized that American Blacks suffered economic, social, and political injustice. Soon other oppressed groups became visible, and by the early 1960s all were encouraged to speak out for reform. Every aspect of American life was scrutinized. Foreign policy and nuclear war and disarmament were major targets of attack, along with discrimination at every level.

This particular reform period is still under way. The oppressed and underprivileged have taken an active role in organizing themselves. Blacks planned and executed the fight for integration in all facets of life in the South; American Indians and Puerto Ricans are raising their voices in anger at injustices they have withstood for centuries. Gay people are banding together for support and going to the public to seek their constitutional rights.

In the 60s, colleges and universities became centers of activity, with the University of California at Berkeley taking the lead, beginning with the free speech movement. Groups were no longer passive, but active and defiant of the system. Protest groups and marches became familiar sights. The media brought them into every American home via newspaper and television. Angry, defiant activists demanded not reform but revolution. More moderate reformers were able to translate these demands into concrete legislative proposals that gradually gained the support of politicians. In 1963 the Equal Pay Act (Public Law 88-38) prohibited discrimination on the basis of sex, in the payment of wages for equal work requiring equal skill, effort, and responsibility and performed under similar working conditions. The Civil Rights Act of 1964 (PL 88-352) was a tremendous breakthrough for all minorities and for women. Title VII prohibits discrimination against people because of race, color, sex, religion, and national origin, by employers, employment agencies, unions, and labor management programs in the private as well as in the public sector. A number of activist feminist groups were formed to monitor the Equal Employment Opportunity Commission (EEOC), whose job was to enforce Title VII (Hymowitz & Weissman, 1978). Affirmative action was launched. (A selected list of laws and executive orders of interest to women is located in Appendix 1.)

In 1966, a third national conference of State Commissions on the Status of Women was held. Women previously involved with the Presidential committee and many who had stood by over the years awaiting some action from the results of the first study grew weary and fearful that nothing more than continued rhetoric would come from more elaborate research. Frustrated with continued sex discrimination in the country, these women banded together in 1966 to form the National Organization for Women. NOW succeeded in becoming a leading national organization.

Much of the leadership in NOW, and the Women's Equality Action League (WEAL), which later split off from NOW, came from well-educated, middle-class White women (and some men). These organizations were structured in traditional ways, with elected officials, conventions, and the specific goal of achieving women's rights. In essence, these organizations, which made up the new women's movement, were established in the same format as those of the first women's movement in the 1800s.

While the traditional women's rights groups were fighting for reform in their way, another group of women was gathering forces. This new group consisted of middle-class women, younger and mostly unmarried, who had participated in the political-protest activity of the 1960s, either in antiwar movements, civil rights marches, or New Left groups on the country's college campuses.

Participation in protest politics had already enriched the lives of these women. Through their experiences and successes with confrontation tactics, they were left feeling courageous, capable, and determined. They had affected change nationwide; established community libraries, parks, and child care services; assisted welfare mothers; supported voter registration; and caused laws to be passed.

As we see, two distinct groups of women emerged in the women's movement during the late 1960s. One group focused on women's rights such as equal pay for equal work, continuation of wives' social security and pension rights after death of the spouse or divorce, equal employment opportunities, and an end to sexual harassment and discrimination against women in general. The other group sought women's liberation through efforts on such issues as universal availability of abortion, equal rights and recognition for lesbians, and the prosecution of rape within marriage. Then in the 70s the two groups moved closer together. Many of the differences that seemed to separate them initially became blurred or lost importance, with the exception of the abortion issue. The movement grew to encompass small and large, structured and unstructured groups, radicals and conservatives, straights and gays, the belligerent and the persuasive. Involved women stood close together. There was a constant interchange of ideas and information. The media—television, radio, newspapers, magazines, books—provided them with complete and constant coverage. The number and the diversity of organizations in the movement multiplied. They spread into states and local communities. A recent study estimated that approximately 80,000 to 100,000 people had participated in these organizations by the early part of 1973 (Papachristou, 1976). In 1966, NOW had 300 charter members, who elected Betty Friedan its first president. By 1974, it had 48,000 members with 700 chapters in the United States. NOW was formed "to take action to bring women into full participation in the mainstream of American society, NOW, exercising all the privileges and responsibilities thereof in truly equal partnership with men" (Papachristou, 1976). NOW also took the stand that women have the right to control their own bodies and therefore should have the sole responsibility for deciding when or whether to bear a child. This stand in favor of abortion was unacceptable to many women, either from personal conviction or because the issue was too controversial. These women split from NOW in 1967 and formed their own group, the Women's Equality Action League (WEAL). They hoped that WEAL would attract business and professional women because of its moderate approach to women's rights, and that the organization could exert a diplomatic and patient influence on legislation (Hale & Levine, 1971).

The National Women's Political Caucus (NWPC) was founded in 1971 by Democratic and Republican women to form a political bloc within their respective parties. The overriding purpose of the NWPC is "to give women the political clout that they deserve." The NWPC seeks to do this in a number of ways:

- by encouraging qualified women to run for elective office
- by lobbying for the appointment of women to policy-making positions in government
- by pressuring the major parties to give equal representation to women in party offices and committees
- by working for the ratification of the Equal Rights Amendment (NWPC, 1979; see the Yellow Pages for NWPC addresses)

The National Women's Conference was held November 18-21, 1977, in Houston, Texas. Two thousand delegates were sent to the convention from 56 states' and territories' International Women's Year meetings, and more than 20,000 people attended. International Women's Year had been declared by the United Nations in 1975, and the UN sponsored an international women's conference in Mexico City. The National Women's Conference passed a Plan for Action, 25 substantive resolutions dealing with such areas as business, battered women, child abuse, child care, credit education, employment, the Equal Rights Amendment, health, insurance, older women, rape, reproduction, sexual preference, women, welfare, and poverty (Braudy & Thom, 1978). Much debate and difference of opinion preceded the adoption of the plan (Van Gelder, 1978). A 26th resolution was passed to monitor the progress of the others and to study the possibility of another national women's conference.

Thus in less than a decade the contemporary women's movement has changed dramatically. It has gone from focusing on limited issues to addressing concerns that encompass all issues affecting women both directly and indirectly. One of these concerns has been to support more women for elected office. As of December 1979, the number of women holding public office in the United States was 17,782, or 10.9 percent of all public offices. This is more than twice the number of women holding office in 1975 (Ms, December 1979).

Another issue that is galvanizing the women's movement is the Equal Rights Amendment. The Equal Rights Amendment (ERA) was initially introduced to Congress in 1923, a few years after women attained suffrage. For over 50 years it has survived Congress' attempt to ignore it, defeat it, or dilute it. On March 22, 1972, it was finally referred to the people through their state legislators (Deckard, 1975). The ERA, as passed by the 92nd Congress, is proposed as the 27th Amendment to the US Constitution and provides that "equality of rights under the law shall not be denied or abridged by the United States or a State on account of sex." To become a Constitutional Amendment, the ERA must be ratified by 38 of the 50 states' legislatures by June 30, 1982. As of the writing of this chapter, ratification by three more states is needed. If these three additional state ratifications are not obtained by June 30, 1982, the ERA will fail and we will be back where we started from. But what does that mean?

Wohl points out some of the ramifications of failure of the ERA. The Supreme Court will continue to await a national mandate to change its position, not withstanding the "equal protection of the laws" clause in the 14th Amendment, that although women are considered citizens and persons they are still "appropriately placed in compartments separate from men" (Wohl, 1979:64). When this separation is eliminated in the eyes of the Court, the burden of ending sex discrimination on the basis of sex will shift from women to lawmakers, where it should be. State laws that discriminate against women, such as those concerned with divorce, owning and retaining property, obtaining credit, and entering into contracts, will have to be repealed under the ERA. Laws concerning equal opportunity for employment and equal pay for equal work will have to be enforced. Under the ERA, homemakers of all classes and races will become equal partners in marriage, and the monetary value of their work as homemakers will entitle them to an equal share of the families' income and property. At present, Social Security laws discriminate against women, especially older women, who have spent their lives as homemakers rather than working outside of their homes. These laws are being rewritten, but without the ERA there is no guarantee that these sex-based discrimination factors will be removed. We strongly suggest that you examine the laws in your own state to see just how equally you are treated under them. What the ERA is addressing is the issue of equality for women before the law, nothing more and nothing less. This chapter has chronicled many of the highlights of the struggle women have gone through in the United States to come this close to real equality, guaranteed by the Constitution.

During the 1980 presidential campaign, the Republican Party and its standard bearer, Ronald Reagan, came out in open opposition to the Equal Rights Amendment. Reagan's election and the shift of the country toward domination by much more conservative elements than has been the case since the 1930s, make the prospect of ratification of the ERA by the needed states in time highly unlikely. Unless women unite and act decisively and soon for our own equal rights, the ERA will die. The National Women's Political Caucus, the National Organization for Women, and their local affiliates, as well as many other women's organizations, are continuing the fight (see the Yellow Pages). We all need to join with them before it is too late. That's June 30, 1982! What happens now to the ERA is up to each of us.

NURSING IN THE 1960s AND 1970s

Entering the 1960s, the expectations of the nurse were similar to those of the housewife. She was to be completely subservient to the physician as wives were to their husbands. She was to participate very little in the more complex technical aspects of patient care. Her primary functions were to serve the physician, to serve the patient, and to clean the hospital, including the equipment and the physical facilities. The male physician was the master of the hospital as the husband was master of the home.

Educators recognized that as theoretical knowledge increased, nursing had the potential to become a science in its own right. In the late 1950s, some educators stated that nursing was not a sex-segregated profession and encouraged men to enter the field. It was hoped that men in nursing would change nursing's image from that of a feminine profession and, therefore, help move it forward. Independent feminist women attempted to advance nursing and were frequently labeled rabble-rousers. Those who dared break out of the cast-iron mold of the traditional "nurse" found themselves unsupported even by their peers. To support these changes was to take a definite stand against traditional nursing roles, against the mystical power of the physician, and against public opinion about both women and nurses. As we enter the 1980s many of these same challenges remain.

Nursing leaders in the 1960s acknowledged that the profession had to move ahead not only in technical knowledge but also in autonomy. Nursing graduates of the 1970s were encouraged to be independent, to make defensible decisions, and to be assertive. Consciousness-raising of the entire profession was and is needed to affect change in the status of female nurses both as women and as professionals. One area in which consciousness-raising is needed is the nurse-physician relationship.

It is the authors' belief that female nurses are not always aware of the type of interaction they have with physicians. The physician has always played a patriarchal role when dealing with nurses. For example, the physician arrives on a nursing unit, and expects the nurse to answer all his questions (which she does), gives her orders (which she follows), and then leaves. If she tries to question him he may give her an inadequate response as he hurries down the hall. Many physicians still demand absolute obedience and even expect unconditional acceptance. The shame of this type of physician behavior is not only that it occurs, but also that nurses allow it and even support it. In addition, nurses are expected to "nurture" physicians. Examples of this include "fixing" mistakes in physicians' orders, protecting them from the possible consequences of their mistakes, and soothing them in stressful situations. The traditional role of the nurse can thus be seen to closely parallel that of wife-mother.

An example of the bind in which female nurses can find themselves is the use of gender differences to obtain power. A young nurse was approached by her head nurse regarding her unprofessional "friendliness" towards the physicians while on duty. Her response was, "It's easier to get what I need from them if I'm nice." Women have for years used their sexuality as their only source of power to achieve their goals. If we continue to use this technique it will defeat us (Levin & Berne, 1972; Thomstad & Cunningham, 1975; Stein, 1968). How can physicians begin to see female nurses as responsible, accountable professional colleagues if they act as playmates?

What of the nurse who assumes the role of an agent of change? Many nurse-administrators view change as unnecessary or unwanted. Even the nurse's peers may find her views threatening as she strives for change. Nurses spend their lives nurturing others, yet too rarely nurture each other.

In the 1960s, nursing became more aware of the need to gain status and legitimacy as an occupation, and perhaps even to emerge as a profession, if nurses were ever to be able to have a real voice in decision making in health and medical care and if individual nurses were ever to attain any degree of autonomy. Education was seen as a vehicle toward these ends. In 1965, the long conflict between academic preparation versus apprenticeship training in health and medical care came to a head when the American Nurses' Association (ANA) issued its first position paper on education for nursing (American Journal of Nursing, 1966). The paper said, in essence, that all education for those who would practice nursing should take place in institutions of higher education, that baccalaureate preparation should be the minimum required for the practice of professional nursing, and that associate degree preparation should be the minimum required for the practice of technical nursing. Whatever the framers of the position paper had hoped it would do for nursing's legitimacy in the outside world was cast in the shadow of the fact that this document essentially dichotomized nursing (Kalish & Kalish, 1978). The lines were drawn for internecine warfare within nursing, the fires of which were fanned by the resolution ANA passed in 1978 at its biennial convention in Hawaii, which included setting 1985 as the deadline for the implementation of the baccalaureate degree as the entry level requirement for the practice of professional nursing. We have obviously not heard the end of that decision.

In the meantime, nursing was making considerable strides toward autonomy and some authority in health and medical care decisions, at least for some nurses. Critical-care specialists and a variety of nurse-practitioners have burgeoned over the last two decades. Their rise has accompanied the ever-increasing specialization and technological sophistication required of all who practice nursing and medicine. Many nurses are proving that they are equal professional partners with physicians in providing services to clients (Kalish & Kalish, 1978). In the 1970s, all of the health and medical care disciplines found themselves facing tremendously difficult questions about cost containment and the kinds and numbers of service providers that will be necessary to serve the needs of the population in the future. Detailed examination of these issues is beyond our scope here, but they remain challenges that nursing and other disciplines will have to continue to address.

A tremendously positive step has been the development of N-CAP, the Nurses' Coalition for Action in Politics, established as the political arm of ANA in 1974. Because of tax and campaign laws, N-CAP is a separate organization from ANA and has its own board of trustees.

N-CAP's purposes are to educate nurses about political activities and to encourage their involvement in politics. In addition, N-CAP raises and distributes money to federal candidates who are favorable to nurses and who support the kinds of health issues they do. N-CAP is a political action committee. There are currently 34 state N-CAPs, which work within their states as N-CAP does nationally. In 1978 N-CAP contributed $98,000 to the campaigns of 231 candidates, 199 of whom were elected (N-CAP Brochure, August 1979; see the Yellow Pages for addresses of your state N-CAP as well as of the Washington, DC, office).

Others were taking and continue to take critical looks at nursing. In 1973, Kushner wrote an article entitled "The Nursing Profession: Condition Critical," in which she contrasts the public image of nurses as saintly servants of physicians, selflessly giving and never asking for anything in return, with the new breed of nurses who are assertive and pushing hard for better patient care as well as their own rights. This latter group is seen as running headlong into nurse stereotypes as well as sex roles and status problems between themselves and male doctors. She quotes Wilma Scott Heide, a former nurse and then president of NOW: "Nursing, in my view and that of feminists and behavioral scientists, reflects the secondary status of women. To the extent that physicians are male and nurses are female, you have the prototype of the male-female relationship of the culture at large. The physician is in charge, the nurse serves" (Kushner, 1973:77).

Beyond that article, there is very little in either feminist or working women's literature, as far as we have been able to find, that says very much for or about nurses. This is a distressing realization. Why are we, the largest group of health care providers and one of the largest single groups of women workers in the country, so little mentioned in connection with politics and the women's movement? Appendix B of this book contains the first report of data from a sample of 88 nurse-practitioners who Archer (1976) asked what impact the women's movement was having upon nursing and upon them as individuals. In January 1980, Ms. magazine published a list of "Eighty Women to Watch in the 1980s" (Sweet et al, 1980), in which only one of the women identifies herself as a nurse. Why so few nurses in this group? Finally, our close reading of working women's publications, such as Working Woman and Savvy, as well as books such as Managerial Woman (Henning & Jardim, 1977), shows no mention of nurses or nursing. Why?

Why are we virtually invisible? Perhaps some of the reasons are the same as those nurse-administrators and deans gave Archer and Goehner (forthcoming) when they were asked if nurses are as politically involved as they could and should be. Ninety-four percent of the sample of 522 said no. Some of their reasons for the lack of political involvement among nurses include:

- Nurses don't know how to participate in political activities (108)
- Apathy (95)
- Lack of time (65)
- Nurses' socialization (58)

All of these reasons can be overcome through education and the reorganization of priorities, which, we suspect, might well follow learning how to participate. The major purpose of this book is to help nurses see the need to participate in political activities and to learn how to do so.

We nurses must end our relative isolation and invisibility. We need to direct some of the energy and effort we are using for battles within nursing (Hott, 1976) to working together to create another and more positive image with the general public as well as with women's groups. We must become more politically active at all levels of government and in all kinds of issues affecting women, especially those having to do with health. As Wilma Scott Heide told the ANA Convention in 1964, we have got to "come out of the booth, in the corner, in the back, in the dark." We hope that this discussion of the women's movement in the United States has raised your consciousness enough for you to reach further and to become involved, particularly with the ratification of the ERA. We hope that the rest of this book will provide you with some concrete guidelines on how to become active, so that female nurses and nursing will no longer be so invisible in the discussions and issues facing all women and, ultimately, all people.

SUMMARY

In this chapter we have presented an overview of the first and second women's movement in the United States. We began with Colonial times and have traced major highlights and activities through the beginning of the 1980s. We have talked a little about some of the changes that have occurred in nursing during these times. We have raised questions about why nursing has such a low profile in so much that is written about the women's movement and about working women. Finally, we have challenged ourselves and you, our female nurse colleagues, to become more involved and active in women's political affairs, particularly in efforts for the ratification of the ERA.

REFERENCES

Acker A, Van Houten DR: Differential recruitment and control: The sex structuring of organizations. *Administrative Science Quarterly* 19: 152–163, June 1974.

Adams A: *Letters.* 1840. 2 vols, reprint. St Clair Shores, Mich, Somerset Publishers, 1972.

Addams J: *Twenty Years at Hull House.* 1910. Reprint. New York, Signet, 1960.

American Nurses' Association's first position paper on education for nursing. *American Journal of Nursing* 66:515–17, March 1966.

American Nurses' Association, House of Delegates: Resolutions. *Nursing Outlook* 26:501–502, August 1978.

Archer SE: Community nurse practitioners: Another assessment. *Nursing Outlook* 24:499–503, August 1976.

———, Goehner PA: Acquiring political clout: Guidelines for nurse administrators. *Journal of Nursing Administration.* Forthcoming.

Aynes EA: *From Nightingale to Eagle: An Army Nurse's History.* Englewood Cliffs, NJ, Prentice-Hall, 1973.

Bird C: *Everything a Woman Needs to Know to Get Paid What She's Worth.* New York, Bantam Books, 1973.

Blackwell E, Blackwell E: *Medicine as a Profession for Women?* New York, New York Infirmary for Women, 1860. Reprinted in Rossi AS (ed): *The Feminist Papers.* New York, Bantam Books, 1973.

Boston Women's Health Collective. *Our Bodies, Ourselves.* New York, Simon & Schuster, 1971.

Braudy S, Thom M: Gazette: The hard-fought resolutions at Houston. *Ms.* 6:52–56, 86–93, March 1978.

Brodie FM: *Thomas Jefferson: An Intimate History.* New York, Bantam Books, 1974.

Brody WH: Economic value of a housewife. *Research and Statistics Notes.* Washington, DC, Department of Health, Education, and Welfare, Social Security Administration, Office of Research and Statistics, August 28, 1975.

Bullough B, Bullough V: *The Subordinate Sex: A History of Attitudes Toward Women.* New York, Penguin Press, 1974.

———: Sex discrimination in health care. *Nursing Outlook* 23:40–45, January 1975.

Butterfield LH (ed): *Adams Family Correspondence.* Cambridge, Harvard University Press, 1963.

Current Population Report: Consumer Income. Series P-60, No 118. US Department of Commerce, Bureau of the Census, March 1979.

Deckard B: *The Women's Movement.* New York, Harper & Row, 1975.

Dickens C: *Martin Chuzzlewit, the Life and Adventures of.* 1844. Reprint. London, Penguin Press, 1975.

The Earnings Gap Between Women and Men. US Department of Labor, Employment Standards Administration, Women's Bureau, 1976.

Ehrenreich B, English D: *Complaints and Disorders: The Sexual Politics of Sickness.* New York, The Feminist Press, 1973.

———: *Witches, Midwives, and Nurses: A History of Women Healers.* New York, The Feminist Press, 1973.

Epstein CF: *Woman's Place: Options and Limits in Professional Careers.* Berkeley and Los Angeles, University of California Press, 1970.

Etzioni A: *The Semi-Professions and Their Organization.* New York, The Free Press, 1969.

Friedan B: *The Feminine Mystique*. New York, Dell Books, 1963.

Grimke S: *The Essential Historical Writings of Feminism*. New York, Vintage Books, 1972.

Grissum M, Spengler C: *Womanpower and Health Care*. Boston, Little Brown & Co, 1976.

Hale J, Levine E: *The Rebirth of Feminism*. New York, Quadrangle Books, 1971.

Heilbrum CG: *Toward a Recognition of Androgyny*. New York, Alfred A Knopf, 1973.

Hennig M, Jardim A: *The Managerial Woman*. New York, Anchor Press, Doubleday, 1977.

Hott JR: Nursing and politics: The struggles inside nursing's body politic. *Nursing Forum* 15:325–340, 1976.

Hymowitz C, Weissman M: *A History of Women in America*. New York, Bantam Books, 1978.

Jones MH: *The Autobiography of Mother Jones*. 1925. Reprint. Chicago, Charles H Kerr, 1972.

Kalish BJ: Of half-gods and mortals: Aesculapian authority. *Nursing Outlook* 23:22–28, January 1975.

———, Kalish PA: An analysis of the sources of physician-nurse conflict. *Journal of Nursing Administration* 7:51–57, January 1977.

———, Kalish PA: *The Advance of American Nursing*. Boston, Little Brown & Co, 1978.

Kilpatrick JJ: ERA: Losing battles, but winning the war. *Nation's Business*, 67:15–16, 1979.

Kraditor A: *Up From the Pedestal*. New York, Quadrangle Books, 1970.

Kushner TD: The nursing profession: Condition critical. *MS* 11: August 1973.

Lash JP: *Eleanor and Franklin*. New York, Norton, 1971.

Lawrence K, Klos K (eds): *Sex Discrimination in the Workplace*. Germantown, Md, Aspen Publications, 1978.

Levin P, Berne E: Games nurses play. *American Journal of Nursing* 72:483–487, March 1972.

Levine L: *The Women's Garment Workers: A History of the International Ladies' Garment Workers' Union*. New York, Huebsch, 1924.

Levine S, Lyons H: *The Decade of Women: A Ms. History of the Seventies in Words and Pictures*. New York, Putnam and Paragon, 1980. Excerpt in *Ms* 8:59–94, December 1979.

Lutz A: *Created Equal*. New York, John Day, 1940.

Mother Jones. Published monthly by Foundation for National Progress, San Francisco.

National Women's Political Caucus: We can end the waste of women's talent. Washington, DC, National Women's Political Caucus, 1979.

N-CAP Brochure. Washington, DC, August, 1979.

Noyes D: *Raising Hell: A Citizen's Guide to the Fine Art of Investigation*. San Francisco, Foundation for National Progress, 1978.

Oakley A: *Sex, Gender, and Society*. New York, Harper & Row, 1972.

Pankhurst ES: *The Suffragette Movement*. Chicago, Academy Chi Ltd, 1977.

Papachristou J: *Women Together*. New York, Alfred A Knopf, 1976.

Riegel R: *American Women: A Story of Social Change*. Rutherford, NJ, Fairleigh Dickinson University Press, 1970.

Rivers C, Barnett R, Baruch, G: *Beyond Sugar and Spice: How Women Grow, Learn, and Thrive.* New York, GP Putnam's Sons, 1979.

Roosevelt E: *It's Up to the Women.* New York, JB Lippincott, 1933.

Rossi AS (ed): *The Feminist Papers.* New York, Bantam Books, 1973.

Rowbotham S: *Hidden From History: Rediscovering Women in History From the 17th Century to the Present.* New York, Pantheon Books, 1974.

Sanger M: *An Autobiography.* New York, Dover, 1971.

Shockley JS: Perspectives in femininity: Implications for nursing. *Journal of Obstetrical and Gynecological Nursing,* November–December 1974, pp 36–40.

Smith P: *Daughters of the Promised Land.* Boston, Little Brown & Co, 1970.

Smuts RW: *Women and Work in America.* New York, Schocken, 1971.

Stein LI: The doctor-nurse game. *Archives of General Psychology* 16:699–703, 1967. Reprinted in *American Journal of Nursing* 68:101–105, January 1968.

Strachey R: *Cause: A Short History of the Women's Movement.* Chicago, Academy Chi Ltd, 1978.

Sweet E et al: 80 women to watch in the '80s. *Ms* 7:35–47, 98, January 1980.

Thomstad B, Cunningham N: Changing the rules of the doctor-nurse game. *Nursing Outlook* 23:422–427, July 1975.

Van Gelder L: Behind the scenes at Houston: Four days that changed the world. *Ms* 6:52–56, 86–93, March 1978.

Wohl LC: ERA: What if it fails? *Ms* 8:64–65, 111, November 1979.

Wollstonecraft M: *A Vindication of the Rights of Women,* in *The Feminist Papers,* Rossi AS (ed). New York, Bantam Books, 1973.

Yates GG: *What Women Want: The Ideas of the Movement.* Cambridge, Mass, Harvard University Press, 1975.

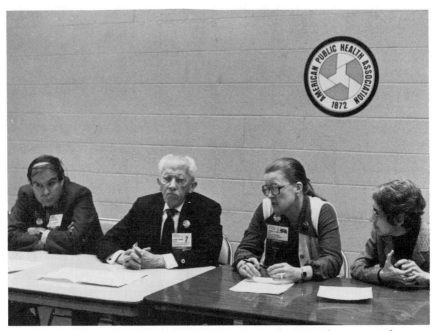

Press conference of Committee for Health in the 1980 Elections at the American Public Health Association's 1980 annual meeting in Detroit. *(Photo by Kathy Foxhall, American Public Health Association)*

CHAPTER 3

Selected Concepts Fundamental To Nurses' Political Activism

Sarah Ellen Archer

IN THE FIRST chapter we described nurse-activism via a typology of political participation. We also expressed our concern for and commitment to assisting nurses to become even more politically active and effective than they are now, regardless of where they choose to demonstrate that activism. In the remainder of the book, we give priority to practical how-tos and to examples of a broad array of strategies for political activism.

In this chapter are selected concepts that are fundamental to nurses' understanding of political participation. This conceptual framework is the foundation upon which the book is built. The concepts addressed here in the order of their appearance are: systems theory applied to political processes, power, decision making, conflict, and change.

SYSTEMS THEORY APPLIED TO POLITICAL PROCESSES

Systems theory provides an excellent means for analysis and understanding of how complicated organizations with many component parts work to attain the organizations' predefined goals. Braden and Herban have developed a three-way classification into which all systems fit (1976:6):

1. Physical or mechanical systems, such as solar systems or the internal combustion engine
2. Biologic systems, such as those that comprise plants and animals

3. Human and social systems, such as families, communities, and political parties

Political organizations are social systems and so fall into the third classification. For those of you unfamiliar with systems theory, I have elsewhere given examples of biologic and family systems, as well as a much simpler political systems model than the one I shall present and discuss here (Archer, 1979a,b). Many other writers have written extensively about systems theory (Churchman, 1968; Buckley, 1967; Emery, 1969; von Bertalanffy, 1968), so I shall not dwell on the rudiments of that theory here. Appendix C contains a number of systems theory terms for your review.

Basically, all political systems, from the United Nations to a rural precinct or district, are composed of interacting and interdependent parts or subsystems. The essential theoretical principles of open systems that apply to all political systems include:

1. Exchange with the environment through inputs, outputs, consequences of outputs, and feedback
2. Interaction and interdependence of the subsystems
3. Concern for systems and boundary maintenance
4. Survival as an absolute priority

The more defined the system's exchanges with the environment, the better its subsystems interact, and the more clearly defined its boundaries—all essential contributors to the system's survival—the more effective and, one hopes, the more efficient the system will be in attaining its predetermined goals and objectives.

The political-systems model shown in Figure 3.1 depicts an open system that interacts with its environment directly through inputs and outputs, and indirectly through the consequences of its outputs. Dahl defines a political system as "any persistent pattern of human relationships that involves, to a significant extent, control, influence, power, or authority" (1976:3). This is a broad definition that has the advantage of encompassing within its framework many systems that might otherwise not be considered to be political systems, such as a professional association, work units, and organizations. A political system's subsystems are interdependent in their interactions within the conversion process that some systems analysts have called "the black box" (see Appendix D). The model in Figure 3.1 is phrased in general terms so that it can be applied to all kinds of political systems, governmental and organizational. This model and my discussion of it are heavily indebted to Almond and Powell's developmental approach to comparative politics (1966) as well as to Easton (1965) and Monsma (1969).

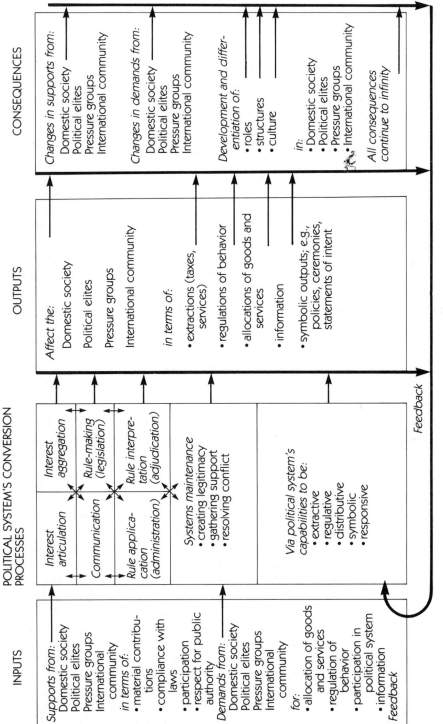

FIGURE 3.1. Political systems model. (Adapted from Almond & Powell, 1966:16–79.)

Inputs

Sources of the political system's inputs from its environment are the four major divisions shown in Figure 3.1. Domestic society includes the general population, much of which is only marginally politically active but whose interests political systems must serve, if not out of philosophical motivation, then out of political necessity in order to survive. A population that is grossly unhappy with its political system's actors will seek new ones through peaceful or other means. Thus, at least to some extent, the political system must respond to the inputs, both supports and demands, that the domestic society makes known.

The political elites are often a far more powerful and concentrated force in many political systems than is the domestic society. These people are themselves politically powerful, often within the political system they seek to influence. Political elites include such insiders as royalty, ministers, legislators, judges, and the very wealthy. Obviously, political elites can wield considerable power and influence over the political system's actions, so their demands and supports receive special attention.

The third sector of inputs, pressure groups, is increasing its power and influence, especially in the United States. Pressure groups have either replaced or subsumed the political elites in our society to a great extent (see the discussion of political action committees (PACs) in Chapter 4) and are becoming a tremendously important component of both partisan and issue-oriented politics. The influence of pressure groups will doubtless continue as a major force on legislators and legislation. Common Cause is continuing to seek legislation to change PACs' influence on the Congress.

The final major source of inputs for the political system is the international community. This is especially pertinent when international opinion and the constraints of already-negotiated alliances result in both supports of and demands upon the political system.

Thus in the United States, elected and appointed officials involved in the conversion processes of government are subject to supports and demands from the people of the United States through a variety of input mechanisms such as voting, lobbying in all its forms, contributing information, and all the other strategies people use to influence others. The political elites—big labor, big banking, big industry, the military, and similar groups—bring the force of their influence to bear on political processes through all the means that the domestic society does, as well as through the sheer weight of their prestige. Pressure groups are aggregates of members of the domestic society and of the political elites, and focus on single issues or a very restricted range of issues, strongly advocating one course of action. The power of such groups, which include anti-gun control groups, right-to-life groups, and the American Medical Association, is awesome. The political action committees are proving to be superbly effective means for the articulation of special interests. Finally, the United States, as are all nations, is subject to the pressures of international opinion as an influence on political decisions. Energy procurement and consumption by the United States is an area where international opinion and pressure will weigh heavily on energy decisions made in Washington as well as in many state capitals.

Supports come from the four constituent groups in terms of material contributions such as paying taxes and serving in the military. Compliance with the laws or rules, and respect for public authority, are also forms of support for the political process. In a democracy such as the United States, participation by as many people as possible through whatever means they choose—as individuals, as members of political action committees, parties, or other pressure groups, and so on—is essential to the health and functioning of our chosen form of government. Demands include those goods and services that the people expect the government to provide: roads, recreational facilities, education, and medical care, to name a few. Constituents also expect that governments will regulate others' behavior for their own protection. Thus we have demands for traffic laws, sanitation codes, antitrust and interstate commerce regulations. Demands for political participation include the right to vote; to speak out, and publish; to be free to assemble, petition, and otherwise to be heard on matters of concern. Informed participation requires information, and so political systems' constituencies demand that the government communicate with them and make known information about issues and policies. Although I am talking primarily about governments here, these same supports and demands are offered to and made upon all kinds of other organizations throughout our society, particularly since the increase in consumer activism and involvement. Each organization has components among its constituent groups that are analogous to those I have described here for governments.

The Political System's Conversion Processes

As Figure 3.1 shows, the political system's conversion processes are many and varied. These are the means that the system uses to transform the inputs it receives from its constituent groups into outputs that it returns to the environment and thereby to these same groups. Each of the six functions is interdependent upon and interacts with all of the others, as well as with those of systems maintenance and adaptation; the two-way arrows connecting these functions illustrate this reciprocal relationship. Let us look at each of these functions.

Interest Articulation. Interest articulation is the process constituent groups use to make demands on a political system and its decision makers. Interest articulation is on the interface, or boundary, between constituents and system, since it is through this process that the people communicate their supports and demands to those in a position to address them. If the constituents' interests do not penetrate a political system to allow the decision makers to know what their constituents want, then these interests are not likely to be addressed. The dissatisfaction that can result may be disruptive to the entire system. Thus if consumers' articulated concerns for restraining the runaway costs of medical and hospital care are not heard and addressed satisfactorily by those in a position to do so within the political system, consumers may begin to take matters into their own hands. Their actions may be constructive or destructive, depending on the mood of the group and the resources available to it. Much of the increase in vested-interest groups and political action committees, with the focus of their power on political processes, is, I believe, substantially due to the failures of decision makers to act upon information they have received from constituent groups in the past. The formation of these powerful groups has enhanced their ability not only to articulate their interests but also to insure that their concerns are heard and that responses are forthcoming.

Interest Aggregation. Interest aggregation is the means by which a political system organizes, sifts, evaluates, and finally converts demands expressed to it through the process of interest articulation into general policy alternatives. In short, it is the process of making some sense out of the myriad inputs it receives from its constituencies—order out of chaos. Three styles of interest aggregation predominate (Almond & Powell, 1966:108-109):

1. Pragmatic-bargaining style is characterized by compromise, negotiating, and the "marketplace" spirit. These attributes make the pragmatic-bargaining style the most responsive of the three, since it is capable of dealing with the empirical data at hand in politically expedient ways. A disadvantage may be a resulting lack of consistency and predictability.

2. *Absolute-value–oriented style* of aggregation cannot compromise its principles, whatever they may be, for the sake of addressing diverse interests. Thus there is thought to be one right way of aggregating articulated interests, and all the other possible ways are unacceptable. Political systems that practice interest aggregation in the absolute-value style are very predictable; however, they fail to be responsive to evolving demands, particularly if these demands come from a value base other than the dominant one.

3. Traditionalistic style. Patterns of the past are the dominant principles for the traditionalistic style of interest aggregation. The motto is: "We've always done it this way; why change now?" Societies whose political organizations practice this style of interest aggregation have little concern or sympathy for interests of groups whose needs differ from those of the traditional culture. Thus minority groups find their needs largely unheard and unmet, a situation that can lead to dissatisfaction and potential disruption. I suspect that there is no political organization that practices only one of these styles of interest aggregation, but rather styles change, to some extent, depending on the nature of the interests being articulated.

Interest aggregation may be carried out by any one or a combination of subsystem groups within a political system, although those systems that are stylistically more traditional or absolute-value–oriented no doubt have an easier time doing so than do systems in which the pragmatic-bargaining style predominates. The bureaucracy—and all systems have one to some degree—is a frequent site of interest aggregation. The difficulty, in situations where the bureaucracy is a major interest-aggregating agency, is in preventing the bureaucracy from being coopted by its client-interest groups. When this occurs, the bureaucracy becomes an instrument of these pressure groups and becomes overzealous in furthering the aggregation of the client groups' interests, often at the expense of the interests of other groups. An example of this problem can be found in relationships between regulated organizations and industries, and the portions of the bureaucracy that are charged with regulation but add interest aggregation to their list of functions. This relationship should be avoided if equitable interest aggregation is to be ensured.

Political parties are examples of agencies that aggregate the interests of their members into political party platforms. As I note in Chapter 4, a real strength of political parties is their potential responsiveness to the diverse interests of their various constituent groups, many of which are small and so represent minority opinions and demands. In two-party systems where the competition is keen, much compromise, negotiation, trade-off, and bargaining occur in the process of aggregating pluralistic interests into a policy statement with which the party members as well as, they hope, a substantial majority of the voters can identify. This demands that parties' statements be broad and general so as to include as many groups as possible. In systems where there are many parties, coalitions are the order of the day. Coalitions are often unstable. A reason for the prevalent instability of these party coalitions is that the small specialized groups that make them up are committed to the aggregation of their own issues. When one of these special commitments is breached, for whatever reason, its interest group is likely to withdraw from the coalition, often taking with it other groups with whom it has developed other coalitions. The purpose of any interest-aggregation group is to transform the array of interests articulated in the first step of the conversion process into a form that will be useful to policy makers' deliberations and decision processes.

Communication. Whether by marathon runner or computer letter, political systems have always devised methods of getting information to and from their constituents effectively and efficiently. All of us are dependent for our decisions upon the quality and quantity of information we receive. In a democratic society such as the United States, freedom of speech, assembly, the press, and petition, to name a few constituent communication processes, must be vigorously protected— even if that means that those we do not like are permitted to speak out. The efforts of political systems' officeholders to communicate with constituents must be encouraged and rewarded with feedback. Communication is a two-way process, and nowhere is it more essential than in political arenas. The quality of decisions made throughout the system is heavily influenced by, if not largely dependent upon, the quality of information communicated among its participants.

The next three subsystems in the political model in Figure 3.1 are those most of us think of when we talk about government: the legislature, the administration, and the judiciary. A major reason we have one branch of government to make rules or laws, one to apply or enforce rules, and one to interpret them, rather than having one branch for all three functions, is that the framers of the US Constitution believed that the political theory of separation of powers would prevent the abuse of power they had seen resulting from the concentration of power. Separation of powers has worked well for this country for more than 200 years. The relative strength of the three branches fluctuates depending on circumstances and actors. Equilibrium is maintained through the checks and balances that the three branches exert against each other, as well as through their mixture of functions. Although each branch, as noted, has a primary role to play, all three engage in communication, interest aggregation, and to some extent interest-articulation functions, as well as having some blurred boundaries separating their primary and interdependent roles. We will look briefly here at the three branches of government; they are examined in more detail in the module on the federal government.

Legislation, or Rule Making. Rule making requires the recognition by constituencies of a body's legitimate right to carry out this function.

In other words, permission, or a charge, must be given to the rule-making body by the people to whom the rules will apply, if the rules are to have any effect. In a democratic society such as the United States, legislative groups at the national, state, and local levels have been given this permission by the people. In other societies the right to make rules has been seized by groups who first make the rules and then see that they are imposed on the people, often against their will. In the latter case, repressive control and enforcement of the rules is necessary; in a system such as ours, people for the most part comply voluntarily, or with only occasional reminders. In other kinds of organizations, the group with the legitimate power to make rules for the organization and its members may be a board of trustees, a board of governors, or a governing body. In any case, the rule-making body must have the power, whether delegated or seized, to carry out its functions.

Rule Application or Administration. Rules must be followed to be effective. It is the function of the administration to ensure that the rules made by the rule-making group are enforced. The better developed and differentiated, or specialized, the administration's branches are, the more effective it can be in rule application, especially in situations where rapid change is occurring in the system's environment. The ubiquitous mechanism for rule application that has evolved is bureaucracy. Weber refers to bureaucratization as the virtual essence of the process of political modernization, by comparing bureaucracies to machines and pre-bureaucracy organizations to manual labor (1958). The bureaucracy, with all its Western characteristics—the division of roles and functions, a hierarchic chain of command, standardized rules, and a merit system for promotion and tenure—serves the administrator, whether he or she be monarch, president, prime minister, or dictator, by providing him or her with information and other resources and by implementing decisions. In addition to enforcing rules made by the legislative branch, the bureaucracy also carries out the rules made by the judiciary as a result of that body's rule-interpretation function. As already noted, the bureaucracy has vital roles to play in interest aggregation and communication within the system. In the United States, the federal bureaucracy is made up of various departments (State, Commerce, Labor, and so forth), the military, the regulatory agencies, commissions, and other special bodies. Although the bureaucracy's primary function is rule application, through the regulatory process the bureaucracy is actively involved in making rules as well. Administrative bureaucracies at other levels of government also perform the primary task of rule application as well as secondary roles in interest aggregation, communication, and rule making or regulation. Usually bureaucrats outnumber both legislators and judges by considerable amounts, making the administrative branch the largest one in government. It is also often the fastest-growing branch as well.

In nongovernmental organizations, the bureaucracy is made up of the administrative and general staffs of the agency. It is their primary role to implement the policies made by the governing body or board. Agency staff and administrators also play roles as regulators, communicators, and interest aggregators between the board and the clientele, and on their own behalf as well. Most agencies do not have a judicial or rule interpretation branch, although the implementation of the ombudsman role provides for this function in some organizations. In these situations, the agency bureaucracy also carries out the rules or decisions made by the ombudsman.

Rule Interpretation or Adjudication. Rules or laws often engender conflict regarding their legitimacy and applicability in given situations. Here enters the judiciary branch to interpret or adjudicate the situation and bring about conflict resolution. Conflict may result, for example, from questioning the substance of a law or rule, as well from the inconsistency of its enforcement. In the first instance, the judicial branch must address itself to the congruence of a given rule or law with the overriding political philosophy of the government. In the United States this supreme authority is the US Constitution, and so the courts rule on the constitutionality of a given law. State supreme courts rule on the constitutionality of laws vis-à-vis the state constitution. Their decisions affect whether laws must be changed to conform with the court's interpretation of the Constitution; if the court finds a law to be already in conformity, it must be enforced. Sometimes, ambiguities in the wording of a law may make it subject to different interpretations. In other conflict situations, the plaintiff may challenge the equity of the law as it applies to his or her given case. The United States Constitution guarantees people equal protection under the law, so if a person can substantiate a claim that the law was unequally applied to his or her situation, and the judicial branch agrees with this claim, then the law is not applied or enforced in that particular circumstance. If the court finds that the law was appropriately and equitably applied, then it may sanction its enforcement. In addition to protecting the rights of individuals from unconstitutional laws or unequal or unpredictable enforcement, judicial interpretations also seek to avoid large-scale conflicts with groups who may feel that laws are discriminating against their group, resulting in the eruption of violent behavior by these groups. Because the interpretation of rules and laws can potentially step on both the legislative and administrative branches' toes to make and enforce rules the courts' autonomy and impartiality, insofar as the latter is possible, are essential—yet another reason for the doctrine of separation of powers.

Most organizations now have some type of grievance or appeals procedure for employees who feel that they have been unfairly treated. Collective bargaining agreements often spell these procedures out in considerable detail. Some accreditation standards also require that a grievance procedure be in place. Ombudsmen, by definition impartial evaluators and arbitrators, also serve an adjudication function in some organizations. Although most organizations do not have separate, identifiable judicial bodies, under grievance and appeals procedures members of the bureaucracy and the administration are constituted as autonomous panels to hear the claims of both sides. This adjudicative role is both extremely important and often very difficult.

Systems Maintenance. Monsma cites three major types of systems-maintenance functions that contribute to the system's ability to exist as a viable entity (1969). They are: creating legitimacy, generating support, and resolving conflict.

1. *Creating legitimacy.* For any political system to remain stable and vital, the people it governs must believe, at least to some degree, that the system has a right to govern them. No group, however powerful, can rule forever by coercion alone. Weber describes three kinds of legitimacy (Gerth, 1953): (a) Legal authority is based on respect for the laws and regulations that a governing body has made. Loyalty under legal authority is based on the laws themselves, not on the individual or group who administers them. Laws are made and changed through prescribed, orderly procedures. Everyone, no matter what his or her rank or title, theoretically, is equally subject to the rule of the laws. (b) Traditional authority's legitimacy rests on a reverence for the past and for preserving the social order. Patriarchal rule represents traditional authority at its epitome. In a traditional society, people are obedient to the wishes of the ruler because of their esteem for him and their heavy dependence on him, not as much as an individual but as the representative or personification of the traditions the society reveres. (c) Charismatic legitimacy evolves from followers' personal and affectual devotion to an individual leader. In this form, compliance with the leader's wishes is based on the peoples' feelings for the individual rather than for either law or tradition. Since the charismatic ruler is not accountable for either law or tradition, he or she is permitted to act as he or she wishes. Charismatic rule is, therefore, often characterized by irrational actions. To survive, a political system must develop and perpetuate in the people it governs a sense of its own legitimacy.

2. *Generating support.* Through its actions, a political system either generates support for itself or loses support. Seeking popular involve-

ment in decisions through public hearings, using the news media to provide the people with information about issues and alternatives, sending members of the government out among the people to provide and/or collect information, and publicizing the manner in which it carries out its interpretation of the best courses of action are examples of the ways government seeks to generate support among the people it rules.

3. *Resolving conflicts.* The more legitimacy a political system has and the more support it generates, the better it is able to resolve the conflicts that inevitably arise when two different groups seek the same resources or when decisions are made that favor, or at least appear to favor, one group at the expense of another. Failure to successfully resolve conflict through such strategies as negotiation, trade-offs, compromises, and, as a last resort, force, would result in disintegration of the political system into increasingly deeper factions, civil war, and, eventually, anarchy. To avoid this destruction, the political system must devise and employ methods that deal with conflicts, if not to everyone's satisfaction, at least to the point that everyone can live with or tolerate the outcome.

Table 3.1 is a matrix of these three systems-maintenance functions as they are carried out by branches of the government: the Presidency, the Congress, the bureaucracy, and the judiciary. As the table shows, each of these branches has specific and relatively distinctive, although interdependent, roles to play in creating legitimacy, generating support, and resolving conflict. The bureaucracy, to a greater extent than the other branches, also is responsible for maintaining the physical functioning of the entire political system: ordering supplies, facilitating information flow, and generally keeping the political system going.

Political Systems' Capabilities. The political systems' capabilities represent examples of what political systems actually do in pursuit of their role as governors of people. Looking at the capabilities of political systems allows for an assessment of their level of activity as well as providing a basis for comparison between political systems.

1. *Extractive capability* refers to the political system's ability to gather human and material resources from its environment, both domestic and international. The success with which the system is able to extract resources is the basis of its ability to function. A bankrupt system cannot long survive without an infusion of additional resources. Some political systems are more able to extract resources than are others. Much of this ability rests on the political system's facility to create legitimacy for itself and its causes and to generate support. Unrest and even revolution may result if political systems carry out their extractive functions in a way that the people feel is confiscatory, inequitable, or

excessive, especially if the people believe they have even a remote chance in bringing about change. Wise political systems develop a variety of sources rather than permitting themselves to be dependent on one. For example, the United States places different tax levies on individuals, businesses, agriculture, imports, and investments. As a result, even if one sector of the economy slumps, others are available for continued extraction of resources. This is in marked contrast to governments who depend for virtually their entire resource base on a single commodity such as coffee or oil.

2. *Regulative capability.* One of the primary responsibilities of any government is regulative, the maintenance of order. Herein lies a system's legitimate right to use coercion to control behavior. Regulations extend from government rules for individual and group contracts to procedures for raising and maintaining military forces. Regulations in the United States, for the most part, serve to protect the individual as long as he or she stays within the boundaries defined by the law. In some other societies, regulation is far more repressive of individual actions. The regulative and extractive functions of any political system are highly interdependent: resources are needed to maintain restraints, and coercion or threat of coercion is often required to make extractions of resources possible.

3. *Distributive capability.* Through its distributive capability, a political system allocates goods, services, appointments, and opportunities of various kinds to individuals and groups within the society it governs. People who feel that they get enough from the government or organization are likely to be relatively supportive of the political system and to feel that it is legitimate. Those who feel that they are being discriminated against and unfairly or inequitably treated are likely to question the political system's legitimacy and either to withhold their support or to foment open rebellion. Political systems can and do use their distributive capability to build coalitions of supporting groups. This is apparent in Presidential campaigns in which large amounts of government resources are distributed to states with crucial primary elections or where political elites come out in support of the incumbent President's bid for reelection. Obviously, judicious use of the political system's distributive capability is an effective means of generating support—for at least as long as the goods last or are valued.

4. *Symbolic capability.* A political system's symbolic capability is measured by the effectiveness of its symbolic outputs into its domestic and international environments. Symbolic outputs include shows of military might through parades and displays: state visits to other countries or the hosting of foreign dignitaries at home; endorsements and statements by political elites affirming values, goals, and the like; and statements of policy or intent by political leaders, such as threats to

TABLE 3.1

Matrix of Systems Maintenance Functions as Carried Out by Branches of the Government

Systems Maintenance Functions	Branches of Government			
	Presidential	Congressional	Bureaucratic	Judicial
Creating legitimacy	Office and activities of the President can be used to create feelings of respect and loyalty. Many Presidential functions can be carried out in formal and traditional ways. Presidents seek to show themselves as charismatic leaders and thus further legitimize their decisions and actions.	The broad representativeness of the Congress and its members' accessibility and responsiveness to the people give it a basis for the peoples' acceptance of the legitimacy of its actions. Congressional traditions add legitimacy to their collective and individual actions in the name of the Constitution.	The bureaucracy's growing role in the formation and oversight of regulatory processes derives much of its legitimacy from the other subsystems whose decisions the bureaucracy carries out. The public prominence of some secretaries, either because of their actions in office or in prior positions, lends some legitimacy to their action.	Because of its role as interpreter of the Constitution and legal precedents, the judicial branch's decisions are cloaked in traditional and rational authority.
Generating support	Because of the President's tremendous visibility and potential as a newsmaker, the President's power as a generator of support for the political system in general and	Congressional accessibility and responsiveness to public demands and interests are not only means to generate support for the political system but also to provide peo-	This is probably the bureaucratic subsystem's most important function, since most people have more contact with members of this governmental branch than with	Respect for and adherence to the laws are tangible demonstrations of support for the political system. The judicial branch's major contribution to generating support for the

as a decision maker in particular is great. To many people, the President is the symbol of the government and, therefore, is a rallying point for support. The President is generally the leader of the party he represents and so can rally partisan support.	ple with an opportunity to be heard and to feel a part of the governmental process—a feeling that engenders and enhances support. Members of Congress can also garner some partisan support.	any other. The quality of these interactions, therefore, has a great deal of influence on how much support a citizen may give the political system.	political system is through the quality and perceived fairness of its decisions.
Resolving conflicts			
Without some conflict little reason exists for the exercise of Presidential leadership. A divided Congress offers an opportunity for Presidential intervention. Much of the President's role involves negotiation or lending the legitimacy of the Presidency to one or the other side. In either case the function is to resolve the conflict before it becomes totally disruptive to the total political system.	Through debate, compromise, trade-offs, negotiation and coalition formation, Congress avoids total deadlock and fosters conflict resolution. By providing the public with a forum in which to be heard, interests can be articulated and aggregated in ways that foster managing conflicts without resorting to violence.	Because of its functions of implementing and enforcing the statutes and orders developed by the other branches, the bureaucracy faces many conflicts. A history of fair and consistent interpretations and equitable enforcement goes a long way to help the bureaucracy deal with present conflicts in ways that are acceptable to the protagonists.	Since the courts' major function is rule interpretation, conflict resolution is a central activity. In fact, the courts rarely become involved in a situation until a conflict has arisen and they are called in to adjudicate it.

Adopted from Monsma, 1969.

impose sanctions, or promises to grant benefits. Symbolic capabilities can expand the value of certain political system activities far beyond their actual effects. For example, the symbolic value of providing a very small increase in Social Security benefits far outweighs the actual financial advantages to the recipients.

5. *Responsive capability.* The relationship between inputs and outputs in a political system is the measure of the system's responsiveness. Much is said about the need for governments and other political organizations to be accessible and accountable to their constituents; this is really a demand for responsiveness. Indeed, an organization's responsiveness may replace other reasons for the allegiance of its constituents, such as custom or religious belief. A key question to ask in analyzing any political system is: "To whom does the system respond?"

The United States' political system is quite responsive to well-developed and well-financed vested-interest groups, now prevalent in the form of political action committees, as we saw in Chapter 4. The major political parties are also able, generally, to obtain some response from the government.

Opinion polls are a mechanism that is increasingly being used to measure public opinion and attitudes toward issues. Elected officials often send questionnaires to their constituents to obtain their ideas and to seek—or at least to appear to seek—guidance from the people who elected them. Newspapers, television stations, interest groups, and a growing number of professional polling organizations also ply their trade, especially during Presidential election years. Often the results of polls taken at the same time and addressing the same issues show very different results. Part of this discrepancy occurs because of poor sampling techniques; some is caused by the way the questions are asked. Thus polls conducted by special-interest groups should be viewed with considerable skepticism. What is important is not the answers to a single question on any given poll, but the kinds of trends that a number of polls taken over a period of time show. During Presidential election years, especially toward the end of the campaign, polls have an effect on shaping opinions as well as measuring them (Baron, 1980). Seeking public input through polls as a basis for political-system decision making, although somewhat questionable, is better than not providing any mechanism for the expression of ideas at all. Another way constituents can try to get their elected officials to respond to them is by writing individual and group letters (see Chapter 4).

In spite of all of these kinds of attempts to foster responsiveness on the part of the political system, a question asked with increasing frequency about the United States government is, how responsive is it to those people who do not vote, are not selected by or do not choose to participate in opinion polls, and who are not active in either political action committees or political parties? In short, how responsive is our government, and other organizations in this country, to a vast number of its citizens? It is regrettable that the answer often must be that our institutions are not as responsive as many citizens would like. In an era of shrinking resources and expanding demands, the abilities of governments and organizations to be equitably responsive to the needs of all the people will be increasingly tested and may be found wanting. Because, as nurses, we often have unique access to many people who feel that they are disenfranchised and helpless, we have both the opportunity and the responsibility to develop and use our political power in coalition with those who cannot alone gain the responses they need. Here is another reason for nurses to become more active and effective in all kinds of political arenas.

The conversion processes—interest articulation; interest aggregation; communication; rule making; rule application; rule interpretation; systems maintenance; and the use of extractive, regulative, distributive, symbolic, and responsive political capabilities—are all vital components of the political system. Through these mechanisms, the political system hears and processes inputs from the domestic society, the political elites, the pressure groups, and the international community into outputs that affect these same groups. We now turn to look at these outputs and their consequences.

Outputs

A political system's outputs, as noted, reflect the system's actions during its conversion processes, in response to the inputs from its environment. The recipients of political systems' outputs are the same groups—domestic society, political elites, pressure groups, and the international community—who furnished the political system with its inputs. Outputs take the following general forms:

Extractions. Examples of extractions from the political system's constituent groups include taxes, tariffs, and required services, such as military. Through these extractions, the political system gathers the resources it needs to run itself. Constituent groups' refusal to permit these extractions, under such circumstances as a taxpayers' revolt or boycott, can bring down a political system in very short order. Other less tangible kinds of extractions that a political system may seek from its constituents include ideas, information, and reinforcement for its actions. Obviously all of these extractions are quickly converted into inputs for the political system to use to maintain itself.

Regulations. Regulations are the results of rule making, rule application, and rule adjudication processes. Laws are examples of the regulatory output of the political system. There are two types of laws: statutory laws that are enacted by a legislative body, and decisional laws that result from rulings made by the courts (Creighton, 1975). Regulations are the rules governing programs set up to implement the intent of laws. These are administered by the bureaucracy with the intent, again, of being sure that the laws are carried out. Many of these regulations infringe upon the behavior of people and groups. For the most part, as long as the people regulated feel that the laws are legitimate, compliance is relatively easy to obtain. In some instances, inspection, monitoring, enforcement, and sanctions for noncompliance are necessary. Examples of the latter set of regulations include monitoring the highway speed limit and issuing citations and fines to people who do not obey it, or enforcement of safety standards in work places by threat of fines or forced suspension of operations.

Allocations. The political system taketh away, but the political system also giveth. The giving is done in the form of allocations: revenue sharing, Social Security benefits, Medicaid assistance, scholarships, and a huge variety of other means for returning resources in the form of goods and services to constituent groups throughout the domestic society. Through foreign aid, the political system also allocates goods and services to members of the international community. Some of the most heated political discussions ensue over the topic of the equity between the amount of money specific individuals and groups pay to the government and the goods and services they are allocated in return.

Information. Peoples' needs for information are increasingly insatiable as technology mushrooms and the pace of living accelerates. Governments, especially that of the United States, put out a staggering array of publications, dealing not only with laws and regulations but also with topics ranging from apricot raising to zoology. Adequate information about regulations is critical to peoples' ability and willingness to conform to them. Thus the information output of the political system must be thorough as well as timely.

Symbolic. Symbolic outputs come in the form of state ceremonies, Presidential addresses, televised Congressional hearings, policy statements, and the like. The actual result of these activities is often far less significant than symbolic power.

All of these outputs from the political system affect and are affected by the environment. Through comprehensive feedback, the political system is able to monitor the effects of its activities on the domestic society, the political elites, the pressure groups, and the international community. Developing surveillance mechanisms for outputs is a constant challenge for the political system. Monitoring the consequences of outputs is even more difficult.

Consequences

Outputs from the political system often have ramifications in their environment far beyond those that are expected and predicted by even the most astute forecasters inside and outside the system. The analogy of the ripple effect is appropriate here: the political system's outputs are pebbles dropped into a calm pool; consequences are the concentric, overlapping, and far-reaching ripples or rings that extend beyond the initial splash. The consequences influence the domestic society, the political elites, the pressure groups, and the international community in relation to their support for the political system as well as their demands of it. Other consequences of the political system's outputs include the development and differentiation of roles and structures as a result of information; the allocations of goods and services; extractions; and regulations. These kinds of changes, consequent to the political system's outputs, continue their interactions and extensions far into the future, indeed to infinity.

Feedback

The political system's conversion processes and their consequences provide myriad opportunities for the political system to develop feedback mechanisms. By so doing, the political system is assured of being provided with information that can assist it to be more responsive to the needs of its constituents. Feedback also helps a system to be aware early of impending changes or problems and, therefore, be able to react appropriately and in a timely fashion. Some feedback occurs naturally, but those in charge of systems should not depend upon this. Rather, concerted efforts need to be made to establish and carefully monitor feedback in a variety of places and with a variety of groups of constituents to insure the rapid reporting of information the system needs to make adjustments. As shown in Figure 3.1, feedback "loops" tie up the loose ends between the system and its environment.

POWER

Power has many definitions, but most of them characterize it as the ability of an individual, group, or organization to cause or constrain actions by other individuals, groups, or organizations (Archer, 1979b). Individuals and groups seek power both as a tool to influence others' behavior and as an end in itself. Seeking power as an end in itself is sheer self-aggrandizement; power, as is money, is only really useful because of what it can help us do. Power can be shared with others, thus enhancing itself. Power can be denied to others and used to keep them in a subservient position.

Because of all of these properties, power is a major ingredient in political activities and of politics itself. Power disparities between groups or individuals within a group can lead to conflict, negotiation, compromise, capitulation, coalition formation, repression, and revolution. Power is sought by those who don't have as much of it as they want; power is defended to the death by those who already hold it. Power is addictive.

"Power to the people" has been a rallying cry to galvanize people who have felt powerless in trying to deal with the Establishment. Many heretofore powerless groups—women, students, ethnic groups, handicapped persons—have experienced brief brushes with power under this banner. Having once tasted this heady wine, they thirst for more. Power remains consolidated in the hands of the political elites and the pressure or vested-interest groups, for the most part. Our society has not seen fit to redistribute power, and many people feel alienated, apathetic, and helpless. We shall see another wave of group effort as more people seek to share the power pie (Alinsky, 1972; Altshuler, 1970; Hawley & Wirt, 1974; Kahn, 1970).

This book is about ways nurses can attain and use power in the political arena. It is about evolutionary change. Many fear that some of the directions that our government is taking, if not changed, will lead to revolution. I believe that revolution will not be necessary if more people learn to participate effectively in government, and government is more responsive. The United States has a 200-year history of being at least relatively responsive to the electorate, however that group has been defined. We are entering another era of crisis, with internal and external threats to our form of government. We must overcome our apathy and find ways to peacefully and effectively influence those who govern us. We must learn to use power as a means to attain just and equitable ends. If we do not, others—and some of us as well—will use power to destroy far more than will be gained. We must get involved before it is too late.

Typology of Power

To understand politics one must understand something about power. What follows is a typology of power drawn from a number of sources.

Legitimate power is authority in a role that is accepted and recognized by an organization's or system's members. In short, the governed have granted the leader or person in authority the right to use that authority over them. In this kind of situation, a minimum of coercion is needed to enforce the leader's decisions and regulations, because people comply voluntarily. Much of the power that the US government exerts over its citizens is viewed by us as legitimate power, and so we permit ourselves to be governed by it.

Reward power is the use of positive sanctions, such as praise, money, and status, to obtain compliance and support. Carried to its extreme, reward power can become bribery. Political action committees that contribute heavily to political campaigns may be seeking this kind of power over the people who are elected as a result (Wieland & Ullrich, 1976).

Expert power is based on knowledge, skills, and abilities in oneself or access to expertise in others. As technology becomes increasingly complex and systems become more interdependent, the power of the expert will become even more accentuated. No one, politicans included, can be expected to know everything, and so the reliance on consultants, counselors, advisors, and others of this ilk will increase. Caution must be exercised to be sure that the experts are not serving their own ends at the expense of the public interest. Conversely, experts must assume the responsibilities for their roles as influencers of public policy (Benveniste, 1972). Thus, a nurse who finds herself in the position of advising a decision maker as a member of a committee staff or as a specially appointed consultant must be sure of her information and of her motives in making the benefits of her expertise available.

Corruptive power is a concept that has evolved from many sources. Perhaps the most succinct statement of this view of power is that of Lord Acton: "Power tends to corrupt; absolute power corrupts absolutely" (1887). Many people seem to see only this aspect of power and to overlook power's many other faces. To be sure, too much power, especially if concentrated in the hands of too few, can be dangerous. The framers of the US Constitution understood this phenomenon from their own experience as well as from their study of history. To avoid the concentration of power, with its high potential for corruption, they devised our government's system of separation of powers and checks and balances.

Referent power is available to the leader who is willing and able to serve as a role model for his or her followers (Wieland & Ullrich, 1976). People see the leader with referent power as one who is attractive and therefore as one whom they wish to emulate and please. Charismatic leaders have a high degree of referent power. Shiflett and McFarland suggest that for leaders to use referent power effectively, they must be sufficiently secure in their own identity and position to make rational decisions and to use their power to see they are carried out appropriately (1978).

Lower-participant power addresses grassroots or "bottoms up" power. The use of such power may be very legitimate and necessary. Indeed it is a basis for community organization and coalition formation. As Wieland and Ullrich (1976) point out, however, lower-participant power can be used in illegitimate ways to bypass or manipulate an organization's hierarchy; thus lower-participant power can also be a basis for revolution and anarchy. Fortunately, needed changes in the health care delivery system in the United States can be brought about without resort to such extreme uses of power. Nurses represent the largest group of health care providers and so we have a tremendous potential to use a variety of kinds of power, including that of lower participants. In addition, I believe that besides the power we can have through organizing ourselves, we have tremendously powerful potential allies in the consumers of health care services. Because we are less likely than many of our colleagues in health care to have vested economic interests in high fees and large profits or excess revenues, nurses and consumers can form effective coalitions to work for changes in the health care provision system such as cost containment and national health service legislation. We will need to form these coalitions and develop strong and well-financed political action committees to offset the tremendous lobbying power of the medical, hospital, and pharmaceutical company cartel. Nurses may take another constructive avenue with lower-participant power by joining with organizations such as Common Cause and working for passage of legislation to require public financing of Congressional and other legislature elections. This legislation would reduce the inordinate power that political action committees now exert over many of our elected representatives through their campaign donations.

Associative power is derived from liaisons with other groups with whom we share our power and from whom we gain power through association (Wieland & Ullrich, 1976). Nurses have many potential resource groups with whom to share power and from whom we can derive it. Traditionally, as Shiflett and McFarland point out (1978), we have sought associative power from physicians, hospital administrators, and other providers in the health care field. Many of us are beginning to realize that our attempts for associative power through these kinds of liaisons have not been terribly fruitful, to say the least, especially since we have pursued this kind of associative power through dependent and "ladylike" means (Heide, 1976). We have become increasingly aware that our colleagues are only too quick to sell us out when it is to their advantage to do so.

I still believe that nurses must seek associative power from others and share their power with others. I am particularly committed to nurses and consumers working together in coalitions to deal with issues and to work for political change. This may put me in Masson's "avant-garde within the assertiveness fringe (that) advocates power politics over change agency. Its members contend that there is no hope for the system or for the nurses trapped within it. Their strategy is to take it by force from outside, preferably in league with disenchanted consumers and ambitious power politicians" (1979:782). So be it. I would say that there is no hope for the system only if nurses continue to do so little to bring about change. A constructive and much-needed first step is for nurses to get their act together within nursing and begin to present a truly united front on critical issues affecting health care as well as nursing. For example if every one of the 1.4 million nurses in the United States were to contribute \$5 to N-CAP, there would be enough money for N-CAP to make a considerably greater impact than it now can. Nurses need to develop associative power within our own ranks as with likeminded others: providers, consumers, and politicians.

Exploitive power, as defined by May, is power taken from or in spite of others (1972). Exploitive power is one of the kinds of power people associate with "dirty politics." It is the kind of power we mean when we accuse systems of using certain people or groups illegitimately for ends other than their own benefit. Much of the rise of organized labor in the health care field and particularly among nurses is a result of feelings of being exploited. We must guard against turning our collective power into exploitive power over others. To use the health care system for our own ends would be an illegitimate use of our power, in my opinion.

Manipulative power is power used over others to suit one's own purposes, often without their knowledge or consent (May, 1972). Manipulation of any kind has come to have a negative connotation for many people, probably because of the possibility that people will be manipulated against their will or without their knowledge. Many seem to think that politics is a particularly manipulative business; this is the source of some of the current negative attitudes towards politics and politicians. To be sure, manipulative power is used in the political arena as it is in all other arenas. But manipulative power's use is not necessarily devious. As is the case with all uses of power, ethical considerations must be borne in mind when we decide to manipulate situations.

Competitive power pits one group's power against that of other groups (May, 1972). Elections are examples of competitive power in that two or more candidates are competing for the same office. Since an election is a zero-sum game, that is, the winner takes the whole office and the loser gets nothing, the use of competitive power is essential to the elective process. One of the pillars of capitalist economies is competition for resources and markets. Thus our cultural values emphasize competition and the use of competitive power as positive attributes. Many women have not been well socialized into the need to compete or in positive, constructive ways to exert competitive power. Women and nurses must learn to compete. Some causes will win, some will lose, and some will continue without resolution for a period of time. Regardless of the outcome of a specific attempt to exercise competitive power, women and nurses must learn to regroup and prepare to compete again. The current status of the Equal Rights Amendment is a case in point. Often competition involves conflict; as we shall see later in the chapter, dealing effectively with conflict is an area in which nurses need different socialization. Whether nurses like it or not, competition and the exercise of competitive power are large components of the political game, and they must learn to play that game well. The remainder of the 20th century will see shrinking resources available to the health and human services sector as other sectors' demands for more resources increase. Thus social needs will be pitted against industrial and defense needs to an even greater degree than is now the case. Within health and human resources agencies, competition between equally justified and needed programs will also increase as resources diminish or at best remain static. Block grants, in place of categorical ones, can only exaggerate this competition. In recent testimony at budget planning meetings for community mental health funding, I discussed the growing needs of the elderly for community mental health services in spite of shrinking allocations for mental health services in general. I was accused of pitting the elderly against the retarded, children, and other population groups. Indeed, as I pointed out in testimony, all population groups and all services are now competing with each other, more than in the past, often for fewer resources. Competition is, and will continue to be, the name of the politics-of-budget game. If nurses are to be effective advocates for any population group or service, we must learn to use competitive power much more effectively. This competitive power must, however, be tempered with distributive justice: the distribution of benefits and costs at least relatively equally to all members of the society (Davis & Araskar, 1978; Nozick, 1974).

Nutrient power is power used for the benefit of others (May, 1972). Advocacy is an example of nutrient-power use. Many of the groups nurses work with are less able than nurses to speak up for their needs and interests. In such situations, nurses can effectively use their power and influence on behalf of these groups. Often spokespersons from outside of a group that stands to gain or lose by the passage of a law or the development of a regulation can be more effective in testimony than can members of the group itself. Classic examples are the *amicus curiae*, or friend-of-the-court, briefs that professional organizations such as the American Public Health Association are asked to prepare to aid the court in making a decision. Other examples include professionals testifying for legislation or regulations that will improve services for Medicare recipients. In both these instances nutrient power is being exercised. Consumers can also use nutrient power to aid health and human service programs. For example, arranging for community leaders not directly involved in the program under consideration to speak with the legislative group about the value of the program combines both nutrient and associative power into one potentially effective package. In all these examples, the groups or individuals providing input are doing so not because they stand to benefit directly, but rather because they want to assist others. That is what nutrient power is all about. Nutrient power is probably the type of power that nurses use most often and with which they are most comfortable. It can be as effective in the political arena as it is on a one-to-one or client group basis.

Integrative power involves sharing power for decision making, planning, and evaluating with others, rather than confining these activities to a small group (May, 1972). Coalition formation, particularly coalitions between consumers and nurses, is an example of integrative power. Integrative power is based on the ideas of shared power and strength in numbers. The ability of a group or an organization to develop a broadly representative support system via which it shares power and thereby also derives added power to deal with issues is a demonstration of the use of integrative power.

Traditional power, according to Weber, rests on established beliefs in the sanctity of the order handed down from the past (1947). Many who have tried to make changes in a variety of kinds of systems have quickly learned that traditional power is strong, especially when we hear things such as, "But we've always done it that way." Much of our political system is firmly rooted in traditional norms and values that are hard to change and sometimes are harder to follow. Those individuals who wield traditionally based power are those to whom these rights have been given because of their fulfillment of traditional roles. Their decisions are generally viewed as final, and their authority is rarely challenged. Under a system of traditional power, decisions are generally made either on the basis of precedent or on the arbitrary decision of the leader. Political parties have been highly subject to traditional power, with the President or the party's candidate being expected to lead as well as to be loyal to the party. As I discuss in Chapter 4, much of this has only recently changed in the United States. Respect for traditional power, again until recently, led to almost certain reelection of incumbents and only rare challenges to incumbent Presidents from within their own party. This is much less the case now, and traditional power may be on the wane.

Rational power rests on the belief in legal rules and the right of people in authority, as long as they conform to those rules, to issue commands and to expect that they will be obeyed. Rational power, unlike traditional power, is highly impersonal, and decisions are based on established rules rather than personal appraisal of and intervention in a given situation. Bureaucratic organizational structure is the result of rational power. Rules govern and are unquestionably enforced by the people appointed to execute them (Weber, 1947). To influence this kind of system from outside, we must know how rules and regulations are made so that we can intervene at the most crucial point in the rule-making process. We can also exercise rational power by enforcing or adhering to rules.

Charismatic power is based entirely on the power an individual wields over others based on his or her exceptional personal characteristics (Weber, 1947). Charismatic leaders can often exert almost limitless power over their immediate followers, but we rarely encounter them on the national scene. Many people lament the paucity of charismatic leadership to be found among candidates for most public offices today. True charismatic power, because it is so closely connected with and dependent upon one individual, is often subject to that individual's capricious whim. Following the passing of a charismatic leader, the problem of institutionalizing what the leader did or wanted done often results in the evolution of either a national or a traditional powerbased organization. Much of the inability of the Johnson Administration in the 1960s to bring the "New Frontier" to fruition was the result of its failure to successfully institutionalize the charismatic power of John Kennedy. The ideas spawned by one group in the clutch of charismatic power can not be adequately explained, much less implemented by that group or others, without the power of the charismatic leader. This phenomenon has much to do with that era so aptly described in *Maximum Feasible Misunderstanding* (Moynihan, 1970). Thus charismatic power is a mixed blessing, but a heady experience, nonetheless.

Sexually based power is traditionally male domination in many cultures, occupations, and societies (McClelland, 1975). As Ashley so well points out, nurses, most of whom are women, have been and continue to be subject to male domination in most work settings (1976). The movement toward more assertiveness and equality for women (see Chapters 2 and 4) is complicating these stereotyped behavior patterns. Women and nurses are learning new games and revising old ones (Thomstad, Cunningham & Kaplan, 1975; Levin & Berne, 1972; Stein, 1968). Sexually based power is not going to go away, at least not in the near future. There are signs, however, that the sexually based balance of power is changing in some parts of our society. Because of the very strong tradition of sexually based power in health care, complicated by disparities in status and income, change may be even slower in our subsystem than it will be in the society at large.

Stages of Power Orientation

Finally, McClelland presents four power orientation stages in terms of an individual's ego development (1975). The four stages are not linear but rather are alternative kinds of actions that give people feelings of power. In stage 1, power is seen as personally strengthening. For such persons, the locus of control is outside of themselves and they are, therefore, dependent upon outside rather than inner resources for support. They probably rarely exercise power themselves but are instead those upon whom power is exercised. They may be able to derive some associative power from others during this stage. Lacking other resources, they may also revert to dependence on sexually based power.

Stage 2 is characterized by the feeling of becoming stronger personally. The locus of control is more internal, and such people feel in control of themselves and of their environment. People in this stage can be assertive and can use legitimate expert, lower-participant, manipulative, referrent, and competitive power effectively.

Feelings of having impact on others describes stage 3. The impact of this stage can be positive in terms of the use of nutrient, legitimate, traditional, rational, integrative, competitive, and expert power. People who become carried away with their feelings about their ability to influence others during this stage may overuse coercive, exploitive, reward, and manipulative power.

In stage 4 the person is moved to do his or her duty based on feelings of power. If the individual chooses to subordinate personal goals to assisting others, the kinds of power that can be used effectively include nutrient, integrative, expert, competitive, and manipulative. If, instead, the person is no longer able to distinguish between his or her personal views and those of the organization or state, the possibility of fanaticism and misuse of power enters. These people are manipulators in the most pejorative sense of the word. Other kinds of power that these people tend to abuse include coercive, exploitive, reward, and competitive. We need to be alert for signs of these various stages of power orientation in ourselves and in others.

Discussion

The typology just discussed illustrates the complexity of the concept of power. To further complicate the subject, none of the types presented are exclusive or discrete. Thus there are great difficulties in defining boundaries between one kind of power and another. My objective in presenting the typology is to show that there are many faces of power, and none is all good or all bad. Power as an end in itself is of dubious value. Power used to further causes that are beneficial to groups who are lacking in resources is legitimate, I believe. This is a reflection of my Robin Hood philosophy of distributive justice and equity—my belief that the have-nots should be helped. That is the easy part. The real dilemma ensues in a situation such as we now face, in which resources are becoming increasingly limited and competition for them is growing. The "truly needy" as well as everyone else, may suffer. Therefore, politics enters the picture, since to give more of anything to one group means taking it from another: yet another illustration of the inseparability of politics, power, and resource considerations.

Nurses are not using our potential power to bring about changes in the health care system through the mechanisms of politics. Part of this is because most nurses are women and have been socialized to be passive and dependent rather than assertive and independent. We have learned to play games, to be passive-aggressive in getting what we want, and to let others do our politicking for us. We can no longer afford to play these roles, nor can our clients afford for us to continue to play them. The politics of health is much too important to leave in the hands of the politicians, the political action committees, and the vested-interest groups that now dominate the scene. We must join forces, learn the dimensions of our power, and use our power to make the health care system and health care in general in this country a right for all and not a privilege. Power is like so many other human capacities: we must use it or we shall lose it.

DECISION MAKING

One of life's dilemmas is that we are generally confronted with far more activities than we can possibly take part in, no matter how much we might like to do so. Making decisions, that is, choosing between often equally attractive alternative activities, is one of the problems nurse-activists must face. There are far more forms of political participation (as shown in the discussion of political-participation typology in Chapter 1) than any one of us can reasonably expect to be active in. Thus we need to learn how to make the best choice we can.

In Table 3.2, I show a rational exercise that can be helpful for making decisions among equally attractive alternatives, or those that seem so at first glance. Let us suppose that each of us has just been invited to become involved in the three different activities listed in the matrix as alternatives. If we are not interested in one or more of the offered alternatives, then we could narrow the field of choice quickly. But, for the sake of discussion, let us suppose that we want to do all three, but we know that that is impossible. How do we decide among them? The first

TABLE 3.2

Decision Matrix: Choosing Among Types of Political Participation, Using Weighted Criteria

Criterion	Weight	Join a Women's Political Activist Group	Take a Seat on the Local Health System Agency Governing Body	Support a Candidate's Campaign for State Legislature
Congruence with personal values	+8	8 × 2 = 16	8 × 2 = 16	8 × 2 = 16
Potential impact on the target system	+3	3 × 1 = 3	3 × 2 = 6	3 × 1 = 3
Opportunity to make contacts	+2	2 × 2 = 4	2 × 2 = 4	2 × 2 = 4
Cost in money	−1	−1 × 2 = −2	−1 × 0 = 0	−1 × 2 = −2
Cost in time	−2	−2 × 2 = −4	−2 × 2 = −4	−2 × 1 = −2
Potential risks or punishments	−3	−3 × 0 = 0	−3 × 0 = 0	−3 × 1 = −3
Personal ability	+5	5 × 1 = 5	5 × 1 = 5	5 × 1 = 5
Professional rewards	+2	2 × 1 = 2	2 × 2 = 4	2 × 0 = 0
Positive subtotal		+30	+35	+28
Negative subtotal		− 4	− 4	− 7
Total		+26	+31	+21

Scoring: 0 = Criterion does not apply or occurrence is not likely
1 = Moderately applicable or likely
2 = Very applicable or likely

step is to clearly understand what each of the alternative activities actually entails. The more we know about each of the possible activities, the better we can understand the relative value of each one, compared to the others. The more we know about each, the more rationally we can apply our criteria, or standards for participation, to each one. Since each of the activities listed as alternatives would vary greatly in terms of local specifics, I shall not describe them here; I leave that to each of you to do *in situ.*

The criteria listed in the left-hand column of Table 3.2 are much more easily described and can be applied to most situations of choice. They are general criteria that many of us would consider appropriate gauges of the relative values of a given set of activities. I suspect that some will think of other criteria to add to the group given here, but these will suffice for this illustration. I have assigned a weight, or loading factor, to each of the criteria on the basis of my own assessment of its relative value for me. Your relative weightings may differ from mine. The principle here is that the value of all of the criteria is not equal; some are more important than are others. The actual weights assigned are arbitrary. To illustrate, I shall discuss each criterion and explain why I have weighted it as I have.

Congruence With Personal Values. This is one of those nonnegotiable factors discussed later under exchange theory. We need to be able to believe in what we're being asked to do. Ideally, an alternative that would get less than a score of 2 on this criterion would not be on our list of alternatives. In reality, we sometimes find ourselves making choices between activities that we do not really agree with or value. This is particularly likely when the activity is something we are told or encouraged to do by people who have power over us. Because of the importance of the activity's congruence with personal values, I have assigned very high weighting to it. To be sure, the weighting is skewed in the direction of this criterion, which is precisely my intent.

Potential Impact on the Target System. This standard addresses the need to assess the effect our participation in a given activity may have on the intended outcome. In some instances, what we can do has the potential to make a great deal of difference; in others, there is little hope for such an outcome. Since all of us have limited resources, it is reasonable for us to consider how we can use what we have to obtain the best results. Many people drop out of activities because they cannot perceive that what they are doing has any effect on the total picture. This is one rationale used to explain the decreasing proportion of eligible voters who make the effort to get to the polls on election day. Because I think it is a relatively important criterion, I have weighted it as $+3$.

Opportunity to Make Contacts.   Increasing and deepening one's scope of contacts is a fringe benefit of many political activities. Its importance should not be underestimated, since in the world of politics, the adage "It's not what you know but who you know that counts" is perhaps even more applicable than in other kinds of activities. Almost all kinds of political participation provide opportunities to meet others, to develop relationships, to see ways to form new coalitions, and to generally widen the circle of people we know. Widening our number of contacts also increases the likelihood that we will be thought of when other opportunities arise and the people we know are casting about for like-minded persons to join their efforts.

Cost in Money.   The relative weight you place on this criterion will be a very personal decision. Since it is a cost rather than a benefit, I have given it a negative weight of -1. I suggest that you find out in advance as much as you can about the possible costs of any political activity: Are expenses reimbursed? How much travel is involved? and so on. Only then can you really put a dollar value on the cost to be expected from participation in a given activity. Know how much you can spend and weigh that amount against what you're told it will cost. My experience leads me to believe that estimated costs are usually too low; remember that.

Cost in Time.   Because I tend to have less time than money, I have rated this factor more negatively than I did money. Your assessment may differ. Again, estimates are almost always too low, so multiply what you are told by some reasonable "fudge" factor. After you have participated in similar kinds of activities, your own estimates of the time required will be better than, or at least as good as, those of others. There NEVER is enough time, so select wisely. The principle of opportunity cost pertains to both time and money costs. What we spend of either of these scarce resources on one activity we then cannot spend for any other activity, and so we must consider not only the costs of the actual activity but also the costs of the other opportunities we have had to forego because of our decision to do one and not another.

Potential Risks or Punishments.   More often than not, this criterion will be scored 0 or does not apply. There are instances, however, where political participation may create risk, such as in the third alternative, supporting a candidate for state legislature (see the discussion of the Hatch Act in Chapter 4). A less obvious potential punishment can ensue, such as the one discussed in Chapter 4, in which the candidate I was supporting in a recent election was opposed by an incumbent supervisor in my county. Since the supervisors have authority over much of the budget for one of Nursing Dynamic's major projects and I am an officer of that corporation, I had to be very cautious in the openness of my support for the supervisor's opponent. Certainly, in a free country we should be and are free to support the candidate of our choice for a given office; nonetheless there are times when prudence must be exercised because of potential negative spill-overs into other areas because of politically partisan activity. The potential for this kind of result should be a criterion in making decisions, particularly in hotly contested elections.

Personal Ability.   This is another of those "bottom-line" criteria, thus the high weighting. The question to be assessed is: can I do what will be asked of me in a given activity? If public speaking is involved, am I good at that? If chairing committees is expected, is this among my repertoire of skills? If soliciting money and votes from strangers is part of the job, can I do these things? If you cannot meet the expectations of the activity, then you should think twice before accepting the invitation. You may not know at the outset what skills and expertise will be needed for some kinds of political participation. Here is another reason to find out as much about an activity as possible before launching into it. Talk with people you know who have been or are involved in the activities you are considering. If possible, observe some meetings or other activities before making a decision. At all costs, make an objective assessment of the requirements and their fit with your skills before making a commitment. Once you are involved, it can be embarrassing to learn that you are simply not cut out for what is expected of you.

Professional Rewards.   Many positions, particularly those on university faculties, have a clearly stated community or public service requirement as part of their criteria for retention and promotion. Service agency nurse-managers are also often expected to participate in community activities as representatives of their nursing service or of the entire agency. Many forms of political participation, particularly at the local level, can fulfill these obligations. If you are in doubt about the relative values of alternative kinds of activities, talk with your employer about them as part of your decision-making process. If the professional rewards are great, you may want to give a particular alternative extra consideration.

Once you have clearly identified what is entailed in each of the alternative activities among which you have a choice, and have set up and weighted your own list of criteria, you can go about the business of completing the matrix and using it as a decision-making aid. This process is illustrated in Table 3.2 for three alternative political activities using eight weighted criteria, or standards. Add up the scores, being careful to keep negative ones negative and positive ones positive, and see what the final score is for each activity. The alternative with the highest score is the alternative of choice.

Although this process is neat and tidy, there are some problems inherent in using this kind of quantitative decision-making tool. First of all, many of the intangible costs and benefits of one kind of political participation over others cannot be readily quantified, no matter how hard we try. Second, we can never have all the information needed to make the best possible decision. Here the alternatives become (a) do nothing until circumstances force the choice—what I call "decision by drift"; (b) keep gathering information; this will keep you busy but you may still end up with an outcome such as the one in (a); or (c) gather as much information as you can in a given period of time and then act on the basis of that information. In this latter kind of quick assessment, a decision matrix such as the one I have just presented can be of real help. Finally, in spite of what the decision matrix shows, you may decide to choose another alternative anyway, or you may manipulate the matrix in such a way that it comes out the way you wanted it to in the first place. That's fine as long as you do these manipulations consciously, that is, you have already made up your mind before going through the exercise and do so only to see what happens. Even then, the exercise may show you some areas of concern that you had not thought of before. In any case, the more rational consideration we can give to choosing among alternative courses of action, whether for political participation or other activities, the more likely we are to understand the ramifications of the decisions we make. That in itself is a positive accomplishment.

CONFLICT

Conflict is the stuff of which politics and change are made. Without conflict there would be little need for political actions; there would also be little change, little creativity, and little progress. Baldridge points out that conflict is a key ingredient and motivating force in political systems, and that conflict theory is part of political activities' basic theoretical foundation (1971). The moment two or more competing individuals or groups want more resources than their "fair share" or than is available, or have different ideas about how something ought to be done, the stage is set for conflict. Indeed, without some degree of conflict in organizations and other political systems, there would be no need for many of a political system's conversion processes, discussed earlier in this chapter.

Conflict, then, is an essential and healthy ingredient in all kinds of political actions. Too little conflict can be almost as detrimental as too much.

Most women and nurses have been socialized to avoid conflict because they have been taught that conflict is categorically detrimental and destructive. This is one of the reasons many women nurses have difficulty dealing with conflict except by passive-aggressive or avoiding/acquiescent behaviors. We tend to personalize conflict, focusing on the persons or personalities involved instead of on the issues. Many people cannot understand how two opponents can fight bitterly over issues upon which they disagree and yet remain friends. A classic example is that of attorneys on opposite sides of a court case. The ability to do this and a background in dealing with conflict may be contributing factors to the overrepresentation of attorneys in US government.

Because of scarce resources and differing values, conflict is inevitable. We must learn not only to deal with it effectively and to use it constructively, but also to stimulate conflict when it is temporarily absent (Lewis, 1976). Speaking to nurse-managers, Lewis notes: "We should visualize a continuum, with too much conflict at one end and too little at the other. At some point between these extremes, the quantity of conflict is functional and valuable. This point is determined by management and will not necessarily be the same for any two organizations" (1976:18). The same can be said about political conflict. No two issues or campaigns will generate the same amount of intensity of conflict. To be sure, if there is more than one candidate for an office or more than one opinion on an issue, conflict will arise. If the political system cannot manage the conflict in such a way as to prevent it from evolving too far toward the excessive-conflict end of the continuum, violence may ensue.

Violence is an aspect of conflict that many people fear and so seek to avoid. Certainly all conflicts do not involve violence; examples are petition, peaceful assembly, nonviolent demonstrations and protests, peaceful elections, speeches, and debates. When these nonviolent means of articulating interests and managing conflict break down, violence often erupts. Violence is a threat to the entire social and political fabric of a jurisdiction. If push comes to shove and the political system cannot resolve the conflict generated by its constituents by peaceful or nonviolent means, it must resort to force or coercion for this control. On the other hand, groups of constituents, feeling that their government no longer hears or responds to their needs, may resort to violence against the government or other groups of constituents in an attempt to attain their desired ends and thus resolve the conflicts they perceive. Violence is at best a zero-sum game, that is, one side wins at the expense of the other. More likely, violence is a lose-lose game: neither side wins as much as it loses or enough to justify its losses. For these reasons, political systems strive to adjudicate and resolve conflicts before they reach the stage where violence is likely to erupt.

At different times and under different circumstances, people may be either conflict prone or cooperative. If individuals and groups are to be able to live in close proximity, they must develop mechanisms to manage conflicts either by themselves or through other, often governmental, sources. Governments can and do permit and tolerate considerable individual conflict without intervening, so long as the people involved do not seriously injure each other, pose a threat to others, or resort to violence to solve their grievances against one another. Some ways to deal with conflict are discussed later in this chapter.

Similarly, the state, especially in the United States, does not interfere with groups engaging in nonviolent conflict, so long as the conflict does not threaten the stability of the country. An example of this is government non-intervention in labor-management disputes so long as they are not so protracted or so severe as to threaten the national economy or security (Dahl, 1976). When this happens, the government intervenes through a variety of means, including compulsory and binding arbitration, to bring the parties into consensus and to end the conflict, at least temporarily.

Stages of Conflict

Pondy suggests several stages in conflict episodes as a framework for examining conflict situations (1967):

Latent Conflict. Latent conflict has numerous underlying causes that Pondy summarizes into three basic types: competition for scarce resources, drives for autonomy, and divergence of subunit goals. He views role conflict as a concept that is useful in the analysis of all three types of latent conflict rather than as a type of latent conflict itself (1967).

Competition for scarce resources is becoming more acute and more widespread through the economy. The health care delivery system is by no means exempt from this phenomenon. Conflict between the health care system and other sectors of the US economy is becoming more overt as the health care system continues to resist efforts at cost containment, consumes almost 10 percent of the gross national product, and contributes little to changes in our relative rankings with other countries on standard morbidity and mortality indices. Competition for scarce resources is intensifying within the health care system as well. Nursing must compete for education and research dollars with medicine, dentistry, and other disciplines. Education and service programs are increasingly at loggerheads as resources dwindle. Service programs compete with one another, and client-advocacy groups become more vocal as they see their special population getting less. These kinds of competition for scarce resources are inevitable and can be predicted to become even more bitter as the amount of resources available for health and human services shrinks. Nursing and other vested-interest groups increasingly will turn to political strategies in the hope of obtaining more than their original allocations.

The notion of nursing as a profession, the desire of nurses to control our own practice, the American Nurses' Association's resolution that a baccalaureate degree is the level of entry into professional nursing practice, and nursing's expanded roles are examples of nursing's drive for increased autonomy. As Davis points out: "Self-direction, or autonomy, is the one condition included in all other institutional elements in most definitions of professions. An occupational group is not self-directing, however, unless it controls the production and especially the application of knowledge and skill in the work it performs" (1979:3). To establish itself as an autonomous profession, nursing must prove itself to be capable of independence and self-monitoring. These are not easy tasks. The situation is complicated by the fact that other disciplines seem to view nursing's striving for autonomy as a direct threat to their autonomy and status. It is almost as though autonomy were a limited resource; for nursing to get more others must lose some. This attitude sets the stage for conflict.

The field of nursing today represents a monument to latent conflict brought about by the divergence of subunit goals: professional nursing versus technical—or whatever the new term will be—nursing; nurse-managers versus nursing staff; education versus service; ANA versus NLN versus the specialty organizations; associate degree versus diploma versus baccalaureate versus graduate preparation for entry into nursing or into certain kinds of practice. Nursing really does not have one voice and is thus exposed to outside forces that seek to divide and thereby conquer it. The fact that nurses seems to prefer internecine inner battles to taking a united stand that would provide us with the clout that our 1.4 million membership should command makes us vulnerable to all sorts of divisive tactics. Unless nursing unites around a defensible position, arrived at through compromise, its internal splintering can bring about its demise. The potential political force that nursing has for implementing change in the health care system will then be lost.

Perceived Conflict. Often, being aware of or perceiving conflict can be the first step to finding ways to deal effectively with that conflict. Sometimes perceived conflict areas, when brought out into the open, turn out to be merely areas of misunderstanding that sound communication can overcome or at least minimize. An example of the effects of perceiving conflicts within nursing is the increasing effort being devoted to improving communication between nursing service and nursing education. In other instances, parties perceiving conflict between themselves will simply agree to disagree and go on about the rest of their business. An example may be the decision of some nurse-administrators to remain active in the American Nurses' Association even though they disagree with the association's emphasis on economic and general welfare matters.

Manifest Conflict. Manifest or overt conflict can take many forms. The most extreme is violence. Because violence is such a threat to the entire social and political fabric of a nation or an organization, as noted earlier, individuals and groups tend to avoid violence and governments tent to intervene quickly when it erupts. As economic conditions in the United States change, the potential for violence in labor-management disputes may increase. Nursing and other occupations with a large pro-portion of women, because of their heretofore relatively low rates of participation in organized labor groups, will be increasingly attractive targets for labor organizers. Thus nurses may find ourselves involved in labor-management disputes where manifest conflict in the form of violence may occur. If this happens I suspect that hospitals will be the first site of this conflict. Many of the symptoms of job dissatisfaction—high turnover, low morale, high absenteeism, low productivity—that hospital nurses demonstrate indicate that there are real problems within many of those institutions (Ashley, 1976). Indeed, as Davis points out, the functional method of patient-care assignment has marked similar-ities to the assembly line (1979). In both situations workers do not have control over their work, often have only a narrow view of health care, and rarely see the outcome of their efforts. These phenomena, coupled with the kinds of latent conflict described earlier, set the stage for alien-ation. Alienated people are ripe for exploitation by those with self-serv-ing ends. Lower-participant power can be used to resist continuation of the present system of things or can be used more aggressively to bring about change. Referring back to Lewis' continuum of conflict (1976), this is clearly too much conflict.

Forms of manifest conflict less destructive to the system can include flight from intolerable situations. New graduates, especially those from baccalaureate programs, may in their first hospital jobs experience man-ifest value and role conflicts aptly called "reality shock" (Kramer, 1974). Because of their socialization as women, many nurses try to cope with manifest conflict in avoiding/acquiescent or aggressive ways, rather than assertively (see Chapter 4). If nurses were better able to assert themselves and stand up for their own and their clients' rights early in the conflict process, they might never find themselves confronting a manifest conflict situation. As yet, women and nurses are not very good at this. Other methods for reducing the possibilities of manifest conflict and for dealing with it constructively appear below.

Conflict Aftermath.   Unless a manifest conflict has been dealt with effectively and resolved to the satisfaction of the parties involved, the underlying causes of the conflict will remain. Although these causes may seem to have disappeared, they will smolder and finally erupt again. Repressing conflict, which is the unsuccessful strategy many people or organizations often use, does nothing to alleviate the latent causes and merely postpones reappearance of the conflict in a manifest form. How and when each conflict episode occurs is influenced by the effects of earlier conflict episodes that have occurred in a group or to individuals as they interact with their present environment (Pondy, 1967).

Strategies for Dealing With Conflict

Below is a brief discussion of a number of strategies for dealing with conflict. Many of these strategies can be effectively applied during early stages of the conflict process and so prevent many of the destructive fallouts of manifest conflict, while making use of the creative and motivational roles conflict can play. The strategies are listed alphabetically rather than in any priority or linear order. None, unfortunately, is a panacea, although combinations of strategies may be more effective than any one alone.

Arbitration.   Arbitration is often the strategy of last resort. As noted earlier in this section, when all else seems to have failed and conflicting groups cannot reach any agreement on their own, there is little recourse but to bring them to arbitration. Arbitration is usually imposed on the parties by an outside, superior force that mandates that the parties involved in the conflict will listen to and abide by the counsel of the arbitrator. If the arbitration is not only compulsory but also binding, the parties must accept the arbitrator's decisions—at least on the surface. That is the rub. Even though labor-management or intra-party disputes are ended as a result of the arbitration, the underlying causes may not have been addressed at all, and so the reasons for the conflict may remain, to reappear at a later time. This phenomenon is particularly likely to occur in winner-take-all situations. Under these circumstances, the losing groups, or those groups who perceive themselves as the losers, may be embittered by the process to the point that they leave the situation, to form a third party, for example; remain in the situation and foment further conflict; or simply withdraw from more than minimal participation in the organization and so become peripheral and less productive. Arbitration, then, although often the only recourse in a conflict situation that threatens the stability and productivity of the entire political or social system, can be a mixed blessing. Its use can be analogous to winning a battle while setting the stage for losing the war.

Avoidance.   Avoidance is a generally unproductive strategy for dealing with conflict. Women, because of their socialization, tend to use this technique rather than confrontation or assertion (see Chapter 3). Avoidance cannot really work, since it makes no attempt to deal constructively and openly with the underlying causes of the conflict. Also, avoidance often interferes with the accomplishment of necessary activities. We can and do pussy-foot around potential conflict-producing topics or areas for a while. But sooner or later, something—often inconsequential—will set off the fireworks, and conflict, long latent and perhaps only recently perceived, will ensue. For many years most nurses avoided the issues of our relative powerlessness in the health care system, our low pay and lack of status, and the denial of our autonomy as professionals. For many of us those days are gone forever because we have realized that our historic pattern of avoiding conflict-producing situations did not and could not work. A major reason for this book is to encourage nurses to confront and to become actively involved with the myriad political and social issues that shape our professional and private lives rather than to continue to avoid them or to let others do their acting for us. We may not do a super job on our own behalf, but at least we will have ourselves rather than others to credit with our successes and to blame for our failures.

Coalition Formation.   Coalitions, as the term is used here, may be permanent alliances or ad hoc groups coming together for a single purpose. In either case, coalitions have real roles to play in dealing with conflict. Relatively powerless groups, which are all too aware of their weak position, are ripe for alienation and manipulation or exploitation by others. They perceive that they cannot do anything for themselves and so often decide it is better to be used by others than to continue their ineffectiveness, to capitulate completely, or to revolt.

A better way, in my opinion, is for relatively powerless groups consciously to form coalitions with other groups, like themselves, who have little power but who want similar changes in the system. The additive, if not the multiplier, effect of this combination of power can be very valuable in setting the stage for constructive change. Nurses' power in the health care system is increasing and can be used to bring about changes, assuming nurses can agree on what we would like to have happen. Consumers are also increasing their power in the health care system vis-à-vis the traditional power brokers: hospitals, physicians, and pharmaceutical firms. Traditionally, because nurses are "semi-professionals" (Etzione, 1969) and as such have different vested interests in the health care system than do hospitals, physicians, and pharmaceutical firms, our potential for coalition formation with consumers, to attain common or at least complementary goals, seems to be great. Changes in regulation and reimbursement mechanisms may pave the way for shifts in relative power among the major actors in the health care system.

Coalitions are often the result of outside threats, or what I call the "sibling phenomenon": siblings tend to fight amongst themselves until a bully comes along; at that point the intrafamilial differences are forgotten and the siblings join together to form a united front against the outside threat. Consider the number of outside threats to nursing: the development of paraprofessionals whose role boundary lines with ours are at best vague; cuts in funding for nursing services, nursing education, and nursing research; proposed changes in some state nurse-practice acts that diminish rather than augment professional autonomy; and the like. These well may cause the various factions that are tearing nursing apart from within to unite and form a viable intraprofessional coalition. Until and unless we as nurses do form such a coalition and learn to speak with one voice, at least on vital issues, we run the real risk of losing what little professional autonomy we have acquired. Such a loss would render our potential for bringing about changes in the health care system remote at best.

Coercion and Repression. Although coercion and repression are different phenomena, they both involve force, and so I have treated them together. Although these strategies may deal effectively with conflict in the short run, they do nothing to alleviate or adjudicate the underlying causes of the conflict. This is another instance, then, of winning the battle only to lose the war. These techniques generally force people to either flee or go underground. In the first instance, good people whom the system needs are lost to it. In going underground, people tend to develop covert ways of undermining a system that has coerced or repressed them. Unless and until all else, including binding arbitration, fails, these are counterproductive strategies for dealing with conflict.

Compromise. Many say that politics is the fine art of compromise. Some find compromise to be anathema, since all they can see is that all sides lose a little and no one position wins out. This is the view taken by those who are so sure that what they want is right and proper that they can brook no idea of any change in their position. These all-or-nothing, zero-sum-game people are deadly to try to deal with in a conflict situation. They are so sure that their way is right that they cannot or will not listen to alternatives, compromises, trade-offs, or anything else. These people create an impasse that is detrimental to all because of the win-lose nature of the situation they create.

Fortunately, most people are able to bargain, negotiate, see alternative ways of reaching goals, and thus reach workable compromises. Such compromises enable movement—to be sure, not as much or as fast as some would like—in the desired direction. The real art of compromise is first to find areas of agreement on principles and goals, and then to address the nitty-gritty of implementation and other details (Bondurant, 1958). This approach to compromise—searching for agreement first on principle, rather than becoming bogged down initially with facts and details—often makes those facts and details more manageable. This approach to compromise does not necessarily entail all sides losing a little. Indeed, once agreement on principles has been reached, often all sides can see how to attain what they want within that framework. Another outcome can be that all sides realize the importance of the principle and so are willing to change, not diminish or deplete, what they want, in order to attain a different or more important goal. The effort here is to turn a win-lose situation into a win-win one. Obviously, reaching agreement or consensus on an overriding principle may be difficult. The key is the willingness of all parties to at least look for such a principle and be willing to talk about the process. The more emotion laden the issue is, the more important it is to find a meaningful compromise, and unfortunately, the more difficult it is to find.

Confrontation and Problem Solving. As does compromise, confrontation and problem solving require open communication and a willingness by all parties to try to resolve the conflict situation. Individuals and groups who chose avoidance as their method for dealing with conflict may be unwilling to function in situations calling for confrontation and problem solving. To use confrontation effectively as a strategy, people must face the reality that conflict exists and be ready to look for and address its underlying causes. Many of nursing's internal conflicts could be dealt with effectively through the strategy of open confrontation and problem solving. The solutions derived would certainly involve some compromise by all concerned, although not as much, perhaps, as many think.

Confrontation, with its forced recognition of and grappling with a conflict situation, can be very threatening. For this reason, many people choose the avoidance mechanism for as long as they can. The fact is, as noted, that avoidance does not work, and sooner or later the conflict will erupt. By the time confrontation is forced, the conflict is often much more deep seated and potentially destructive than it would have been if people had communicated with each other about it earlier. Often the sooner we confront a conflict situation and begin mutual problem solving to deal with it, the more successful we are in resolving the cause as well as dealing with the symptoms.

To be effective confronters, we must learn to focus on the issues, not on the personalities, involved. This depersonalization, although difficult, is essential if we are to be able to focus on the conflict without feeling that our personal survival is at stake. Women seem particularly prone to personalizing conflicts. Perhaps it is because we seem to be more concerned with being liked by and liking those with whom we work, than are men (Hennig & Jardim, 1977). We must become more skillful at communication and confrontation, even with people we may not like very well. In short, we need to be assertive rather than either aggressive or avoiding. Many of us need to practice these behaviors. Support and self-help groups composed of others who have similar needs can provide experiential learning in confrontation and problem solving. Explore the possibility of setting up such a group with members of your own network and give yourself a chance to practice this very effective conflict-resolving strategy.

Cooptation. Cooptation involves taking other competitors for scarce resources into one's own ranks. For example, we were recently preparing a grant proposal for submission to a local foundation. As soon as we got an inkling that another organization was also planning to submit a competing proposal, we invited this other organization to join forces with us in our proposal. The two organizations have now reached a mutually acceptable agreement for subcontracting services. As a result, only one proposal, ours, went forward.

As another example, political parties may seek to retain or attract dissident factions into the party's ranks through the inclusion of a compromise plank in the platform or putting a faction member on one of the nominating slates. Cooptation, then, is a useful strategy early in a potential conflict situation, since its purpose is to draw factions together and thus provide a relatively united front rather than to compete and to invite open conflict.

Divide and Conquer. Failure of a group, such as nursing, to unite its many internal factions through compromise, cooptation, confrontation, and problem solving, or coalition formation, into a solid front, sets the group up for outside forces to use divide-and-conquer tactics on the group. Indeed, this is what is happening in nursing now. A number of nursing-specialty groups have evolved, either because the American Nurses' Association and the National League for Nursing (themselves originally amalgams of multiple nursing organizations) have failed to meet these nurses' needs, or because these nurses seek to institution-alize their own uniqueness—or both (see the Yellow Pages). In any case, most nurses now have a number of organizations competing for the scarce resources of their membership dollars and participation. This range of choice can be viewed as either healthy or divisive. Now that resources for nurses and nursing are shrinking, the trade unions are eyeing nurses as potential new members, and the health care system in general is under considerable scrutiny and faced with change, nurses need to present a united front. Otherwise, numerous factions outside of nursing, all very attractive and with compelling promises, will increas-ingly draw off nurses into their ranks, thus weakening nursing at the very time when it has the most potential to use our collective and co-hesive power for change. I have heard it said, but hate to believe, that nurses are other nurses' worst enemies. If we permit our internal divi-sions to become deeper and seek allies against other nurses outside of nursing, then this saying may prove to be true. This should be avoided at all costs.

Exchange or Trade-off.   The trade-off is a standard part of political life: you do something for me and I will do something for you. It is an example of the change theory in action. Often time elapses between favors given and favors offered or required in return. In this way, an individual or group can build up a backlog of outstanding "debts" that can be called in when they are needed. Thus, nurses who support a political candidate may not want anything in return for that support at the time it is given. At a later time, however, when the elected person's assistance is needed, it is asked for with the expectation that such help will be forthcoming as a result of the previous favors or support. Thus the trade-off process greases the wheels of politics. Nurses are becoming more skilled at using this kind of influence. N-CAP and state N-PACs now contribute money to selected political campaigns on the national and state levels (see the Yellow Pages). Through this mechanism, orga-nized nursing has joined the ranks of other business, professional, and labor vested-interest groups whose political action committees are increasingly influential in political exchanges.

Increase of the Amount of Resources Available.   This used to be an easy way to avoid or reduce conflicts deriving from competition for scarce resources. Today, virtually no sector of the economy can lay claim even in its wildest dreams to augmentable, much less unlimited, resources. The health care provision system is beginning to wake up to this reality. For many years, we providers went our merry way, assuming that, since we were in a life-saving business, no matter what we asked for in the way of new facilities, technology, and staffing, it would be forthcoming from a grateful and dependent society. If this state of affairs ever pertained, it no longer does. Extramural funds are increasingly hard to obtain, and we are having to learn to live within lower budgets. These budgets, particularly in the public sector, are being eroded by inflation and Proposition 13–like tax cuts. About the only way to increase resources at this juncture is to cancel out some programs and services in order to make room for others to expand or to be developed. While this redistribution of resources may reduce conflicts between some groups, it is bound to increase competition and, therefore, conflict between others. The cuts in the federal Health and Human Services Department's budget are a prime example of this phenomenon. Health-professional schools are competing with each other for training grant and capitation monies; service programs are forced into conflict with research and professional education programs for shrinking funds. Unfortunately, this scenario will probably become fairly routine as economic priorities continue to shift.

Role Clarification.   Much conflict in the health care system results from role ambiguity. This problem has been intensified by the large numbers of new kinds of providers that have developed in the last few years. Questions about where one role ends and another begins contribute to the development of latent conflicts that can become manifest unless they are dealt with quickly and carefully. One of the reasons health care provider teams often have difficulties arriving at an efficient and effective division of labor is that role boundaries are unclear.

As specialization becomes more marked within the health care system, greater attention must be paid to the development and communication of role identity. Oda suggests three steps in the role-development process: "(1) clearly identifying the role purpose and function for oneself and others; (2) implementing the role through goal-directed interactions; and (3) achieving recognition and support of the role" (1979: 506). Following these steps can facilitate the reduction of role ambiguity and increase acceptance of the role. Nurses who choose to become politically active and visible often spend a great deal of time convincing others that political activist is a legitimate and necessary role for nurses to play. Then energy must be directed toward the attainment of specific goals, while communicating these goals to others. As more nurses become effective political activists, the role will gain legitimacy both inside and outside nursing.

Values Clarification.   As I discuss in Chapter 4, values are fundamental and vital components of life. Women are socialized into one set of values; citizens of the United States acquire another set of values;

nurses are professionally indoctrinated to yet a third set. Many of the specific values within each of the three sets are highly congruent with values in the other two; others are much less so. Potential value conflict is intensified by the current social and political changes that are remolding some of our most fundamental values. Thus we need to examine our values and see if they are still the values we wish to follow. As with role clarification, values clarification involves the clear definition of values for ourselves and others as well as adherence to those values we hold dear. In this time of change, frequent examination of our values as they relate to those of others can help us to understand our own behavior and that of others. The rising popularity of bioethics provides us with another chance to examine fundamental values and come to grips with what we think about them. It is vitally important that we know what our values are and be able to explain them and live by them. For many of us, such values as the right to free choice, equity, and distributive justice are so fundamental as to be nonnegotiable, regardless of the situation. Other values may be less important and so can be modified as times and circumstances change. Knowing our own values will make us better able to confront, solve problems, compromise, and form coalitions; it will also reduce the need for us to practice avoidance as a strategy for conflict management.

This discussion of conflict stages and ways to deal with conflict is intended to make us more comfortable with conflict situations. No matter where we live or work, conflict will be present. The more politically active we become, the more we will have to deal with conflict. Knowing ourselves and our personal and professional roles and values will make us better able to interact effectively and comfortably with others in all sorts of conflict situations. The more effective and comfortable we become in dealing with conflict, the more we will be able to appreciate its constructive attributes and to anticipate and often avert many of its destructive ones.

CHANGE

The desire for change is a motivating force behind most political activities and is an almost inevitable outcome of such activities. Conflict, as noted, plays a major galvanizing role in political processes and change. If we are to be effective in our endeavors, whether in the internal politics of our own organization or in a larger arena, we cannot be content to permit change to occur at random. Instead we must develop strategies that will enable us to predict, plan, implement, control, and evaluate change in our environment (Hersey & Blanchard, 1977). In this section,

I will briefly summarize Watson's stages in the change or reform cycle (1969) and three types of change strategies described by Chin and Benne (1969). Throughout I will provide examples from the political arena to illustrate the change processes being discussed.

Stages of Change

Watson succinctly describes the change or reform process as four stages in a cycle (1969). In the first stage, only a very few people are serious about the reform or change, and so resistance seems to them to be massive and undifferentiated. No one knows, at this point, exactly what form the change process will take.

During the second stage, pro and con forces become clearly identifiable. The ramifications of the proposed reform for the social system and the relative strength of the reformers' support and opposition can be seen. People and organizations begin to take sides. This differentiation of forces previews the third stage.

In the third stage, the forces in power, assuming they are not the ones proposing the reform, mobilize to stamp it out. If the reformers are to prevail they must generate enough power to overcome this opposition. This third stage, then, is usually a winner-take-all, zero-sum game. If the reform movement survives stage 3, in stage 4 the reformers are the group in power. They must now consolidate and institutionalize their position and power not only among their opponents, but also within the ranks of their supporters, some of whom may be developing ideas of their own. Some of the supporters may be disenchanted with the real or perceived slowness in bringing about the reform they worked so hard to achieve. They may also feel that the reform leaders may be, now that they are in power, less enthusiastic about the reform than when they were in the trenches. Thus, reformers, having won their cause, find themselves defenders of a new status quo against would-be change agents from inside as well as outside their own ranks. And so the cycle begins again. If the reform or change fails during the third stage, its supporters may be totally annihilated and the reform may die. In other instances, the reformers may retreat and retrench to build a better power base for another try at stage 3 at a later time.

A serious mistake that many reformers make—often with disastrous results—is the failure to assess adequately their opponents' strength. As you support changes in any organization or arena, you should take great care to know who your opponents are and how much strength they have relative to yours. This assessment process is essential, whether you are seeking to produce change in your own institution, local community, state, or nation. You cannot afford to have any surprises from unknown opponents or from groups whose strength of opposition you have miscalculated. Smart and effective change agents learn to recognize opponents and to compromise with them or coopt them early in stage 2. In this way they can go into stage 3 with virtually all of the battles already won.

A microcosmic example of these change stages can be found in a committee context. Let's say that you and another committee member are interested in changing the committee's position supporting legislation that would permit profit-oriented adult day care facilities to become eligible for federal funds. You two prepare your facts on both sides of the issue and make the case for your preference as part of state 1. Then you carefully assess the other members of the committee to try to determine who is a staunch and probably intractable opponent. These people you leave alone for the time being. You concentrate your efforts on those committee members whose position on the issue of profit-oriented adult day care is uncertain or waivering and who could be helped to waiver in your direction with some well-planned and well-executed educational lobbying (see Chapter 6). The goal of your lobbying is to persuade some of the members whose commitments are not fixed to lend their support to your position. You must do your homework well and present a convincing case, using normative and reeducative strategies, in order to be sure that the people you seek as supporters are truly committed to your position and so do not desert you in stage 3. You need to be prepared to make some concessions and some compromises to win their support. Also, you must anticipate being asked for trade-offs in terms of your later support on issues that the people you want to help you feel strongly about and hope to pursue. These demands are highly reasonable ones that you should anticipate and understand as part of the negotiation and coalition-formation process.

Stage 2 begins when you and your opponents become aware of each other's positions, and differentiation on the issue is clearly drawn. If you have done your lobbying well in stage 1, you should have the number of votes you need to make your position on the issue prevail when the final tally is taken. If your lobbying efforts have not assured you that you have sufficient votes to carry out your proposed reform, try to prevent the issue from coming up at all on the agenda or, if it does come up, find some way to stall for time until you can solidify your power base. This is vital since in stage 3 the opposition will do all it can to defeat your cause and prevail. That is why if you are the committee chair or have influence over the chair, your best move is to be sure the issue is not brought to a committee vote before you have the needed votes to win.

The competition, both behind the scenes and on up front, can be very fierce in stage 3, since your opponents will be employing the same strategies that you are in an attempt to retain the prominence of their position on the issue. When the final tally is in, stage 3 ends, since, assuming there is not a tie, one side will have won and the other will have lost. If your position loses, then the other position will remain dominant, and you will have to figure out another strategy for making the change you desire. This may take time and requires that you try to influence the selection of new committee members whose position on the issue is supportive of yours.

If your position is supported by the majority of the committee members at the end of stage 3, then you enter stage 4 as the group in power, at least relative to this issue. You then have the happy chore of trying to persuade the committee members who opposed the position to now support or at least not openly oppose implementation of the majority's vote on the issue. Also some of the supporters of the issue may now decide they want to see implementation done differently than previously agreed to, and so dissension within these ranks will appear also. More negotiations, trade-offs, and shifts in coalitions will be needed before the change can be institutionalized, that is, made pervasive and operational. You should not become too carried away with the elation of having won the vote in support of your position, because the most interesting, and often most trying, part of the change process is yet to come as you seek to implement the change.

In the process of working for change or reform, it is well to remember that you are involved in a highly political and potentially conflict-ridden activity. Unless the change or reform you seek to bring about is literally a life-and-death issue, try to view the process as a game and so to keep some perspective on the situation. It is well to remember that, as are games, some reform movements are won, some are lost, and others are rained out. Throughout the discussion of this example of the reform process, the focus has been on the issue as the point of disagreement between your side and the opposition. For your own sake, keep the focus on the issue and do not permit opposition to it to become personalized to you—either in your own mind or in others'. Remember, the issue is what is at stake, not your own integrity or personality. This perspective is what enables political figures and attorneys to debate and argue viciously over issues about which they disagree without letting their disagreements spill over into their personal relationships with each other. This is a hard but essential lesson to learn if you are to be an effective nurse-activist and change agent.

An interesting phenomenon may occur even if one's cause is not successful. A case in point is Norman Thomas and the Socialist Party in the United States. Much of the Socialist platform on which Thomas and other Socialists ran for President of the United States has been incorporated into our political system—even though neither Thomas nor any other Socialist ever won that office. Perhaps the Democrats made some of the Socialist's issues their own because they sought to coopt the Socialist vote, or because they believed that some of what the Socialists wanted was appropriate, or because these ideas were ideas whose time had come. At any rate, the game of reform and change need not always be a totally zero-sum, winner-take-all game, after all.

Strategies for Change

Chin and Benne describe three types of strategies for bringing about change: empirical-rational, normative-reeducative, and power (1969). Each of these types of change strategies can be applied in political activities.

Empirical-Rational Change Strategies.   These strategies are based on the assumptions that people are rational and that they will pursue their own self-interests once they know what they are (Chin & Benne, 1969). Empirical-rational strategies rely on the power of knowledge. Thomas Jefferson and many other political thinkers since him have expressed the necessity of having an informed electorate if participative government is to have any hope of success. Education in the United States has tried to address this necessity for an informed and literate electorate, with varying degrees of success. Certainly, the press, mail campaigns, posters, buttons, flyers, and other written campaign material are predicated on the assumption that the electorate will be able to understand them and will be motivated by them to vote for a particular candidate or issue. Sometimes this is indeed the case; in other circumstances, voters may prove how fickle—and often apparently irrational—they can be by their choices. Perhaps rationality, like beauty, is in the eye of the beholder.

On a number of occasions, I have lamented to active political figures that the electorate is acting irrationally and illogically, only to be told that I should not expect people to act rationally. Perhaps this is true and acounts for why many of the best-laid political plans go astray. But the rational, factual approach to educating people for effective political change by pointing out how such change is in their best interests or the interests of those they hold dear or esteem, does work. For example, in June 1980, the people of California by a 60-40 percent margin defeated Proposition 9, which would have cut state income taxes in half. A progeny of the Proposition 13 property-tax-cut measure that passed in 1978 and initiated a nationwide taxpayer revolt, Proposition 9 would have been disastrous for all kinds of state services, with the poor, the elderly, the students, and the handicapped hardest hit. Many of us campaigned vigorously against Proposition 9, using as our major tool an appeal to people's self-interests in terms of the threat of reduced fire and police protection, as well as the greatly increased fees for all kinds of services. We pointed out to the best of our ability the consequences that the passage of Proposition 9 would have had for the people of California, especially for those groups who could least afford to have their services cut and their fees raised. The proponents of the proposition denounced us for using scare tactics. We assiduously avoided such moves, having learned that they will backfire, from our experience in opposing Proposition 13 two years earlier. The proponents used the arguments that halving state income taxes would get rid of government interference and inefficiency. For the most part, the proponents on both sides of the issue were rational and tried to summon up empirical data to back up their statements. As evidenced from the election results, our rationale in opposing Proposition 9 prevailed. Again, both sides depended heavily on appeals to the voters' self-interests in their campaigning, on the assumption that people would listen and vote in a way that best served their own perceptions of what the issue meant for them. The same process has been reenacted with regard to the Federal budget in 1981.

Normative-Reeducative Change Strategies. These strategies are built on the assumption that commitments to socio-cultural values undergird peoples' actions. Change occurs, according to proponents of these strategies, only when people are persuaded to abandon their old commitments and to adopt new ones. Problem solving and training, or retraining, are suggested normative-reeducative strategies that can be applied to individuals, groups, and systems (Chin & Benne, 1969). Providing individuals, groups, and systems with data and feedback from outputs and their consequences enables them to be better problem solvers as they examine alternative kinds of commitments. This is basically the decision-making process discussed earlier in this chapter. These strategies rely on the power produced by understanding individual and aggregate behavior.

Lobbying, presenting testimony, educational campaigning, and similar activities are all efforts to alter peoples' thinking and to persuade them to "be reasonable and to do it our way." Fundamental normative beliefs are hard to change. Some normative beliefs, such as the citizens' rights to bear arms and the right to life, can be all prevailing. These issues can and have become very powerful single-issue focal points that carry considerable weight in the political arena. Other commitments are not so strongly held and may be open to more change. Learn to recognize the symptoms of political flexibility as well as those of closed-mindedness in individuals, groups, and systems you attempt to change. Use your energies where they can do the most good, that is, with those with the potential to change. For example, in our campaign against Proposition 9, we worked very hard with groups of the elderly, many of whom pay little state income tax and so had little to gain from the proposed tax cut. What we tried to educate them about was the effect that such a tax cut would have on the services on which they depend heavily: subsidized transportation; supplemental income and medical benefits; community service programs such as meals-on-wheels, adult day care, home care and the like. Because the elderly almost always vote in disproportionately large numbers, we felt that they were a particularly fruitful group to direct our educational efforts towards. Another target group we chose were students in the state's public higher education programs, all of which have been historically tuition free. Passage of Proposition 9 would have inevitably brought about the imposition of tuition. Again students are a group who pay little state income tax and so would accrue little direct benefit from the measure's passage; they had a great deal to lose, however. We carefully pointed these realities out to them. Obviously, normative-reeducative change strategies also rely heavily on empirical-rational strategies, since a major objective of educational campaigning is to show people what direct effects alternative courses of action will have on them.

Power-Coercive Change Strategies. These strategies rely heavily on the compliance of the less powerful with the wishes of the more powerful. The power used in some instances is legitimate power or authority; in other situations the power may be illegitimate and coercive. Political and economic sanctions in the form of laws, taxes, and fines are common examples of legitimate power means to bring about changes. Sanctions can be imposed for failure to follow laws or to pay taxes or fines. Change agents seeking to use these kinds of strategies try to mass political and economic power behind the changes they want. Coercive and illegitimate strategies include force, threats, bribery, and extortion. These latter strategies are generally implemented at the expense of the people involved, that is, the strategies force change on the people rather than winning their participation and consent. The use of any of the power or coercive change strategies can and often do result in divisiveness and polarization (Chin & Benne, 1969).

Chin and Benne go on to identify three kinds of power-coercive change strategies: nonviolence, political institutions, and recomposition and manipulation of the power elites (1969). Nonviolent change strategies seek to alter the situation through peaceful means such as Thoreau's civil disobedience, Ghandi's boycott and refusal to function, and King's peaceful assembly and demonstrations. All of these nonviolent strategies depend heavily on the moral coercive effects of these actions on the people or groups in power.

Political institutions are also instruments for promoting and enforcing change, with legislation as an obvious example. However, it is one thing to make a law; it is quite another to enforce it. The 55-mile-an-hour speed limit and the prohibition of marijuana are two cases in point. Without a combined normative-reeducative and power-coercive strategy approach to this kind of change, results are less than policy makers hope for.

Recomposition and manipulation of the power elites as a means of instituting change has as a fundamental example the Marxist ideology of a classless society, free of private vested interests such as ownership and control of the means of production of goods and services. Marx saw this kind of society coming about through the development and ultimate dominance of the working class as a counter force to the traditional power elites. Other strategies have sought to manipulate and reconstitute power elites via reeducation and/or rational approaches in order to bring about changes without building countervailing and potentially destructive forces. It is interesting that in their discussion of change strategies, Chin and Benne do not include violence, except perhaps as it is implicit in power-coercive strategies. As shown in the section of this chapter on conflict, violence can be an effective, albeit fearsome change strategy, and one that is usually undertaken only as a last resort.

SUMMARY

In this chapter, selected fundamental concepts for nurses' political activism have been presented. A political-systems model (Figure 3.1) shows systems theory as applied to the political arena: inputs, political systems conversion processes, outputs and their consequences are discussed. Particular attention is given to the political system's conversion processes as a vehicle to illustrate some of the major functions of government as they relate to each other and to their environment. These conversion processes are interest articulation, interest aggregation, communication, rule making (legislation), rule application (administration), rule interpretation (adjudication), and systems maintenance. A glossary of systems terms is found in Appendix 4.

Power is characterized as the ability of an individual, group, or organization to cause or to constrain the actions of others. A typology of power, including legitimate, expert, corruptive, referent, associative, exploitive, nutrient, rational, charismatic, and sexually based power, is presented. Each type of power is briefly discussed as it applies in political arenas and to nurse activists. Finally, a four-stage power orientation is presented.

A decision matrix (Figure 3.2) is discussed as an adjunct to decision making, a major political function. In the process of developing and using the matrix, decision makers must define and develop plausible alternatives and weigh each against a set of specific criteria. The process enables a decision to be made in rational and qualifiable terms. Although the policy makers may choose another alternative than the one the matrix process indicates, they can use such a matrix as a rational and quantifiable assist to their final selection process.

Conflict occurs whenever two or more parties compete for scarce resources. Thus conflict will be an increasing component in all facets of health care and in nursing as well. The stages of a conflict—latent, perceived, manifest, and conflict aftermath—are discussed. A number of strategies for dealing with conflict are included: arbitration, avoidance, coalition formation, coercion and repression, compromise, confrontation, cooptation, divide and conquer, exchange or trade-off, increase in the amount of resources available, role clarification, and values clarification.

Watson's stages of the change or reform process introduce the section on change (1969). An example of these stages of change or reform in a committee setting is given. Finally Chin and Benne's three types of change strategies—empirical-rational, normative-reeducative, and power-coercive—are discussed (1969).

REFERENCES

Alinsky SD: *Rules for Radicals: A Pragmatic Primer for Realistic Radicals.* New York, Vintage Books, 1972.

Almond GA, Powell GB Jr: *Comparative Politics: A Developmental Approach.* Boston, Little Brown & Co, 1966.

Altshuler AA: *Community Control.* New York, Pegasus, 1970.

Archer SE: Selected community health processes, in Archer SE, Fleshman RP (eds): *Community Health Nursing: Patterns and Practice,* ed 2. North Scituate, Mass, Duxbury Press, 1979a, pp 57–90.

———: Politics and economics: How things really work, in Archer SE, Fleshman RP (eds). *Community Health Nursing: Patterns and Practice,* ed 2. North Scituate, Mass, Duxbury Press, 1979b, pp 277–312.

Ashley JA: *Hospitals, Paternalism, and the Role of the Nurse.* New York, Teachers' College Press, 1976.

Baldridge JV (ed): *Academic Governance: Research on Institutional Politics and Decision-making.* Berkeley, Calif, McCutchan Publishing Co, 1971.

Baron A: The slippery act of polls. *Politics Today* 7:21–25, January–February 1980.

Benveniste G: *The Politics of Expertise.* Berkeley, Calif, The Glendessary Press, 1972.

Bondurant J: *Conquest of Violence.* Princeton, NJ, Princeton University Press, 1958.

Braden J, Herban NL: *Community Health: A Systems Approach.* New York, Appleton-Century-Crofts, 1976.

Buckley W: *Sociology and Modern Systems Theory.* Englewood Cliffs, NJ, Prentice-Hall, 1967.

Chin R, Benne KD: General strategies for effecting changes in human systems, in Bennis W, Benne KD, Chin R (eds): *The Planning of Change,* ed 2. New York, Holt Rinehart & Winston Inc, 1969, 488–498.

Churchman CW: *The Systems Approach.* New York, Dell Publishing Co, 1968.

Creighton H: *Law Every Nurse Should Know,* ed 3. Philadelphia, WB Saunders Co, 1975.

Dahl RA: *Modern Political Analysis,* ed 3. Englewood Cliffs, NJ, Prentice-Hall, 1976.

Davis AJ: Nursing's influence on health policy for the eighties, in *Nursing's Influence on Health Policy for the Eighties.* Proceedings Scientific Session American Academy of Nursing, September 8, 1978. Kansas City, Mo, American Nurses' Association, American Academy of Nursing, 1979, pp 3–12.

———, Aroskar MA: *Ethical Dilemmas and Nursing Practice.* New York, Appleton-Century-Crofts, 1978.

Deutch M: Productive and destructive conflict. *Journal of Social Issues* 25: 7–42, 1969.

Diers D: A different kind of energy: Nurse-power. *Nursing Outlook* 26:51–55, January 1978.

Easton D: *A Systems Analysis of Political Life.* New York, John Wiley & Sons, 1965.

Emery FE, ed: *Systems Thinking: Selected Readings.* Baltimore, Md, Penguin Books, 1969.

Etzioni A: *The Semi-Professions and Their Organization.* New York, The Free Press, 1969.

Gerth H: Weber's three types of legitimacy. *Berkeley Journal of Sociology* 187:1–12, 1953.

Hawley WD, Wirt FM: *The Search for Community Power,* ed 2. Englewood Cliffs, NJ, Prentice-Hall, 1974.

Heide WS: Introduction, in Ashley JA (ed): *Hospitals, Paternalism, and the Role of the Nurse.* New York, Teacher's College Press, 1976, pp v–viii.

Hennig M, Jardim, A: *The Managerial Woman.* New York, Anchor Press, Doubleday, 1977.

Hersey P, Blanchard KH: *Management of Organizational Behavior: Utilizing Human Resources,* ed 3. Englewood Cliffs, NJ, Prentice Hall, 1977.

Kahn S: *How People Get Power: Organizing Oppressed Communities for Action.* San Francisco, McGraw-Hill, 1970.

Kalisch BJ: The promise of power. *Nursing Outlook* 26:42–46, January 1978.

Kramer M: *Reality Shock: Why Nurses Leave Nursing.* St. Louis, CV Mosby Co, 1974.

Leininger M: Political nursing: Essential for health service and education systems of tomorrow. *Nursing Administration Quarterly* 2:1–16, Spring 1978.

Levin P, Berne E: Games nurses play. *American Journal of Nursing* 72:483–487, March 1972.

Lewis JH: Conflict management. *Journal of Nursing Administration* 6:18-22, June 1976.

Masson V: On power and vision in nursing. *Nursing Outlook* 27:782–784, December 1979.

May R: *Power and Influence: A Search for the Sources of Violence.* New York, WW Norton and Co, 1972.

McClelland DC: *Power: The Inner Experience.* New York, Irvington, 1975.

Monsma SV: *American Politics: A Systems Approach.* New York, Holt Rinehart & Winston, 1969.

Moynihan DP: *Maximum Feasible Misunderstanding: Community Action in the War on Poverty.* New York, The Free Press, 1970.

Nozick R: *Anarchy, State, and Utopia.* New York, Basic Books, 1974.

Oda DS: Community health nursing in schools: Developing a specialized role, in Archer SE, Fleshman RP (eds): *Community Health Nursing: Patterns and Practice,* ed 2. North Scituate, Mass, Duxbury Press, 1979, pp 495–511.

Pondy LR: Organizational Conflict: Concepts and models. Administrative Science Quarterly 12:296–320, September 1967.

Power: Nursing's Challenge for Change. Kansas City, Mo, American Nurses' Association, 1979.

Shiflett N, McFarland, DE: Power and the nurse administrator. *Journal of Nursing Administration* 8:19–23, March 1978.

Stein T: The doctor-nurse game. *American Journal of Nursing* 68:101–105, January 1968.

Thomstad B, Cunningham N, Kaplan BH: Changing the rules of the doctor-nurse game. *Nursing Outlook* 23:422–427, July 1975.

Von Bertalanffy L: *General Systems Theory.* New York, Braziller, 1968.

Watson G: Resistance to change, in Bennis W, Senne KD, Chin R (eds): *The Planning of Change,* ed 2. New York, Holt Rinehart & Winston, 1969, pp 488–498.

Weber M: The Theory of Social and Economic Organization. New York, The Free Press, 1947.

———: *From Max Weber: Essays in Sociology,* Gerth H, Mills CW (eds). New York, Oxford University Press, 1958.

Wieland GF, Ullrich RA: *Organizations: Behavior, Design, and Change.* Homewood, Ill, Richard D Irwin, 1976.

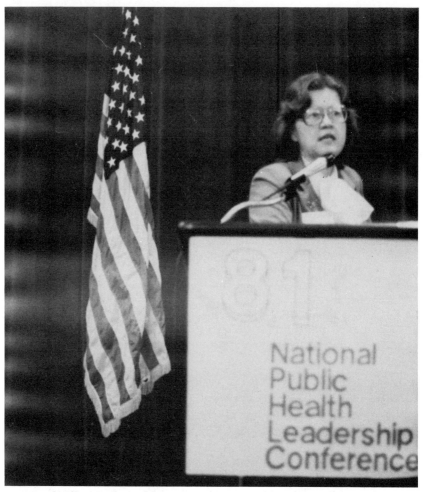

Sarah Ellen Archer addressing American Public Health Association's
1981 National Public Health Leadership Conference, Washington, D.C.
(Photo by Barbara Wilcox.)

CHAPTER 4

Political Strategies for Nurses' Involvement

Sarah Ellen Archer

THIS CHAPTER IS a selection of strategies and means of involvement that nurses can use to increase their political activities. Assertiveness is a prerequisite of effective involvement in many arenas, and politics is no exception. The chapter begins with a basic discussion of assertiveness, with references provided for those who need more depth. Specific efforts are made to tie assertiveness to political participation. And as in all endeavors and fields, the importance of role models and mentors must be increasingly well understood and utilized in nursing. Networking is another essential ingredient for information-sharing and professional support. The "getting involved" section of the chapter focuses on campaign work for both candidates and initiatives, as well as on other ways to influence public policy. Many view the Hatch Act as a total prohibition against public employees being able to participate in political activities. The discussion of the act highlights the kinds of activities public employees can and cannot carry out. Finally, political parties and political action committees are discussed briefly because of their importance as vehicles for political participation.

ASSERTIVENESS

Why Assertiveness?

As nurse-activists, we must be assertive in standing up for our constituents and in the presentation of our positions on political issues as well as on our rationale for taking those stands. The objective of this discussion is to assist nurse-activists, to look at our own behavior, the effects of our behavior on others and on their behavior towards us. If we are satisfied with our assertiveness skills, we can continue to interact as we have been. If we do not feel that our present behavior patterns are as effective as we wish they were, then we can use the guidelines presented here to make the needed changes. Assertive nurse-activists are better nurse-activists because we are better able to communicate effectively with others—peers, constituents, labor leaders, lobbyists, elected officials, staff members, regulatory agency personnel, attorneys, and the public—and most important of all, because assertive people are more comfortable with ourselves. I present assertiveness, aggressiveness, and avoidance/acquiescence as three prototype behaviors. A few applications of assertiveness for nurse-activists are explored, and ways to help other nurses to become more assertive are considered. After looking at our own behavior, if we are not satisfied with our ability to be as assertive as we would like to be, we must find an assertiveness training course and get further help. As nurse-activists we will need all the assertive behavior we can muster.

Exercise: Clarifying Your Values

Values are fundamental components of life towards which we have high regard, whether we are aware of them or not. Women have been socialized into a set of values about our roles in this society. As nurses, women have acquired another set of values as part of our development. Much of these two kinds of socialization is coming under increasing scrutiny (see Chapter 2). Along with this scrutiny there is a new emphasis on examining and clarifying values (Simon, Howe, & Kirschenbaum, 1972). Table 4.1 provides an opportunity to examine selected values about yourself and your relations toward others. Read through the value statements and note your level of agreement with each one before reading further.

Value statements 1a through 1e address the notion that others' feelings are more important than your own. We chose the actors in these value statements because of their relevance to nurse-activists. If you found that you answered differently with regard to your feelings about constituents and peers than you did about elected officals, staff members, and regulators, perhaps you need to examine your perceptions of your own relative power and worth. Also, if you agreed, and particularly if you strongly agreed, with any of these statements, you may need to reexamine your feelings about your own worth. To assertively insist on being treated as an equal or peer, you must first believe that you are equal with others.

TABLE 4.1

Clarifying Your Values as a Nurse-Activist

The following are value statements about nurse-activist activities. Check your level of agreement with each of these value statements.

Value Statements	Strongly Agree	Agree	Disagree	Strongly Disagree
1. Others' feelings are more important than are mine, so a. I should give less importance to my own feelings when they are at odds with those of elected officials.				
b. I should give less importance to my own feelings when they are at odds with those of staff members.				
c. I should give less importance to my own feelings when they are at odds with those of my peers.				
d. I should give less importance to my own feelings when they are at odds with those of regulatory body members.				
e. I should give less importance to my own feelings when they are at odds with those of my constituents.				
2. I should tell others about my achievements.				
3. I should take a stand on what I believe, even if this is in opposition to the stand taken by my supporters.				

TABLE 4.1
Clarifying Your Values as a Nurse-Activist *(continued)*

Value Statements	Strongly Agree	Agree	Disagree	Strongly Disagree
4. I should take a stand even if it is in opposition to my peers.				
5. I should take a stand even if it is in opposition to those in power.				
6. It is more important to be liked than to accomplish a task.				
7. It is better to be acquiescent than to risk rocking the boat.				
8. I would rather work late to get my work done than to limit others' interruptions.				
9. Other vested-interest groups' needs are more important than are nursing's and so they should be given priority.				
10. I am responsible for my constituents and so I must stand up for their rights.				

Adapted from Simon et al: *Values Clarification: A Handbook of Strategies for Teachers and Students.* New York, Hart Publishing Co, 1972.

We have to learn to be comfortable telling others about our achievements. Women and nurses are socialized to believe that we should be modest and retiring about what we have done and can do. We are not advocating that we become braggarts about our accomplishments. Somewhere in between these two extremes is a healthy pride in our ability, which is appropriate to share with others. The reality is if we do not wave our own flag or blow our own horn, no one else will do it for us, either.

Items 3, 4, and 5 deal with the willingness to take a stand—even if you are wrong and your stand is unpopular with others. These are examples of risk-taking behaviors—another area in which nurses and women have not been socialized to excel. These three value statements focus more on interpersonal risks than on organizational risks. Nevertheless, if you can run the risk of displeasing your colleagues and perhaps even finding that you are not liked (the focus of value statement 6) because you have acted on the basis of your beliefs, then you should be able to weather the consequences of your decisions. At least you will be able to look yourself in the eye.

Value statement 6 focuses on the very realistic value of wanting to be liked by your colleagues. The problem arises when the nurse-activist must take a stand that is unpopular with some of these colleagues and therefore risk displeasure, possible dislike, and potential backlash. We all should be adult enough to separate our reactions to individuals from our reactions to their behavior, but such is not always the case. It is not in your job description that you must be liked by everyone; you were appointed, or your volunteer efforts were sought, because of your abilities, not to run for a popularity contest. But don't become an unbenevolent despot who would rather be right than popular—particularly since the two are not mutually exclusive. Be aware of the risks of having close personal friends among those you work for. Seek your friends and support system outside of your work place. In this way you will not be dependent on people in your immediate work setting for the meeting of your social and personal needs. Seek out other activists—nurses and nonnurses—and form a peer group so that you can share experiences with knowledgeable others who are not directly involved in your situation. Nurse-activists, like others experimenting with new and less traditional roles, need support systems composed of others who are having similar experiences.

Many nurse-activists are constantly told: "Don't rock the boat; things are bad enough already." The problem here is that unless actions are taken—and taken consciously with planning and design—things are not likely to get better of their own accord. To be sure, we do not advocate nurse-activists rocking the boat just for the fun of watching other people get seasick. There has to be a reason for change. After planning and considering alternative actions, if it still looks as though the boat should be rocked, then rock it and do it well—but do not sink the boat, since that is permanent and devastating.

Statement 8 deals with those of you who cannot assert yourselves by saying such things as, "I have to have this report done in 20 minutes and so I can't stop to talk to you now. Please call me later when we can make an appointment." Obviously, if the person who wants to see you is in a distressed state, then you should make necessary arrangements to deal with the situation. That kind of crisis situation is not what this value statement seeks to have you consider; rather it is the everyday, usually unannounced or at best very short-notice demands that others make on time that you have already scheduled for other things. It's a matter of old-friend priorities. The nurse-activist will find that there are endless demands on her time: meeting with constituents; researching issues; preparing testimony, letters, and statements for constituents; working on coalition formation with activists from other organizations and interests. All these things take time, and scheduling becomes a monumental task. You simply have to draw the line on interruptions in order to accomplish the important things. Set aside some specific time for working on issues, telephoning, doing correspondence and other tasks, as well as giving some time to new business, contacts, and interruptions. During this time you can return calls or meet with people who sought to reach you while you were busy with your other tasks. If a nurse-activist is to survive, she must set and enforce limitations on her time.

Giving priority to other vested-interest groups at the expense of the needs of your own constituents, value statement 9, is similar to statements 1a through e. What is under consideration here is the ability to assert nursing's worth. If nurse-activists do not assert our position, we cannot count on anyone else assuming this function for us. At some point, this responsibility to assert your position relative to other vested-interest groups may smack of territoriality; to be sure sometimes it indeed will be boundary maintenance. That's a vital component of the job as a nurse-activist. As we saw in Chapter 3, if any subsystem is suboptimized to the point of weakness, all of the other subsystems and ultimately the entire system will suffer. Territorial battles may be waged over space, budget, personnel, priorities, or any number of other considerations. The nurse-activist must have her rationale clearly thought out, her documentation organized in a convincing way, and the areas in which she can compromise clearly defined in her own mind. And then she has got to stick to them. Compromise is the name of the game. Compromise, however, does not mean that the nurse-activist has to sell out and get nothing. Never is assertiveness more important than in negotiations.

It follows that nurse-activists must also interpret and stand up for the rights of their constituents assertively and in a mentoring fashion, avoiding the "compassion trap" (Adams, 1971). Nurse-activists have a responsibility and an obligation to stand up for those they represent—assuming that they need and warrant defending—even if so doing means that we get our knuckles rapped (see editors' note, Chapter 7).

What Is Assertiveness?

To understand what assertiveness is, we must first compare and contrast three prototype kinds of behaviors: assertiveness, aggressiveness; and avoidance/acquiescence (Bakdash, 1978; Clark, 1978; Rohrbaugh, 1977). Phelps and Austin add a fourth behavioral type, indirect aggressiveness (1975), which we will subsume under aggressiveness, on the premise that avoidance/acquiescence and aggressiveness are two sides of the same coin (Rohrbaugh, 1977). We demonstrate all three of these types of behavior patterns in our interactions with others; thus no one is an "aggressive type" or an "assertive type" all of the time. Indeed, there are situations where one of these behavior modes may be far more appropriate than either of the others. The art is to know why and when to use what kind of behavior, and then to employ it effectively.

Assertiveness is the ability to say what you mean and mean what you say in a clear and concise manner, while respecting the rights of others to do the same and considering the consequences of your behavior. Components of assertiveness that are critical for nurse-activists include:

- Admitting and accepting your own strengths and weaknesses
- Recognizing and exercising your own rights and respecting others' right to do the same
- Setting long- and short-range goals for yourself in a clear and consistent manner
- Being ready to accept and deal with the consequences of your decisions and of the positions you take
- Being secure enough in your own beliefs and values that you do not have to shrink back into passivity or avoidance or boil over into aggression
- Conveying clearly to others what you expect from them and what they can expect from you (Clark, 1978)
- Being able to stay comfortably in your "adult" instead of lapsing into your "parent" or "child" (Chenevert, 1978). Because of the "compassion trap" (Adams, 1971) female nurse-activists must be extremely careful to avoid assuming the parent role with subordinates or the child role with superordinates—particularly male superordinates
- Being ready to deal with conflict as a positive force in the overall change process
- Realizing that you are a role model for other nurses and other women and enjoying the opportunity to model positive, assertive behavior
- Being willing to take reasonable risks in order to achieve your goals

- Using "I" communications: "I think that . . ."; "I appreciate your position, but I do not agree . . . "; "I have confidence that you can do . . ."
- Developing and using the ability to say "no" so that others do not take advantage of you (Chenevert, 1978)
- Identifying those areas where compromise and negotiation are not possible and those areas where they are, and then being able to stick to your decisions
- As Kipling said: "If you can keep your head when all about you are losing theirs and blaming it on you. . . . " (Williams, 1952:738)
- Standing up for your rights and those of the people and organizations you represent

Aggressiveness is a behavior aimed at seeing that the actor achieves his or her objectives regardless of who may be hurt in the process. Aggressive people seek to have their own way through:

- Control, threat, manipulation, and/or punishment of others
- Disregard of others' rights
- Failure to assume responsibility for the outcomes of their behavior (Clark, 1978)
- A view of conflict as a zero-sum game in which the winner takes all by force, rather than as an opportunity for constructive compromise and change
- Retaliation; getting even
- Making progress at others' expense
- Attacks on other people rather than problem solving; blaming others for problems
- Masking, or at least seeming to mask, feelings of insecurity behind hostility and attack
- Passing the buck to others rather than accepting responsibility
- Using "you" communications: "You never do anything right!" "You're always trying that sort of thing with my budget"

Avoidance/acquiescence is behavior where the person allows himself or herself to be overpowered and dominated by others. Acquiescent people tend to:

- Let others dominate them while maintaining a passive exterior, although they may be seething inside
- Allow others to define their rights and goals and then go along with these imposed definitions
- Turn hurts inside, which results in depression, self-blame, self-punishment, and resentment

- Avoid conflict and risks and not rock the boat—at least not obviously
- React rather than act; turn to other people for answers rather than setting own goals and then doing own problem solving
- Rarely be open in their communication; evade situations instead of meeting them head on
- Be respectful of others' rights but not respect their own rights; have low self-esteem and self-devaluation

As mentioned earlier, aggressive and avoiding/acquiescent behaviors are very similar (Rohrbaugh, 1978). Both are reactive rather than goal directed; both reflect underlying insecurity and failure to take responsibility for one's own actions, feelings, and their consequences; and both use indirect patterns of communication. As Clark points out, aggressive behavior is often an eruption of pent-up anger, resentment, and embarrassment that the person's usual avoiding/acquiescent behavior pattern has not permitted to be expressed (1978).

Discussion

A common problem with assertive behavior is that while you may believe that you are being assertive, you are seen by others as being aggressive or nonassertive. Aggression may indeed be in the eye of the beholder. For many people, any woman who does not act in an avoiding/acquiescent manner is automatically seen as being aggresive. One of my male colleagues pointed out that most men react to women as though they were either aggressive or passive, but never assertive. He asked, why don't woman just act aggressive and be done with it, since that's the way in which their behavior will be interpreted anyway? My response was that one of the most rewarding things about being assertive is that it feels good to the person being assertive. We cannot be held responsible for, nor can we control, how others respond to us. We can, and must, however, be honest with ourselves and with others.

I do not endorse the catch phrase I have heard directed to those who are unable to cope with people who are newly assertive: "That's their problem." If we are truly concerned about our own rights and those of other people, we cannot write off others' responses to our behavior—assertive or otherwise—as their problem. Besides, we may well find that "their problem" can indeed be our problem, depending on how they choose to interact with us. If you are able to be comfortable with your response in a given situation and are able to understand the reasons behind your action, then you are in a good position to cope with the other person's reactions and their probable consequences.

You must learn to be prepared for what, in your opinion, are over-reactions to your assertive behavior. You must also learn to handle the hostility you will feel when others misinterpret your assertive behavior as aggression. Meeting hostility with hostility is often a futile undertaking. You must learn other, more productive, coping mechanisms. You must develop your own behavioral style. Whichever style or mix of styles fits you—assertive, aggressive, avoiding/acquiescent—develop it carefully and use it consistently, so that you, at least, are comfortable with it.

I cannot urge you strongly enough to do all that you can to anticipate actual situations before they occur and to role-play your chosen response pattern before you confront the situation. You need to think through possible confrontations with those who oppose your position, and to anticipate as many of their moves and your countermoves as possible, rather like a game of chess. Think through alternative scenarios for the kinds of actions and reactions you can expect. The better you know your fellow players in the politics game, the more likely you will be able to think through their probable responses to your behavior. Also, give some serious thought as to how you can use such stress-diffusing techniques as deep breathing and other relaxation exercises, so that you can keep your own fear and anxiety under control during a confrontation. Practice these kinds of techniques so that they are instantly available to you when you need them.

Think through the answers to these kinds of questions before you face the real situations: On what issues will you be assertive to the point of confrontation? With whom is this confrontation likely? What is his or her style? How do you react to it? On what issues are you willing to negotiate? With whom are these negotiations likely to occur? How do you react to his or her style in negotiating? How will you react if your boss says your demand is unacceptable? How do you wish you could respond? The questions that any given situation raises are endless. It has often been said that the best defense is a good offense. Learning to keep your head, to anticipate others' behavior, and to plan your own assertive responses ahead of time is insurance against guilt feelings that can result from losing your temper and becoming aggressive, or being passive. Again, you must do this mental role-playing beforehand, since in the heat of the situation you may well respond in a manner that is contrary to what you want.

Assertiveness puts "me" on an equal footing with everyone else, which is very difficult for many nurses and women to do because of their socialization (see Chapter 2). Others may try to make you feel guilty or selfish when you are assertive; in reality, assertiveness is not selfishness, it is rather an attitude that discourages selflessness. Clark points out that two of the most frequent questions about assertiveness behavior that she is asked by nurses in her workshops are: "Isn't asser-tiveness manipulative?" and "Isn't it uncaring and unfeminine for nurses to be assertive?" (1979:21). The answer to both questions is no. Fortunately, socialization patterns are changing gradually, and young nurses are more likely to be assertive than are older ones. Many people who have not learned to be assertive may accept assertive behavior in others. This incongruity of behavioral styles can create and perpetuate some serious personnel problems. Assertive behavior can also be per-ceived as threatening, especially by men dealing with assertive women. Be alert for unexpected reactions.

People who use avoidance/aquiescence as their major behavioral style can also create real interpersonal problems. They generally refuse to confront and will not discuss feelings, desires, or beliefs openly so that they can be dealt with. Instead, these people brood, pout, withdraw, or agree until at some point a last straw comes along and they blow. The nurse-activist needs to be aware that under many apparently passive exteriors lurk very aggressive characteristics. To deal with these kinds of behavioral patterns, nurse-activists need the counsel of experienced colleagues. Once again, a peer support group can be a tremendous help in developing and perfecting one's own behavioral style, as well as cop-ing with the styles of others.

Table 4.2 summarizes the kinds of behaviors that are associated with assertive, aggressive, and avoiding/acquiescent styles and relates them to variables such as leadership style, decision making, attitude toward conflict, and risk taking that are components of nurse-activists' roles. The stereotypes in the table help us to compare and contrast the three behavior styles. See if you can identify some of your own behaviors and those of others in the table.

ROLE MODELS AND MENTORS

Those who are risk takers often can go off more or less on our own, pursue our own course, make our own mistakes, and finally develop our own style of behavior in all kinds of arenas with a minimum of guidance and help. The majority of people, however, need and welcome examples and advice that they can follow, especially in the area of political participation. Role models and mentors are tremendously helpful in this situation. Role models are people who are doing the kinds of things we would like to do or need to do; they provide us with a pattern we can either follow closely or adapt to what feels comfortable for us. Ideally, role models for women nurses should be both women and nurses. Most of us can name several women we admire and from

TABLE 4.2
Assertive, Aggressive, and Avoiding/Acquiescent Behaviors in Response to Selected Personal Variables

Variable	Behaviors		
	Assertive	Aggressive	Avoiding/Acquiescent
Leadership style	Democratic and participative	Autocratic, "Vesuvian"	Laissez faire and management by default until pushed too far; then becomes autocratic, aggressive.
Self-perception	Knows strengths and limitations. Self-confident; goal directed.	Often insecure and masks this with over-confident, almost arrogant behavior. May refuse to recognize own limitations.	Insecure. Often knows some of own limitations but not what to do about them. Discounts own abilities and strengths.
Characteristics as leader	Supportive, open, self-directing and expects others to be also. Straightforward. Leads by example and consultation.	Volatile, hostile, and often hurtful of others. Directs others and leads by sheer force.	Weak, other-directed, passive, until totally overloaded, then explodes. Does not lead; drifts until circumstances make decisions inevitable.
Decision making	Solves problems, considers alternatives and their consequences, seeks input but makes own decision. Accepts consequences of own decisions.	May act hastily without sufficient information and counsel. Blames others for unwanted consequences.	Avoids decisions. Lets others or circumstances make decisions for her and then blames them for unwanted consequences.
Risk taking	Takes risks after careful consideration of probabilities.	Takes risks often without adequate consideration of probabilities.	Avoids risk taking. Gathers data forever and uses this as excuse for inaction.

Communication pattern	"I believe that . . . "; "I am pleased that . . . "	"You are always . . . "; "Why don't you ever . . . ?"	"What do you think ought to be done . . . ?"; "The situation doesn't seem to warrant . . . "
Body language	Appropriate for what she or he is saying. Open and relaxed.	Appropriate for what she or he is saying. Closed and tense or overtly threatening.	Gives a message at odds with what she or he is saying, thus creating confusion.
Perceives conflict	Sees conflict as a positive part of solving problems and the negotiating process. Considers others' feelings when exerting own rights.	Says she or he loves a good fight. Goes to any extreme to win, regardless of others' feelings.	Avoids direct conflict, but may do a great deal behind the scenes to foster conflict. Shies away from confrontation. When pushed explodes into aggression.
Concern for others' rights	Concerned for others' rights, but not at the expense of own.	Others' rights are second to own.	Greater concern for others' rights than for own—or so they say.
Concern for own rights	Stands up for own rights and meets conflicts head on.	Demands own rights regardless of the consequences to others.	Views own rights as less important than others'.
Preferred game strategy	Win-win.	Win-win or win-lose — as long as she or he wins.	Avoids overt games but may complicate them for others.
Willingness to negotiate	Goal-directed and willing to negotiate; knows on what she or he will compromise and on what she or he will not. Listens to others, but makes own decisions.	Reluctant to negotiate. Wants things own way or else. If people do not like it they can get out. Uses others.	Either avoids negotiating or is so passive that she or he tends to give everything away rather than to negotiate. Lets herself/himself be maneuvered and used.

whom we have learned a variety of possible roles. Few of us can hope to be a Barbara Nichols (president of the American Nurses' Association), Sister Rosemary Donley (who spent her Robert Wood Johnson Foundation Fellowship working with Congress), or Connie Holleran, (formerly of the American Nurses' Association Governmental Relations Office in Washington and now Executive Director of the International Council of Nurses), but each of these three women is a splendid example of a style of participation on the national level. Other nurses, such as Jean Moorhead (see Chapter 7) and Rosalie S. Abrams (D-Md State Senate), can provide role models on a state level. These and other women nurses who have chosen to be nurse-activists in a variety of political arenas provide an array of role models for almost all of us.

Some of us were fortunate to have excellent role models for female political participation very early in our lives, and to grow up assuming that these kinds of behaviors were not only normal but expected. Many of us who chose nursing as a profession were influenced to some extent by a concern for people, often, no doubt, fostered by our early observations of other helping people. This latter characteristic gives us something in common with the agitators and activists of the 1960s, whom Keniston has described as tending to have "an unusual capacity for nurturant identification—that is, for empathy and sympathy for the underdog, the oppressed, the needy. Such a capacity can have many origins, but its most likely source in upper-middle-class professional families is identification with an active mother whose own work embodies nurturant concern for others" (1968:309). My own experience fits this description. We children early on dubbed both our parents, but especially our mother, "crusader rabbits," because she and other women she knew were eternally advocating for those less fortunate and articulate. Her lessons have been of inestimable value to me, and this book is dedicated in part to her. I have had many role models, female and male, but she was the first and most influential. The validity of Keniston's observations is also borne out in the social-reform efforts of women such as Jane Addams early in this century (see Chapter 2).

Many women nurses have not had this sort of early role model and so have to learn about these kinds of involvements later in life. Fortunately, there are an increasing number of women and nurses who are visible advocates and activists; however, there are not nearly enough. One of the purposes of this book is to provide our readers not only with the information that we have to share, but also to provide role models by describing our own and others' political involvement. We feel very strongly that as women and nurse-activists develop power, and skill in using it, they have an obligation to share what they have learned and to serve as role models for others (Kelly, 1978).

Mentors are those people, generally already established in an organization or in another kind of position, who help younger people or those newer to the system to understand the system and to move upward in it. A mentor is one who facilitates another's growth and progress towards his or her own goals. Often a faculty member or a superior at work plays a mentor role for many of us. Mentors can be, and probably usually are, role models. A major difference is that the mentor is actively involved with the other person, while role modeling need not involve any direct interaction between the role model and the follower. The mentor role is an extremely satisfying one, in that mentors can take pride and personal pleasure in helping to launch others on their way and so have the reward of watching them take off. Nowhere can this mentor function be more useful and more fruitful than in the area of political participation.

Staff and students, as well as other colleagues, are interested in what nurse-faculty and nurse-managers do. Therefore, we who are in these kinds of positions have superb opportunities to be both role models and mentors. Both what we say and what we do, as politically involved nurse-activists, can influence those around us to follow suit. To provide this kind of example is an integral, although often unwritten, part of our responsibilities as nurse-managers and nurse-faculty.

NETWORKING

Most dictionaries have not yet caught up with a recent change in our American language: the usage of "network" as a verb as well as a noun. Networking is the process of linking people together for mutual support and aid to attain goals. We can network for professional, political, social, personal, and a variety of other reasons. Networks and networking are ideas whose time has definitely come for women. Female nurses need to network as much as, if not more than, other working women; we need to develop what Kelly calls "the good new nurse network" (1978).

My first network experience was in 1964 after finishing the master of public health program at the University of Michigan and going into my first teaching job. My classmates and faculty from the public health nursing program were a network I relied upon for consultation and support. This network has now broadened to include many members of the public health nursing section of the American Public Health Association (APHA). We see each other regularly at the APHA's annual meetings, as well as at other meetings such as the Federation of Graduate Faculty in Public Health/Community Health Nursing, American Nurses' Association (ANA) and National League for Nursing (NLN) conventions, and a variety of other meetings across the country. At other times, my colleagues are only as far away as my telephone or mailbox, depending on how fast I need their input. The network is also a means for being asked to give papers, run conferences and workshops, and serve as a consultant. Some of these opportunities even involve getting paid! These activities provide a chance to see old friends and to make new ones all over the United States as well as abroad. To some extent, we all "use" and are "used" by our friends; we know each other's strengths and interests, and so when the need arises, it's logical and effective to call on each other. Similar kinds of networks can exist in other nursing-specialty organizations (see the Yellow Pages) as well as within the ANA's sections and the NLN's councils. Although none of these organizations are in and of themselves networks, they all have the potential for helping their members to meet and form networks. I was delighted to see the listing of women's networks (First National Directory 1980) in *Working Woman*, but dismayed not to find any nursing organizations in it or in Welch's book (1980). I sent off a letter to the editor and have written to Welch suggesting that the ANA, NLN, the nursing-specialty organizations, and their state affiliates be included. Kleiman (1980) lists the ANA as a network under Medicine. She does not list any other nurses' organizations.

Why network? Welch lists three reasons (1980*a* and *b*): (1) Working women can understand other working women better than men can, because women have problems men simply don't have. (2) Men tend to leave women out of their informal communication patterns, and so women often do not have access to the information they need. Information is power, women need to find ways of broadening their communication networks to gain increased access to information. (3) The higher a woman goes in the organizational structure, the fewer women she will have around her for peer support and counseling. She will have to go outside of her organization to find women peers with whom she can relate. This is a variation of the old "it's lonely at the top" routine. Networking is also a terrific source of opportunities for short- and long-term job information.

Ideally, at least some of the networks that we belong to should include men as well as women. For too long men's networks excluded women; we should not make the same mistake. A network that has been invaluable for me developed through the American Public Health Association because of its interdisciplinary makeup. This is particularly true as a member and then chair of the Executive Board. In this network, I have access to colleagues in all disciplines related to public health all over the world. These contacts are invaluable both professionally and personally. I think, however, Welch is correct that many men cannot understand some of the problems women face in business as well as in politics, and that we do need to have a women's network upon which to call. Actually, an essential component of political and business involvement is to be a part of as many networks as possible in order to gain access to as much information and as many contacts as possible. That's both the name of the game and the bottom line, especially in political participation and business.

Information Networks. An information network's purpose is to supply its members with the kinds of reliable information they need, in time for them to use it effectively. For example, Born describes a network, Newmyer's in Washington, that does nothing but gather and transmit information to its business clients (1980). The staff is composed of former investigative newspaper reporters. These people work very hard at developing and maintaining contacts in key places. Newmyer's staff works closely with staffs of other information-gathering networks, and many trade-offs take place. For example, in the course of gathering information for one of its own clients, a network may also pick up a good deal of data that would be of value to the client of another network. By passing this information along, the exchange is built up. At some later point the second network will return the favor, and so it goes. The whole objective of the process is to see to it that client organizations receive information about legislative, administrative, and regulatory decisions in as timely a fashion as possible. The better the information network's contacts with people in government, the more timely and accurate the information to which they have access.

The charge of manipulation is often an objection raised about participation in networks. In reality, the people who are involved in formation brokering expect to be used. People in the kinds of jobs that provide them access to information assume that they will be asked for that information. Making information available to interested people is part of their jobs. Sometimes they cannot give information or make comments. When this is the case, they will say so. The process of information sharing is an exchange and a two-way street. People give information out with the expectation that they will get other information of use to them in return. This payoff can either be immediate or delayed. N-CAP and state N-PACs (see the Yellow Pages) are examples of real or potential information networks in the political arena for nurses. As other nurses' organizations develop political action committees and hire lobbyists, they too can serve this function.

A very effective network is the telephone tree. I belong to such a network through Common Cause. I am called by my contact person, who describes the issue and the action desired. I then call my six contacts, each of whom has a list of people to call. In this way a number of people can be reached in a very short time and with very little effort on any one person's part. As a vehicle for getting telegrams, letters, or telephone calls to legislators to express a position on a pending bill, this kind of network is very efficient. The telephone tree network can be used effectively by nurses' groups to mobilize support or opposition on a given issue. Again, the point is to get information out to as many people who need it as quickly and reliably as possible.

An important duty of members of information networks is to learn the areas and issues in which other members of the network or their clients are interested. In that way we can be alert to gather and pass on information useful to other members of the network even if these data are not pertinent to us. As others begin to provide this same kind of service for us, the information exchange begins to function most effectively.

Credibility is essential in all facets of political participation, including networking. The importance of developing and guarding one's reputation as a reliable source of information cannot be overemphasized. You must learn that if you do not know something, it is OK to say so—far better than trying to bluff your way through. Once people begin to suspect that an information source is not credible, they begin to alter their networks in such a way as to cut out the unreliable individual. This is tantamount, in both political participation and business, to being ostracized. Beware that it does not happen to you. You are only as effective as your information permits you to be. If you lose your place in an information network, you are lost.

Professional and Political Networks. Professional networks can serve a number of purposes, including the exchanging of information on professional and political issues and concerns, and acting as support systems. I mentioned that I have been part of a professional network since 1964. Obviously this network has grown and changed over the years; this is true of all networks, since they are living things. I have become a member of a number of other formal and informal professional networks as well. At this point, I can and do get the help and consultation I need on almost any professional or political problem with three phone calls or less. These calls may be to colleagues all over the country and in some instances abroad. If the person I call does not have the information I need, she or he is almost always able to refer me to someone who does know where to get it. Obviously, if there is sufficient lead time this gathering of information can be done by mail; however, a real advantage of phone or face-to-face contact is the strengthening of personal relationships.

All of the professional and political organizations listed in the Yellow Pages (Chapter 10) are or could become networks for our use. Being in close contact with as many of these networks as possible broadens our scope of sources of information and support. Likert's "linking pin" concept (1976), where a member of one group is also a member of another for the express purpose of fostering communication and exchange between the groups, exemplifies what I mean here. As we learn to network and consciously to form linking-pin relationships, we can greatly expand our involvement in the web of networks that is growing among women in the United States.

Networking, as noted, is particularly crucial in the political arena, and, as nurses seek to become increasingly active and visible in politics at all levels, they must learn to develop, expand, and use professional organizations as information and contact networks. N-CAP and the state N-PACs, as well as nursing-specialty organizations and the national and state Leagues for Nursing (see the Yellow Pages) are ideal beginnings for networks. Many of these organizations are already networking on a variety of professional and political issues. While nurses must not confine themselves to networks of nurses only, nursing organizations are an excellent place to start.

Some of the organizations, such as the National Women's Political Caucus (NWPC) and the National Women's Education Fund (see the Yellow Pages) are increasing women's participation and clout in political affairs at all levels of government. It is essential that nurses become more involved with these kinds of organizations, too. Through them we can expand our network of contacts and sources of information into other arenas and learn strategies that will help us to deal with issues related to health and nursing from other points of view. For example, I recently participated in a workshop, sponsored by our local chapter of NWPC, entitled "Don't Fight City Hall, Run It." Speakers were women who hold a variety of county and city offices and who discussed running a successful and efficient election campaign. Since I was working on several other women's campaigns at the time, I found the session a great opportunity not only to learn from the formal presentation, but also to meet and exchange cards with a number of politically active women whom I had not met before. The League of Women Voters is another organization that educates people on political issues. If your local area does not have organized affiliates with these and other political organizations, get a group of your friends and colleagues together, write to the national office of the organization of your choice, and start your own group locally. None of us nurses can hope to have much impact on the systems we seek to change as long as we act alone; our strength is in collective and concerted action as a group. Remember, nursing is the largest discipline among all of the health providers. If we were truly organized, there is very little we could not do. Coalitions with consumers, especially female consumers, could greatly increase our clout. We must learn this lesson and learn it soon.

Getting Into a Network. As I indicated at the beginning of this section, my first and still most effective network is the one that evolved from my master's program in public health nursing at the School of

Public Health. This network is now greatly expanded through the public health nursing section of the American Public Health Association. It serves as an information and professional network as well as a support system. I tell every incoming group of graduate students that their classmates and faculty are a ready-made network that they can call upon for the rest of their careers. I encourage graduate students in my management classes to form professional and support networks with other nurse-managers in their work settings, to exchange information and to obtain peer consultation. They, like all the rest of us, will need it.

Professional organizations and many of the other groups listed in the Yellow Pages (Chapter 10) are ready-made networks. Which one or ones you choose to join will depend on your interests and, to some extent, the organization's proximity to you. Read through the descriptions of the national organizations and then send for additional information from those whose purpose may be particularly congruent with your needs or objectives. Both Welch (1980a) and Kleiman (1980) provide extensive listings of networks all over the country. You will have to be selective, since there are many networks, and each of us only has so much time and other resources to give. A rule of thumb might be to belong actively to at least one professional and one political network. For example, I am most active in the public health nursing section of the American Public Health Association and in the National Women's Political Caucus. Obviously, you may make other choices.

If you cannot find a ready-made network, then you and a group of like-minded colleagues and friends can form your own, at least on a local level. Again, the issues you address—professional, political, and/or support—will determine much of how you organize and structure the network and how it functions. Again both Welch (1980a, c) and Kleiman (1980) provide guidelines for the do-it-yourself network. They concentrate on rather elaborate and more or less permanent networks. To be sure, these kinds of networks are most helpful. I believe, and my experience has helped establish this belief, that we also need to have ad hoc networks—networks that form for a specific reason and for only as long as that reason continues to exist. For example, many of us who worked to defeat California's tax-cutting initiative, Proposition 9, in the 1980 elections, were active members of a short-lived issue-related network. Once we had won our fight against that initiative, we all went our separate ways. We may well have no further contact with one another unless a similar issue appears on the horizon again. I am not advocating exclusive "ad hocracy" in networking, but I am convinced that this approach is valid and effective.

Whatever kinds of networks you choose to become affiliated with, I think that you will find them useful and rewarding. Just knowing that you can almost always get the information or help you need in three phone calls or less is very reassuring. Networking is nowhere more important than for those who choose to work in politics.

GETTING INVOLVED

The opportunities for nurses to become involved in political processes are endless. The discussions of the typology of political participation (see Chapter 1) developed for our studies of nurse-leaders' activities illustrates what many of our colleagues are already doing. In this section I will focus on some of these processes in more depth. Some of the kinds of participation discussed require a great deal of time and effort both for initial entry as well as for on-going participation. I have already discussed networking as a means for gaining information and contacts. The better your networks are the more contacts and sources of information you will have, and the easier will be your entrée.

Volunteer Work for a Candidate. Every election year offers a wealth of opportunities to get involved with campaigns at all levels of government. Many local elections are nonpartisan, and so support of a candidate does not involve any of the political parties. Most state and federal races are partisan. Whatever kinds of campaign involvement you choose, you will learn a great deal about politics, with often relatively little investment of time and money.

The reasons for supporting one candidate rather than another vary greatly. You may know the candidate already from previous work in politics or other arenas. Your friends may recommend the candidate as one whose views and stands on issues are congruent with yours. Endorsements by people you respect may sway your thinking to one candidate. Never underestimate the power that an endorsement from the right people at the right time can have. Remember this when you are asked to give endorsements; you are laying a very precious commodity on the line: your credibility. You may select a candidate, at least initially, because you do not like the other candidates. To really commit support to a person though, I think you should be working for that person rather than against another. Use your contacts (networking, again) to check out all the candidates carefully before making a selection.

Gaining entrée into a campaign is facilitated if members of one or more of your networks are already active workers. If this is the case you will not have to try to gain entrée on your own, you will be recruited! But don't let your lack of acquaintance with a candidate or with someone already involved in the campaign hamper you. Just call up—either the candidate's home or headquarters, depending on the stage of the campaign—and volunteer. When you do this, be realistic about the amount of time you offer and the kinds of tasks you agree to take on. Don't over-extend yourself or agree to do things you really don't know how to do, unless you can work with someone who does know how. Above all, when you've made a commitment, keep it. Again, the importance of building and maintaining credibility cannot be overemphasized. If people find they cannot count on you, they will soon cease to count on you at all. A good strategy is to volunteer to work in the campaign headquarters or another area on a regular schedule throughout the campaign. In this way people will learn that they can count on you. This can lead to your being asked to get involved with more interesting things: writing speeches, handling problems, and eventually being in on elections. This beats being consigned to stuffing envelopes and making phone calls. Although these are vital activities in any campaign, they are far less riveting than are others.

As I write this, my colleagues and I are gearing up for a most interesting campaign for our state legislature. The woman we supported in the contested party primary won, and now faces an opponent in the general election who is a conservative male physician. I have known our candidate since we worked together on another person's campaign several years ago. When I heard she had filed her candidacy in the primary, I called to inquire how I could best help her. She asked that I organize a network of nurses who could contact other nurses, health care providers, and interested voters. I gathered a group of influential nurses in our county, and we met with the candidate to discuss issues with her. In this way we not only had the opportunity to learn about her beliefs on issues of importance to us but also to influence these beliefs. We continued to meet with members of her staff and, just before the primary, sent endorsement letters to our nurse colleagues in the assembly district. As I indicated, she won the primary, and our hopes are high for the general election.

Now we are meeting again with members of our candidate's staff to work out and clarify some of her positions on issues and to compare them with those of her opponent. We will be sending another endorsement letter to nurses just before the election. In addition, we are planning to mobilize our nurse colleagues to do door-to-door precinct work for our candidate, explaining how her positions differ from those of her opponent on health and other issues, and urging that they, too, support her with their votes. We obtained the names and addresses of all of the nurses in our district through a member of the planning group, who is also a member of the board of a local organization that had purchased the list from the Board of Registered Nurses for use in their continuing education program. We bought the mailing labels, and another member of the group volunteered her firm's photocopying machine to make the mailing labels. (Networking, again.) The planning group of nurses is paying for the postage and duplication of the letters as a monetary contribution to the campaign. The whole process has been a valuable learning experience and has enabled us to get to know many of the nurses in our area better. Because our candidate's opponent is a physician, some of us see this race as a test of nurses' abilities to successfully support a political candidate in our area.

We are finding a number of rewards through working in political campaigns at the local level. Working at the local level on political campaigns can present problems, however. In a recent election, I supported a candidate whose opponent was then a sitting member of the board of supervisors of the county in which I live. Because I am an officer of Nursing Dynamics Corporation, and because that corporation receives a great deal of its funding for services from various county funds, my support for the supervisor's opponent had to be less vocal and public than might otherwise have been the case. I discussed my predicament with my candidate; he was very understanding and supportive. I had no indication that the supervisor would have penalized the agency because of my political opposition to his candidacy, but I decided not to take the risk. It may be easier to work on political activities on the local level because you know more about the situation; conversely, it may be more difficult for the same reason.

Campaign work is fun and rewarding. Precinct walking for your candidate even gives you an opportunity for some fresh air, sunshine, and exercise. A number of the organizations listed in the Yellow Pages (Chapter 10) have publications and other materials to help you be a more effective campaign worker. Two I have found invaluable are the National Women's Political Caucus, both nationally and in my own county, and the National Women's Education Fund, which puts out a splendid *Campaign Workbook*, a step-by-step guide to running a campaign. These aids will be invaluable to you, whether you are running someone else's campaign or administering your own. More nurses should run for office; public policy is much too important to be left in the hands of politicians, attorneys, and bureaucrats.

Work for a Ballot Initiative.   Much of the previous material about working on an individual's campaign also applies to working for the passage of a ballot initiative or referendum. Some states have limitations on the numbers and kinds of issues that can be submitted directly to the voters for their decision. California is among the states with the most liberal and far-reaching citizen initiative process. In fact, a California state legislator told me recently that he doubted that any really significant legislation would come from the legislature in the future; it would come through the initiative process, instead. California has already demonstrated this tendency by the passage of the property-tax-cutting initiative, Proposition 13. Proposition 9, which appeared on the primary ballot in spring 1980, would have cut state income taxes by 50 percent. This initiative was soundly defeated at the polls, but not without considerable effort by both proponents and opponents.

In developing a ballot initiative, you must have an issue that commands sufficient public interest to enable your sponsoring group to amass the thousands of registered voters' signatures that are required for the measure to qualify for placement on the ballot. This is much the same process that candidates from parties that are not officially recognized and independent candidates must go through to get their names on the ballot. You must also be sure of your state's requirements and regulations on the initiative process before you proceed. No point wasting a lot of time and effort doing things wrong. Making mistakes that should have been avoided can jeopardize the whole effort. So if you think you have an issue that could become a ballot initiative, be sure that you also know the procedures your state requires you to follow.

As in supporting candidates for office, a major objective in supporting an initiative is to be sure that the issue is recognized by the voters. Name recognition is terribly important. In our work to defeat Proposition 9, we sought out groups that we believed would be particularly hard-hit if the measure passed. Our first step was to be sure that they understood what the proposition actually said. One of the tough and costly lessons that we learned too late in working against Proposition 13 was that scare tactics can and often do backfire. This time out we talked about possible effects—reductions in city and county services to the elderly, young, needy, handicapped, and poor—all of whom can least afford to have already depleted services further reduced. Since we had some evidence of the effects of Proposition 13, we could point to it in saying that things would get worse if Proposition 9 were to pass.

Much has been written about voting behavior and the changes it has undergone in recent years (Broder, 1971; Silbey & McSweney, 1972; Nie, Verba, & Petrocik, 1976). Fewer people vote, people no longer can be expected to vote along party lines, and people seem increasingly to vote for their own interests even if that means that others' interests may be compromised. Some groups, such as the elderly, vote in disproportionately large numbers; such groups can be fruitful targets for educational presentations that seek to influence voting behavior. We concentrated heavily on the elderly in our campaign against Proposition 9. Most of California's elderly pay little or no personal income taxes; thus they could be advised that their personal savings from the initiative's passage would be small. On the other hand, since many elderly depend on numerous public services, they stood to lose a great deal if the proposition passed and these services were further reduced. Apparently our presentations paid off, since the final election result—a smashing defeat of Proposition 9—was the reverse of what the polls had been predicting only a few months before the election.

However you choose to work in elections, whether for individual candidates and/or for initiatives, the effort provides many learning opportunities. Friendships can be made and broken in political campaigns: part of the art is to learn to separate personal feelings from feelings about issues. Losing is a sad experience but we must learn to bounce back and try again. Nobody wins every election, not if the elections are really free and fair. Many people try politics and, if they lose, never try again. Others, the ultimately successful ones, learn from their mistakes as well as from their successes and come back to try again. These are the people who enjoy the game for its own sake as well as for its outcome. Nurses, as well as many other special-interest groups in the electorate, need to learn to be more willing to play the game.

Influencing Policy.   Many people prefer not to campaign either for candidates or for issues. There are many other ways to influence public policy. Writing letters to legislators and regulators is an effective way to make your ideas known, as well as trying to get others to see things your way. Obviously, a legislator's constituents have some clout, since when the next election comes around they are the people who will be able to vote for or against reelection. We should make more use of our power as constituents, particularly on issues where we can bring large numbers of constituents together in a concerted effort to influence events (see Chapter 6 for a discussion of lobbying).

Letters, then, are a useful tool not only for expressing opinions but also for exerting clout. Letters should be personally and individually written; avoid using Xeroxed copies of others' letters that you merely sign. Rewrite the letter in your own words and send it in its own envelope. Many elected officials are not as impressed by petitions or letters with multiple signatures as they are with individual letters. When you write, refer to the bill, law, or specific issue to which you want to direct attention; don't be so obscure in your references that the official cannot figure out what you want. Give the reasons for whatever stand you take. If you are for it, tell why. If you oppose it, give specific reasons. Also tell the official what it is you want him or her to do: to vote for or against a bill or law, co-sponsor specific legislation, etc. Some officials say that telegrams and mailgrams have more impact on their thinking than do letters; others treat them all the same. Find out from the people you may want to influence what kinds of correspondence have the most impact on them.

Personal contact, either in the official's office or in the district when he or she makes visits, can be tremendously important. This is particularly true if you have taken the effort to get to know the official before you need his or her help. Having been sufficiently active in the most recent campaign to be remembered by either the official or members of the staff helps too. Do not be discouraged if you have an appointment to see the official and you see a staff person instead. Often the staff knows more than the elected official does and will write the bill, analysis, memo, or whatever results from your visit. As with written communication, be clear about what you want to talk about and what you want done. Giving the official's secretary or other staff person an idea of what you want to talk about when you make the appointment gives them a chance to gather whatever materials they may need before you arrive and so use everyone's time most effectively.

A frequent and effective way that we as professionals can use our expertise to influence policy decisions is through the vehicle of testimony. Testimony should be short, sweet, and to the point. Make a real effort to say everything you have to say that is really important in the first two or three minutes. Don't belabor the points. Make them clearly and go. Rather than repeat what previous speakers have said, either say that you concur or confine your remarks to content that complements or amplifies what has already been said. Nothing turns policymakers off as much as having people insist on reading repetitious and boring testimony. In fact, this kind of behavior by witnesses can actually change policymakers' minds and lead them to vote against a measure they originally favored. Try to put yourselves in the policymakers' position. Most have done their homework and are well prepared on the issue at hand. They do not want to be lectured to, but, instead, want to hear new and convincing information about the issue. Try to give this information to them in an interesting and succinct manner. Again, credibility is all-important. If you make a glaring error in any part of your testimony, everything you say may be discounted. Have your facts as well organized and as well documented as you can.

Other Ways to Be Involved. As we noted in the discussion of the typology of political participation in Chapter 1, there are many ways to become politically active and involved. I have touched on several here in some depth. Others are dealt with at even greater length by other contributors to the book. Jean Moorhead describes what it is like to be a candidate; Dona Cutting talks about lobbying; Cheryl Beversdorf shares her early experiences as a member of the staff of a Senate committee; Ruth Fleshman discusses grassroots organizing and influence. These women, all nurses, speak from their own experience and can serve as role models to help us to increase our involvement and to develop new styles of participation. Elsewhere, Moorhead describes the process she went through, as a nurses' association lobbyist, to get a bill written, carried, and passed (1979). As is stressed throughout the book, nurses have power, but they must learn to use it effectively. This book seeks to help us be better able to do just that.

THE HATCH ACT

In 1939 Congress enacted Public Law 76-252, an "Act to Prevent Pernicious Political Activities," commonly know as the Hatch Act. In essence, the law states that any person employed in any administrative position in any department of the US government may not "use his official position for the purpose of interfering with, or affecting the election or the nomination of any candidate for the office of President, Vice President, Presidential elector, member of the Senate, or Member of the House of Representatives, Delegates or Commissioners from the Territories and insular possessions" (PL 76-252, Section 2). The law goes on to say: "It shall be unlawful for any person, directly or indirectly to promise any employment, position, work, compensation, or other benefit, provided for or made possible in whole or in part by any Act of Congress, to any person as a consideration, favor, or reward for any political activity or for the support of or opposition to any candidate or any political party in any election" (PL 76-252, Section 3).

This law was enacted to protect civil servants from having to contribute money or to vote the way their boss wanted them to out of fear of losing their jobs. Most states now have adopted similar laws covering governmental employees on local, county, and state levels. If you are a public employee, you need to be familiar with your state's version of the Hatch Act to be sure of what you can and cannot do in the political arena. This awareness will not intimidate you or preclude your political involvement, but rather help you to be aware of what restrictions, if any, exist for you. Even if there are restrictions under your state's version of the Hatch Act, they apply to you *only* in your capacity as a public employee. What you do as a private citizen cannot be restricted; however, you must make it clear that your political actions are undertaken as a private citizen and not as a public employee. Be sure others know you are speaking and acting on your own behalf rather than on behalf of the agency you work for. Absolutely do not use agency or institutional stationery, other supplies, or equipment, and do not use work time for political activities.

Common Cause provides a helpful list of political activities government workers are permitted to engage in under the Hatch Act. Such workers may:

—make partisan campaign contributions;
—join political parties;
—work for or against ballot measures (initiatives)
—serve as election judges;
—wear political buttons (off duty) and display bumper stickers;
—take part in nonpartisan activities, such as running for election to a nonpartisan local school board (about three-fourths of local elections are nonpartisan (Who Is Hatched? 1979:17).

Prohibited activities include being an officer in a political party, collecting funds for a partisan purpose, being a delegate to a party convention, and circulating partisan nominating petitions (Who Is Hatched? In Common 10:17, 1979).

From these listings, it is apparent that the main focus of the prohibitions under the Hatch Act is partisan activities. Such prohibitions preclude government workers from using any government resources in at most only three of the types of political participation that we discussed in Chapter 1: working for the election of local, state, or federal candidates known to be in favor of health care and nursing issues by sponsoring fundraisers and so on; participating on political parties' committees; and persuading others to vote for specific candidates. This latter activity, persuading others to vote, needs to be emphasized. For example, as a supervisor you may not use your line authority in any way to influence or coerce your subordinates to vote the way you want them to. If the elections are nonpartisan, as most elections at the local level are, then activities in them are not prohibited under the Hatch Act. Again, be sure that you are familiar with the specifics of your own state's version of the Hatch Act. Do not let supposed restrictions of the Hatch Act interfere with your rights and responsibilities to participate fully in a variety of political activities.

POLITICAL PARTIES

Every four years the two major political parties go through their courting ritual with the voters, the Presidential election process. There were 16 Presidential primaries in 1960; in 1980, there were 35, more than ever before. As a result, approximately 75 percent of the total number of delegates to the major parties' national conventions in 1980 were selected through primaries, thus increasing the voters' direct participation in the Presidential nomination process and decreasing the importance of roles traditionally played by the parties. This change is but one of the many symptoms of the public's increasing distrust of and disdain for political parties in the United States.

A December 1979 poll asked 1,047 people whether they were satisfied or dissatisfied with specific components of the Presidential nominating process. Seventy-nine percent of the respondents indicated that they were satisfied with the primaries; 18 percent were dissatisfied, and 3 percent had no opinion. Sixty percent were satisfied with party conventions, 34 percent were dissatisfied, and 6 percent had no opinion. Political parties ranked lowest, with only 53 percent of the respondents satisfied with them, 46 percent dissatisfied, and 1 percent undecided (Skelton, 1980). Another indicator of the parties' waning appeal is the trend for up to 75 percent of the voters in some states to register as independents. Since there is no Independent Party, this refusal to declare affiliation with a major party means that these people cannot vote in primary elections if their state has a closed primary. A high price to pay for avoiding party affiliation. This situation may change if John Anderson and Barry Commoner are at all successful in their third party movements.

These and other trends show the weakening of political parties' traditional roles as objects of identification and affection and as guides to electoral choice and candidate evaluation. "Party affiliation, once the central thread connecting the citizen and the political process, is a thread that has certainly frayed" (Nie, Verba, & Petrocik, 1976:73). Even if people have remained affiliated with a political party, that party affiliation is much less influential in the 1980s than it was in the 1950s. Some people, who agree with George Washington's warning in his farewell address about the danger parties pose to internal security, view this decline in party power as a good thing. Others voice equally strong concerns about the loss in organization and continuity that accompanies weakened political parties. Still others do not understand enough about the major parties to know what the changes may mean. The following discussion of political parties is to help you make an informed decision about whether you want to register and participate in one.

What Are Parties and What Do They Do?

Political parties are nothing more than voluntary associations of voters whose purpose in organizing is to select and control government personnel and policies. They provide opportunities for ordinary people at the grassroots level to get involved in the political process; they select and nominate candidates for public offices; they support nominated candidates (see Chapter 7 for a description of how helpful a party can be to a nurse running for office). Parties organize the electorate into more efficiently functioning groups. Parties serve a watchdog function for other parties, so that neither can get too far out of line and so provide for their one form of separation of powers through their competition with one another. Parties supply a forum for the establishment and articulation of issues. They offer people a choice in each election, perhaps not as clear a choice as the parties once did or as the electorate might like, but a choice nonetheless. Parties provide an opportunity for minority groups' needs and opinions to be heard and to become part of the party platform. The party in power tries to gain favor with the public through its choice of personnel and policy decisions. The party out of power is quick to criticize and to make alternative proposals in an attempt to unseat the party in power, all through peaceful and relatively rational means. In this process, the public is shown more than one facet of the issues, which fosters better informed decisions. This list of functions indicates that political parties are useful devices in a pluralistic society such as ours.

A detailed history of the evolution of the major and minor political parties in the United States is beyond the scope of this book. The reference section for this chapter contains a number of sources for those of you interested in reading more (Broder, 1971; Chester, 1977; Fairlie, 1978; Nie, Verba, & Petrocik, 1976; Saloma & Sontag, 1973; Silbey & McSeveney, 1972). The United States followed the English tradition of a political system with two major parties rather than a multiparty system as found in many European countries, or a single-party system as found in more controlled societies where single party is an organ of the government instead of a voluntary association of the electorate. In the biparty system there are two major parties of relatively equal size, as well as a few minor parties that tend to focus on limited issues, such as the Peace and Freedom Party in the United States. Generally, third parties do not attain sufficient power to supplant a major party, although such situations have occurred.

Despite the emphasis given in the media to national political activities, US party organization tends to give greater emphasis to local interests, with the most vital organizations being at the grassroots. In addition, in contrast to vested-interest groups and political action committees (PACs), political parties address a broad range of interests and issues. For these reasons, parties offer excellent opportunities for people who want to become involved in general rather than special or single-issue politics. To be sure, many local elections such as school and hospital boards, mayoral and judicial races, are at least nominally nonpartisan. Legislative and congressional elections, however, are decidedly partisan (see Chapter 7). Thus party involvement offers the chance to work for and with people who will eventually make state and national policies. Some people may choose to work on the party platform or other party committees rather than in support of individual candidates. The state party conventions determine party rules, nominate candidates in states where there are no primaries, develop and adopt the party platform, and appoint the committees that run party candidates' campaigns. Committees are also appointed to handle the party's business between elections. Delegates from the state conventions go to the national conventions to nominate the party's Presidential and vice-presidential candidates and to articulate the party's national platform. Because of the size and complexity of the national convention, much of the real work is done outside of the convention setting, an opportunity to exert considerable power behind the scenes. Each party appoints three national-level committees to carry on campaign functions after the convention. These committees assist the Presidential nominee's campaign and plan the next national party convention; the congressional campaign committee focuses on the election of party candidates to the House of Representatives. The senatorial campaign committee assists party candidates for the United States Senate. In some states, representatives to these and other committees, as well as to the party's national convention, must be elected at the primary election. In other states, these committee positions are filled by appointments made by the party's state hierarchy.

Because of the unwieldy nature of the conventions as well as past abuses of power by a few bosses in smoke-filled rooms, the present system of primary elections has evolved. In this system, candidates and some convention delegates and committee members are chosen by the electorate in a process that is much like the election itself. A few states have an open primary in which each voter receives a ballot listing all of the parties' candidates. This enables voters to choose from any party they wish in the primary without regard to their own party affiliation. Most states have a closed or party primary in which only registered party members may vote, and then only for the candidates seeking their party's nominations. Thus Republicans vote for Republican candidates and Democrats for Democratic candidates. The winners of pluralities in these primaries become their party's candidate for a given office in the general election.

An advantage of the primary system of candidate selection is that it puts much of the power for the selection of final candidates into the hands of all of the party members who choose to vote in the primary. It enables a majority of the party members to break the hold that bosses and machines may have had over the party's candidate selection. Perhaps these are some of the reasons that almost four out of five people in the December 1979 poll were satisfied with the present primary system (Skelton, 1980). Some of the disadvantages of the primary system include its expense for the candidates, who, if their primary is contested, must in essence run two campaigns for each office they seek. Some voters object because they must go to the polls twice, once to choose their party's candidates and a second time to vote in the general election. Internal weakening of the party may occur as a result of rival factions running opposing candidates and splitting the party so badly that the opposing party's candidate is elected in the general election. Finally, there is little doubt that the primary election has weakened the party system by removing much of the power from the party itself and from those who run, or seek to run, it. Ward bosses such as Tammany Hall's Plunkitt would not have approved of the primary election system (Riordon, 1963).

Another function of the party mechanism is to help organize the party's members of Congress and state legislatures. Thus elected members of a party form the party's legislative caucus in each chamber of the state legislature and of Congress. The legislative caucus chooses the party leadership for the next legislative session. The majority party chooses the speaker of the lower chamber and the president or president pro tempore of the upper chamber. Minority party leaders in both chambers are generally referred to as the minority leaders. Both parties in both chambers have floor leaders, or "whips," and a variety of other elected leaders to manage the party's business and to try to organize members to vote along party lines on crucial issues. I say try, because increasing numbers of legislators are pursuing independent paths—or at least paths that are independent of their party's wishes—and so party legislative caucus power, beyond electing its publicly acknowledged leaders, is very limited. This is yet another symptom of the erosion of the parties' former power and organizing force in US politics.

What Has Happened to the Major Parties in the United States?

Events such as Watergate, Koreagate, and Abscam have undermined the public's faith in politicians and, to some extent, in political parties as well. In the December 1979 poll, only 7 percent of the respondents indicated that they respected officeholders (Skelton, 1980). Not a smashing endorsement! The last four Presidential elections have seen decreasing numbers of voters going to polls; in 1976, 54 percent of those eligible to vote for President of the United States chose to do so. President Ronald Reagan was elected in 1980 by 27 percent of the American population of voting age. He got 43,901,812 votes to Jimmy Carter's 35,483,820 and John Anderson's 7,127,664 (U.S. News and World Report, 1981). Another indication that political participation is at a very low ebb. Both parties are suffering from this phenomenon.

Another set of factors contributing to political parties' decline in influence with the voters include the blurring of party positions. The fact that it is often hard to tell party lines and party candidates apart is a large part of the problem. Time was when, at least theoretically, the Republican party stood for business, free enterprise, high tariffs, and minimum government. Its members were predominantly wealthy businessmen and rural aristocrats who were definitely conservative. Democrats, on the other hand, were thought to stand for big government, welfare and labor rights, low tariffs, and big spending. Its members were predominantly urban proletarians with liberal ideas.

Now is not the first time, nor will it be the last, that blurring of party identities has occurred. After the Civil War, the Republicans were pushing for new state constitutions in the reconstruction of the South. Blacks and white carpetbaggers supported these reform efforts, while whites of all classes banded together to vote against them. The Republican Party became so hated in the South by the people who wielded power that only recently could a Republican be elected to any political office there. Hence we have had the "solid South," led by Southern Democrats who were often indistinguishable from conservative Republicans.

In their desire to woo and win voters, major political parties today tend to avoid controversial—and alienating—issues, leaving these for the more strident single-issue groups and the minority parties to artic- ulate. Candidates try to remain as uncommitted as possible, tending to become more and more alike. It is little wonder that many people cannot tell what the parties stand for; sometimes one wonders if the parties themselves really know.

Peoples' opinions about what parties stand for also change, even though the parties themselves may not have changed their ideological stance. For example, in April 1981, the Gallup Poll found that for the first time in ten years, respondents perceived the Republican Party as the party that was more likely to keep the country prosperous. The same poll also found that the Democratic Party was perceived as being the party more likely to keep the United States out of World War III, another reversal of opinion since 1970 (Gallup, 1981).

Political parties are victims of the same changing values and con- flicting ideologies that are weakening so many other institutions in our society. Vested-interest groups, now personified by political action com- mittees and single-issue lobbies such as the anti–gun control or the right-to-life groups, are gaining inordinate power over legislators at all levels of government. As discussed earlier in this chapter, these groups can bring tremendous pressures and resources to bear to impose their position. Who needs parties for issue clarification and articulation with these kinds of powerful vested-interest groups? An interesting debate could be held about the relationship between the decline of political parties and the rise of political action groups: I suspect that they are closely related. At any rate, political parties are in something of a catch 22, since people see them as relatively ineffective and so put their ener- gies into other organizations inside or outside of the political arena; as a result the political parties are weakened further.

A related phenomenon is the very high number of voters who are registered as independents. Apparently many people either do not wish to be affiliated in any way with either major party, or they think that registering as an independent means that are joining the Independent Party. There is no Independent Party, and so often all these voters are doing is preventing themselves from participating in their state's pri- mary election and receiving party-generated information about candi- dates and issues. The price for their independent status is partial disen- franchisement and isolation from an information source.

Most of the minor parties are relatively ineffective in getting can- didates elected, although they do play a very important role in address- ing controversial issues, such as the Vietnam War, that the major parties do not want to touch. If the issues and positions that the minor parties take prove to be useful, acceptable, or even popular, one or both of the major parties may incorporate all or part of these issues or positions into their party platform. This is one of the reasons that minor parties either come and go, or remain minor parties such as the Socialists. Again, this may change.

Because political parties seek middle-of-the-road positions to avoid alienating their increasingly heterogeneous and tentative adherents as well as the great number of independent voters, they can neither lay down platforms that their candidates must follow nor hold their candidates, once elected, accountable to and for the party line. Recent US Presidents have not been the real leaders of their party; indeed it is often questionable who, if anyone, are the leaders of the major political parties in the United States. Not so with the British, as well as the Canadian and the Australian systems. In these systems the prime minister can be turned out of office by his or her own party if the party is not happy with his or her actions.

Why Bother With Political Parties?

After all this, I suspect you are asking this question.

No democracy has been able to survive without strong political parties to carry out essential political functions. Because parties have the capability of dealing with broad issues, as opposed to the narrow interests of political action committees and other vested-interest groups, they offer us a chance to learn about the entire political and electoral process from the inside. This can be done in our own communities, since parties have strong grassroots organizations in most parts of the country. In the Yellow Pages, you will find the addresses of the major parties in your state; contact them for the address of your county's or city's organizations.

As working members of a party, we have opportunities to influence the choice of candidates for many offices and to help shape the state and national platforms on a variety of issues, including those dealing with nursing and health. It is true that political parties in the United States today are relatively weak; the remedy for this is for more people like us to become involved in the party of our choice to see that it becomes stronger. Single-issue and reform groups typically fade away when they achieve or are defeated in attaining whatever limited goal they have set for themselves. Political parties, however weak, tend to continue. I suspect that when Common Cause and other organizations working for public-financing legislation for congressional as well as Presidential elections are successful, the influence of such political action committees will greatly decrease, and political parties will rise to fill the void. In the meantime, the routine of work in keeping party organizations together can also help us to learn the vital tools of cooperation, compromise, coalition building, and policy development.

For those nurses who have ambitions to run for elected office, a strong background of experience with the political party of their choice can pay off tremendously well; in fact, party mechanisms are the gatekeepers for many offices (see Chapter 7). Precinct-level work is a relatively sheltered workshop in which to learn how politics work and to find out if you are really interested in becoming a nurse-activist. Party work is a golden opportunity for nurses to form coalitions among themselves as well as with other people. None of us can do what needs to be done alone. Finally, we should try to avoid situations in which one nurse competes with another for a position. Nurses should run against nonnurse candidates so that more nurses can be elected. This must be a major objective for nurse-activists. Politics is much too important to leave to those outside the field of nursing (see Chapter 7).

POLITICAL ACTION COMMITTEES (PACs)

The federal Election Campaign Act of 1976 (Public Law 94-283) is administered by the Federal Elections Commission, created in 1971 (PL 92-225). The purpose of these statutes, as with earlier fair-campaign-practice acts, is to make individual and group campaign contributions a matter of public record by requiring meticulous reporting of names of the contributors and the amounts contributed. In addition, there are some restrictions on contributions by groups, for example, persons or firms who do business with the government are prohibited from making campaign contributions to candidates for federal offices (President, Vice President, electors, members of the US Senate or House of Representatives). Many states have also enacted similar fair-campaign or campaign-disclosure laws that apply to candidates for state and local offices. You can find out the exact provisions of your state's campaign laws by contacting your secretary of state or comparable state officer.

Under the present federal Election Campaign Act, no one individual may contribute more than $1,000 to any one federal candidate during a single election. Prior to the passage of this act there were no such restrictions on campaign contributions by individuals, nor was reporting of all contributions strictly required. While this restriction may have controlled some of the political influence individuals bought—or at least thought they bought—with their massive campaign contributions previously, it also gave impetus to the formation of an increasing number of political action committees (PACs).

PACs are special organizations set up by organizations, corporations, and other vested-interest groups to collect money and influence public policy through campaign contributions and lobbying efforts. PACs are particularly attractive to otherwise tax-exempt organizations, which would lose their tax-exempt status if they engaged in large amounts of partisan political activities. Thus the American Medical Association, the American Nurses' Association, and other organizations have chosen the PAC route to be able to use their political clout without losing their very favorable tax status. Some corporate and single-interest PACs have non-committal names such as the Sunbelt Good Government Committee (Winn-Dixie Stores, Inc), the Citizens for the Republic (a Ronald Reagan organization), and Civic Improvement Program (General Motors Corporation). Unless you knew by whom these PACs are sponsored, you would not know whose interests they serve.

Organizations have long sought to influence elected officials through their campaign contributions. The American Medical Association (AMA) has one of the longest and most successful histories of this kind of activity because of its early recognition of the influence government has on health issues in general and medical practice in particular. A recent example of the AMA's effectiveness is to be seen in the defeat of hospital cost containment legislation in late 1979. (AMA $ key in hospital vote. *Frontline* 5, 1979). Common Cause's review of data on campaign contributions made by AMA PACs during 1976 and 1978 congressional elections showed that House members who voted against the cost-containment bill received almost four times more money in campaign contributions (an average of $8,157 per member) from AMA PACs than did members who voted for the bill. The American Nurses' Association has followed the AMA's lead in establishing their own PAC, N-CAP (see the Yellow Pages). N-CAP, however, like other professional vested-interest groups' PACs, has nowhere near the financial clout of the AMA.

According to Common Cause, PACs "are the growth industry of the political world" (PAC money mushrooms. *In Common* 10:7, 1979). In 1974 there were 608 PACs registered with the Federal Elections' Commission; in 1979 there were over 2,000. Figures for the 1980 elections will be much higher. The big surge came after Congress repealed the prohibition, in force since 1940, against firms that do business with the government being able to contribute money to political campaigns. Businesses and groups are now free to form PACs and to seek to influence legislators via their campaign contributions. Clearly this is a conflict of interest. Individual PAC contributions are limited to $10,000 per candidate per election on the federal level. State restrictions on PAC contributions vary.

In 1978–1979 the 10 largest PACs in terms of gross receipts were:

- Citizens for the Republic (a Ronald Reagan organization)
- National Conservative PAC (in 1980 elections sought to unseat five senators it targeted as being too liberal)
- Committee for the Survival of a Free Congress
- Realtors' PAC
- American Medical Association PAC
- Automobile and Truck Dealers Election Action Committee
- Gun Owners of American Campaign Committee
- AFL-CIO COPE Political Contributions Committee
- UAW Voluntary Community Action Program (United Auto Workers)
- National Committee for an Effective Congress (PAC money mushrooms. *In Common* 10:12, 1979).

PACs are and will continue to be a fact of political life in the United States. Before you become involved with or contribute to a political action committee, be sure you know who or what are vested interests the PAC serves and that you want to be associated with such interests.

SUMMARY

In this chapter I have discussed a number of strategies for involvement in political activities. I start out with a value-clarification exercise, followed by a discussion of assertiveness, aggressiveness, and avoidance/acquiescence. These three types of behaviors are then compared and contrasted in terms of such personal variables as leadership style, decision making, risk taking, and perceptions of conflict.

Role models and mentors are increasingly being recognized for their essential value in helping others to develop their potentials. This is a fairly new idea for nurses, but one whose time has definitely come. The same can be said for networking, the process of linking people together for mutual support and aid. I describe some professional and political networks as well as how to get into a network.

Because others in this book have dealt with nurses as candidates, lobbyists, grassroots organizers, members of Senate staffs, and participants in collective bargaining, I confine my discussion in the getting-involved section of the chapter to working on campaigns for candidates and initiatives as well as on some suggestions for influencing policy.

The discussions of the Hatch Act, political parties, and political action committees are designed to provide the reader with an introduction to these political entities. The Hatch Act discussion is included to make us aware of the act's existence, as well as explaining what it covers and what it does not. Thus public employees can make informed decisions about the kinds of political participation they can engage in. Political parties and political action committees are both vehicles for political involvement that we as nurses need to understand better. Such understanding will enable us to participate in these important entities more effectively.

REFERENCES

Adams M: The compassion trap, in Gornick V, Moran AK (eds): *Woman in a Sexist Society*. New York, Basic Books, 1971, pp 555–575.

AMA $ key in hospital vote. *Frontline* 5:9, November–December 1979.

Assertive Nurse, Herman S (ed). 10012 Woodhill Road, Bethesda, Md, 20034 ($3 for six bimonthly issues).

Bakdash DP: Becoming an assertive nurse. *American Journal of Nursing* 78:1710–1712, October 1978.

Bloom LZ, Coburn K, Pearlman J: *The New Assertive Woman*. New York, Dell Publishing Co, 1976.

Born RC: Corporate CIA: In Washington it helps meet business' need to know. *AMA Management Digest* 2:9–12, January 1980.

Broder DS: *The Party's Over: The Failure of Politics in America*. New York, Harper & Row, 1971.

Campaign Workbook, National Women's Education Fund, (1532 16th Street, NW, Washington, DC 20036. $15 for single copies; $10 each in lots of ten or more; updated regularly).

Chenevert M: *Special Techniques in Assertiveness Training for Women in the Health Professions*. St. Louis, Mo, CV Mosby Co, 1978.

Chester EW: *A Guide to Political Platforms*. New York, Anchor Books, 1977.

Clark CC: Assertiveness issues for nursing administrators and managers. *Journal of Nursing Administration* 9:20–24, July 1979.

————: *Assertiveness Skills for Nurses*. Wakefield, Mass: Contemporary Publishing Co, 1978.

Fairlie H: *The Parties: Republicans and Democrats in this Century*. New York, St. Martin's Press, 1978.

Fesler JW (ed): *The 50 States and Their Local Governments*. New York, Alfred A Knopf, 1967.

First national women's network directory. *Working Woman* 5:26–40, March 1980.

Gallup G: How the parties are perceived. *San Francisco Chronicle*, May 4, 1981, p 8.

In the running: Careers in politics. *Working Woman* 5:65, 72, 76, February 1980.

Jacobsen GA, Lipman MH: *Political Science*, ed 2. College Outline Series. New York, Barnes & Noble, 1979.

Kelly LY: Endpaper—The good new nurse network. Nursing Outlook 26:71, January 1978.

———: Endpaper—The mentor relationship. Nursing Outlook 26:339, May 1978.

Keniston K: Young Radicals. New York, Harcourt Brace & World, 1968.

Kleiman C: Women's Networks: The Complete Guide to Getting a Better Job, Advancing Your Career, and Feeling Great as a Woman Through Networking. New York, Lippincott & Crowell, 1980.

Likert R, Likert JG: New Ways of Managing Conflict. New York, McGraw-Hill Book Co, 1976.

Lipset SM: Marx, Engles, and American political parties. Wilson Quarterly 2:90–104, winter 1978.

Moorhead JM: Community health nurses' involvement in legislative processes, in SE Archer, RP Fleshman (eds): Community Health Nursing: Patterns and Practice, ed 2. North Scituate, Mass, Duxbury Press, 1979, pp 566–591.

Nie NH, Verba S, Petrocik JR: The Changing American Voter. Cambridge, Mass, Harvard University Press, 1976.

PAC money mushrooms. In Common 10:7—12, Fall 1979.

Paizis S: Getting Her Elected: A Political Woman's Handbook. Sacramento, Calif, Creative Editions, 1977.

Phelps S, Austin N: The Assertive Woman. San Luis Obispo, Calif, Impact Publishers, 1975.

Riordon WL: Plunkitt of Tammany Hall: A Series of Very Plain Talks on Very Practical Politics. New York, EP Dutton, 1963.

Rohrbaugh P: Assertiveness, acquiescence, and aggression: An alternative model. Assert 14:5, June 1977.

Saloma JS III, Sontag FH: Parties: The Real Opportunity for Effective Citizen Politics. New York, Vintage Books, 1973.

Scaring D, Schwartz J, Lind A: The structuring principle, political socialization, and belief systems. American Political Science Review 67:415–432, 1973.

Silbey JH, McSeveney ST: Voters, Parties, and Elections: Quantitative Essays in the History of American Popular Voting. Lexington, Mass, Xerox College Publishing, 1972.

Simon SB, Howe LW, Kirschenbaum H: Values Clarification: A Handbook of Strategies for Teachers and Students. New York, Hart Publishing Co, 1972.

Skelton G: What U.S. voters think of the political system. San Francisco Chronicle, February 13, 1980, pp 5–6.

Welch, MS: Networking: The Great New Way for Women to Get Ahead. New York, Harcourt Brace Jovanovich, 1980a.

———: How to start a women's network. Working Woman 5:82–83, March 1980b.

———: Networking on the job. Ms. 8:85–88, March 1980c.

Who is hatched? In Common 10:17–18, Fall 1979.

Williams O (ed): A Little Treasury of Modern Poetry: English and American, rev ed. New York, Charles Scribner's Sons, 1952.

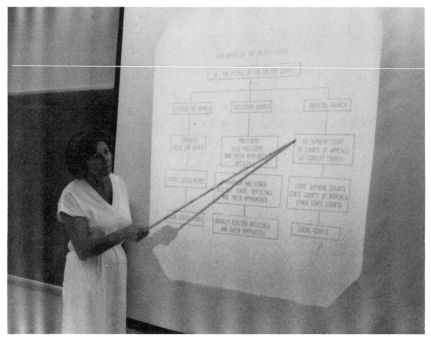

Patricia A. Goehner teaching the structure of the U.S. government to graduate legislative processes class at School of Nursing, University of California, San Francisco. *(Photo by Katherine McInerney)*

CHAPTER 5

Legislatures and Legislators

Patricia A. Goehner

LEGISLATION IS FREQUENTLY proposed that affects the nursing profession and health care. Such legislation places new challenges in nurses' pathways. Nurses must become knowledgeable about the political process. As you read this chapter you will gain an understanding of the legislature and of the steps a bill takes in becoming a law. Such knowledge will enable you, as a nurse and as a member of a professional group, to provide timely input that will have an impact on the legislative process.

Your input into the political process is important and can be given in various ways. Nurses have the power to elect officials who are concerned with health issues and with nursing. Nurses also have the power to influence a bill to law by taking a stand on an issue and presenting testimony during committee hearings, by talking with and writing letters to legislators. By applying your knowledge of the political process and utilizing the strategies mentioned above, you will influence the direction of a bill and thus determine the future of nursing and of health care.

LEGISLATURES

A legislature is an institution within which individuals deliberate, debate, and decide matters of policy affecting those whom they represent. Making public law in this fashion might be called the characteristic function of a legislature in the American system (Crane & Watts, 1968).

Each of the 50 states possesses lawmaking power. Each state has a legislature whose task is the making of laws for that state. However, the federal government, within the scope of its constitutional powers, may pass legislation effective in every state. The laws passed by the federal government are the supreme law of the land, and state statutes passed in contradiction to them are unenforceable.

Occasionally, when conflicts occur between state law and federal law, the Supreme Court of the United States is the final arbiter. Both state and federal courts are obliged to refuse to enforce a state statute contradicting federal constitutional or statutory law. Also, the Supreme Court of the United States may review state legislation and decide whether or not it conflicts with the Constitution of the United States or with legislation passed by Congress.

State legislation must comply with the provisions of the state constitution. Final decisions in regard to compliance are vested in the state courts.

However, legislatures are not lawmakers exclusively. The legislature shares its lawmaking authority with many institutions and groups such as the governor, other executives, courts, and citizens. Citizens can participate directly in the lawmaking process through the practice of initiative and referendum. Two thirds of the states allow for the initiative, a procedure whereby a certain percentage of voters may by petition propose a law to be placed on the ballot for voter approval or rejection. Circumventing the legislature, the voters draft the proposal, circulate petitions that must usually be signed by 5 to 10 percent of the registered voters, and campaign for its passage. Referendum, practiced in 29 states, provides for the submission of legislative and state constitutional measures to the voters for their acceptance or rejection. In nearly all states a referendum is required to approve amendments to the US Constitution.

Election of Legislators

There are various election systems used to choose the members of the 50 state legislatures. (Primaries are used in all of the states to nominate state legislators.) Forty-eight states elect their legislators on a partisan basis. Two states, Nebraska and Minnesota, elect their legislators on a nonpartisan basis. Primary elections vary among states. Six states—Alaska, Michigan, Minnesota, Montana, Utah, and Wisconsin—use the open primary, where voters receive ballots of both parties. The other 42 states use a closed primary, in which voters are required to declare their party affiliation at the polls and vote the ballot for only that party's primary.

Our laws provide that any citizen who is 18 years of age is entitled to vote provided that he or she is mentally competent and not in prison. In most states a person who is on parole for the conviction of a felony cannot vote.

As a voter you need to know the candidates. Knowledge of a candidate must include their awareness and understanding of health care issues and of the nursing profession. Also, you need to know what committees and subcommittees they serve on: health committee, finance committee, and so on. If a candidate is an incumbent, look carefully at how he or she voted on health care and nursing issues. Use this information as the basis upon which to cast your ballot.

Apportionment

The principle of the apportionment of both houses of state legislatures on a population basis is the established principle of the American constitutional system. Reapportionment was established to produce equitable distribution of state monies, more liberal welfare programs, more progressive tax schemes, and increased inter-party competition. According to Crane and Watts, "reapportionment may have political consequences affecting the distribution of political power within a state and thereby indirectly influence the nature of public policy although its influence does not show up in the analysis of welfare expenditures and the like. These consequences will differ from state to state" (1968:38).

Structure of Legislatures

The structure of each state legislature is set forth in the state constitution. Forty-nine states have bicameral legislatures, and Nebraska has a unicameral legislature. In a bicameral legislative system, power is shared by two coordinate legislative bodies, although often one of the bodies is referred to as the upper house and the other as the lower house.

Official Names

The dual legislative bodies are called the legislature in 25 states. Terms used in other states are general assembly, legislative assembly, and general court. The upper house, a term used merely for clarity, is called the senate in every state including the unicameral Nebraska legislature. Names for the lower house, a term also used merely for clarity, are house of representatives, assembly, general assembly, and house of delegates. For details, see Chapter 11.

Number of Legislators

The number of state legislators vary. In all states, the senate is smaller than the other house. For details for each state, see Chapter 11.

Sessions

In most states, annual sessions of the legislature were common until the late 19th century. Because of a distrust of legislatures, biennial sessions were established as a means of preventing the legislatures from doing very much. Now, most states have annual sessions, though a few still have biennial sessions. Some of the states with annual sessions consider only budget or necessary revenue acts during the off-year session.

All states have regular sessions and special or extraordinary sessions; in most states however, the governor decides when to call a special session. The length of the sessions is restricted by the individual state constitutions; consequently, some states have no restriction, while others are limited to 30 days. For details for each state, see Chapter 11.

Committees

Because of the complexity and large number of measures (bills and resolutions) introduced in the 50 state legislatures, committees have become an essential part of the legislature. It is impossible for each legislator to be aware of and knowledgeable about each individual measure. Committees, therefore, provide a division of labor as well as an area of specialization. In state legislatures, committees are not the powerful, independent, decision-making bodies that they are in Congress (Crane & Watts, 1968). All bills that are introduced are generally referred to a committee by the speaker of the house or presiding officer of the senate.

The number of committees varies within each state government. The median number of senate committees in state governments is 16, whereas the number of house committees in state governments is 18 (Smothers 1977–1978). Committee proliferation is best demonstrated in North Carolina, where the house has 45 standing committees and the senate has 32. Many state legislatures have more committees than does Congress.

Joint Committees

In addition to the standing committees in each house, many states have joint committees. Joint committees are composed of members of both houses and are generally used to reconcile differences that occur between the houses.

Conference Committees

Many states have conference committees composed of members of both houses. Conference committees are created to adjust differences between houses when a legislative proposal passes one house in one form and is amended in the other house. A bill or resolution cannot be sent to the executive unless it has passed both houses in identical form. This three- to nine-member committee works out a compromise acceptable to both houses; if reconciliation of viewpoints is impossible, however, the bill dies in conference.

The size of each committee varies. Each committee has a name. Listed below are the names of the standing committees of Congress. Similar committee names are used in each state. Also, for details for each state, see Chapter 11.

House

Agriculture	Interstate and Foreign Commerce
Appropriations	Judiciary
Armed Services	Merchant Marine and Fisheries
Banking, Finance, and Urban Affairs	Post Office and Civil Service
Budget	Public Works and Transportation
District of Columbia	Rules
Education and Labor	Science and Technology
Foreign Affairs	Small Business
Government Operations	Standards of Official Conduct
House Administration	Veteran's Affairs
Interior and Insular Affairs	Ways and Means

Senate

Agriculture, Nutrition, and Forestry	Environment and Public Works
Appropriations	Finance
Armed Services	Foreign Relations
Banking, Housing, and Urban Affairs	Governmental Affairs
Budget	Judiciary
Commerce, Science, and Transportation	Labor and Human Resources
	Rules and Administration
Energy and Natural Resources	Veteran's Affairs

Joint Committees (Made up of Senators and Representatives)

Joint Economics Committee	Internal Economics
Fiscal and Intergovernmental Policy	Priorities and Economy in Government
Economic Growth and Stabilization	Energy

The assignment of members to committees and committee chairmanships is important. Committee membership and chairmanship is based on seniority in Congress, but this is not the case at the state level. In most states, it is customary for the speaker of the house and the presiding officer of the senate to appoint members and chairman of each committee. In some states a committee-on-committees serves this function, and in the California Senate, appointments are made by the committee on rules. In this selection process, it is not uncommon for the speaker of the house and the presiding officer of the senate to assign legislators of his or her party to important committees and legislators of the opposite party to minor committees. Also, the office of chairman, even of the lowliest committee, confers status upon its occupant. In committee membership, consideration is given to individual expertise; for example, the health committee is composed of legislators who are nurses, doctors, and other health professionals.

The major function of committees is that of lawmaking, which involves studying, sifting, sorting, drafting, and reporting legislation that has been referred to it (Crane & Watts, 1968). The process of studying a particular legislative issue includes allowing groups and private individuals to present their views at hearings. These legislative hearings must be open to the public, and are intended to provide a bridge to public opinion. All citizens have the right to attend hearings and may submit written testimony and/or request to address the committees. Presenting testimony is an effective way to influence legislation and legislators. For details for each state, see Chapter 11.

At the state level, legislative proposals are heard in one committee at a time; in Congress, however, it is not uncommon for a legislative proposal to be heard in more than one committee simultaneously. The politics of committees is important everywhere, because committee decisions are usually upheld on the floor.

Staff Services

With the growth of the amount of material set before legislators, and the need for technical knowledge, came the need for professional staffs to provide assistance. These legislative councils assist legislators by providing them with research, information, and expert counsel. This expert help is needed to write and to clarify legislation. The majority of states now employ attorneys who specialize in statutory revisions, a highly technical field concerned with eliminating archaic provisions in statutes and making certain that old conflicting sections are removed when new legislation is enacted (Crane & Watts, 1968). Also, standing committees now have access to research and technical assistance in about three fourths of the states (Keefe & Ogul, 1973).

Calendars

Legislators handle a large number of bills. A bill proposes a change or an addition to a state law. After a bill has been passed by the committee, the proposed legislation is scheduled for consideration by the parent chamber, and it is placed on the calendar. All bills must be placed on the calendar prior to the second and third readings. The most complex calendar arrangement is that of the United States House of Representatives, which has five different calendars: union, House, private, consent, and discharge. Money bills are placed on the union calendar, while public bills are placed on the House calendar. Bills of a private character such as an individual claim against the government, are placed on the private calendar, and the bills on this calendar are considered on the first and third Tuesday of each month. Noncontroversial bills, which appear on the union and House calendar, can be then placed on the consent calendar and are taken up on the first and third Monday of every month. The bills on the consent calendar are reported by title and passed, one by one, without the formality of a vote, if there is no objection. The discharge calendar lists motions to discharge bills from committee and is taken up the second and fourth Monday of each month.

In addition to these five calendars, other special calendar days exist. The House considers measures from the District of Columbia on the second and fourth Mondays in each month. The second special day is calendar Wednesday, which permits a standing committee to call up for immediate floor consideration proposals listed on the House or union calendars that have been sidetracked for lack of privilege status (Keefe & Ogul, 1973). The Senate has a less complicated calendar system.

Unlike the federal government, most states have only one calendar. Noncontroversial bills can be placed on the consent calendar at the request of the author, however, and are considered by unanimous consent. Thirty-five of the states currently use the consent calendar.

Sources of Law

Before proceeding into the steps a bill takes toward becoming a law, you need to know that there are four sources of law relevant to the legal boundaries of nursing. These four sources are statutes, regulations, court decisions, and attorney general opinions (Anderson, 1978).

Statutes are laws enacted by a state legislature or the United States Congress to deal with specific problems (Anderson, 1978). The state legislature enacts statutes that give regulatory agencies, such as the Board of Registered Nursing, the power to make regulations. Regulations make statutes more specific and workable by covering areas the statutes do not address (Anderson, 1978).

Court decisions affecting the boundaries of nursing vary. Courts interpret statutes and regulations pertinent to nursing practice.

Finally, the attorney general, who is the chief lawyer for state government, must at times define the tasks and procedures a registered nurse may or may not perform. His or her opinion, which has the same impact as a statute, regulation, or court decision, is necessary because statutes defining registered nursing practices are often vague.

STATE LEGISLATIVE PROCESS

An idea can become a bill, and that bill can eventually become a law; however, this process involves many steps. The legislative process described below follows the California procedure (see Figure 5.1). The steps are generally applicable to all states. If a state's legislative process is significantly different than the one described below, this difference is described under that state in Chapter 11.

Bill to Law

Many ideas for new bills or for changes of old ones come from constituents such as nurses, lobbyists, pressure groups, legislators, and the governor. An idea for a bill is in essence a problem statement. This statement must be based on the study of the problem and on the people involved. If you have an idea, you must find a legislator who is interested in it and who is willing to introduce it in bill form, since only legislators can formally introduce bills. The legislator's staff of aides, who are knowledgeable of the legislative process, provide assistance so that the problem statement is clear and concise. The problem statement, or proposal, then goes to the legislative counsel, the legislative reference bureau, or a similar committee composed of lawyers. The legislative counsel puts the idea or proposal into bill language; he or she also incorporates all of the existing codes that will affect the proposal. The bill is introduced by the legislator when he or she submits it to the clerk during the designated time on the daily calendar. This introduction is known as the first reading. In some legislatures, bills can be introduced only at the beginning of the legislative session. Even if a bill can be introduced any time during the legislative session, however, it is preferable to introduce it early in the session in order to avoid losing it in the hectic closing days when the calendars may be cleared imprudently (Crane & Watts, 1968).

The bill is numbered and assigned to a policy committee by the speaker of the house, if introduced in the house. If a bill is introduced in the senate, the presiding officer of the senate, or the rules committee, or the committee-on-committees performs this task. Committee assignment is important; health issues, for example, should go to the health committee because of that committee's interest and expertise in the

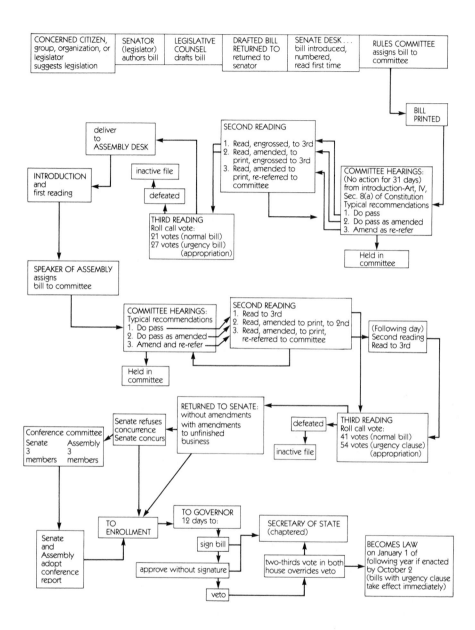

FIGURE 5.1.   How a bill becomes law—a simplified chart showing the route a
bill takes through the California Legislature. (From Archer & Fleshman,
1979:573. Reprinted with permission from California State Senator Peter Behr.)

health field. Another committee might not be interested in a health issue and might not act upon the bill, so the bill might die in committee. Or, a committee that is not interested in a bill might vote against such a bill, which would mean that the bill would no longer be viable. In most state legislatures 50 percent of the bills introduced die in committee; this means they are never reported out of committee. According to Babcock (1962), most of the bills "pigeonholed" in this fashion probably ought to die, and some may even have been intended for that fate, because legislators occasionally introduce bills at the request of constituents whom they do not wish to offend but for whose bill they want no responsibility.

After the first reading, the bill is sent out to be printed, and a period of 31 days must elapse before a bill can be heard in committee. This is an opportune time for the public to find out that the bill has been introduced. Such information can be obtained by reading the newspaper, or calling a professional organization that monitors all new legislation.

Committee Hearings

Committee hearings occur after the 31-day waiting period, and the hearing dates are published in the daily file or in a similar state publication. The daily file is published every morning for both the house or assembly and the senate. A notification that a bill is scheduled to be heard must be printed in the daily file for at least three days in advance of the hearing. However, it is not sufficient to just monitor the daily file. The author of the bill is allowed to pull the bill off the committee's calendar twice before the bill must be heard. The author does this if he or she feels there is an insufficient number of votes for passage. Or, the author may stall as a tactic to dissipate any opposition. Another monitoring device, therefore, is to call the author's office prior to the scheduled hearing.

At the committee hearing, the author describes the bill and his or her reasons for writing it. The author then presents the witnesses he or she has gathered to testify in support of the bill. Committee hearings thus afford groups an opportunity to record their positions on legislation and to submit opinions and data in support of a bill. Opposition to a bill is also heard. This is the time for individuals and groups to voice their legitimate concerns. Equal testimony time is given to opponents as well as to proponents of the bill.

During a committee hearing, one of the initial questions asked those testifying for the opposition is whether or not they have notified the author of their position. Protocol demands that this courtesy be extended to the author and if it is not, the committee is less interested in what a witness has to say (Moorhead, 1979).

Upon completion of the testimony, the committee votes on the bill, and it either passes or fails. A quorum must be present for the committee to vote. If the bill passes committee, it proceeds to the floor of the legislature for a second reading. In California, if the bill fails in committee it is dead for the duration of that session of the legislature. Some legislatures require committees to report all bills, some have no provisions for forcing a bill from committee, and others do not require all bills to be reported but can force a bill from committee.

Floor Action

If a bill that has been passed by committee involves an appropriation of money, it must go to the ways and means committee in the house of representatives, or the finance committee in the senate, or a similar appropriation committee. Generally the author of the bill and fiscal experts testify before this committee. When the bill passes the appropriation committee, it is placed on the calendar and proceeds to the floor of the legislature, either house or senate, for a second reading. After the second reading the bill is "engrossed," which means the enrolling clerk compares the printed bill with the original bill to detect and correct any discrepancies.

In California, as in some other states, the second reading is merely a formality; often just the title of the bill is read, and then the bill is placed on the calendar for the third reading, which marks the final passage of the bill. In most states, the second and third reading cannot take place on the same day (see Chapter 11 for details).

The second reading, and in some states the third reading, is the time when the author reads the bill. The author discusses the bill, and a floor debate by the members of the legislature takes place. Also, there is an opportunity at this time for members of the legislature to offer amendments, and these amendments must be voted on. Most state legislatures have limits on the length of time a member can speak. There is generally a limit on the number of times a member might speak on a bill, which is usually once or twice. Unlike the United States Senate, filibusters are rare in state legislatures. A favorable report by a committee does not mean that a bill will automatically pass. A final vote is taken, and the majority of members of the house or senate must vote affirmatively for passage of the bill. Generally, votes are recorded. Once a bill has passed the house of origin, it is sent to the other house, except in Nebraska, which has a unicameral legislature. A bill proceeds through the second house in the same manner as it did in the house of origin.

If a bill passes the second house in the same form as it passed the first house, it is ready to be sent to the governor. If the second house amends the bill and these amendments are not agreed upon by the house of origin, the bill is sent to conference committee. This committee, composed of members of both houses, works out a compromise. After the conference committee has reported, each house may either accept or reject the report as is; they cannot amend the conference report. If the conference committee's amendments are not accepted by both houses, the bill is dead. However, let us assume the bill is passed and is sent to the governor. If the governor does not veto a bill it becomes law in 12 days, either with or without his signature. In all states except North Carolina, the governor has the power to veto. Once the bill becomes law, it goes to the secretary of state to be chaptered. To "chapter" a bill means that the bill is entered into the appropriate place in the state's legal codes (Moorhead, 1979). Once the bill is chaptered, it is known by its chapter number, and the bill number is dropped. The bill numbering system begins all over again at the beginning of the next legislature.

Often in state legislatures bills are passed at the end of the session, giving the governor an opportunity to use the pocket veto. "Pocket veto" means that the governor of a state or President of the United States withholds his or her signature from a passed bill until after the legislature adjourns, which automatically kills the bill. With a pocket veto, the governor does not have to explain his or her action by sending the bill back to the legislature. The bill merely fails to become a law because the governor did not sign it. Some governors also have an item veto, which the President does not have, over appropriation measures. An "item veto" means that the governor may approve part of a bill and reject other parts (Crane & Watts, 1968). Most states require an extraordinary majority of both houses to override a veto, making passage difficult (for details see Chapter 11).

As I mentioned earlier, these steps may vary slightly from state to state, but remember, this normal legislative process takes days, weeks, or even months. There are many opportunities to provide input during this process, and input is essential if nurses are going to affect change in proposed legislation.

Legislative Documents of Assistance

A variety of booklets are published by the legislative staff so you can keep track of a bill's progress. The names of these publications may not be the same in each state; however, the content is similar and each state publishes this information.

Daily File. The daily file provides the reader with a list of the membership of all standing committees of each house as well as a schedule of their committee meetings. This daily file also contains the dates the different bills are scheduled to be heard in committee, a list of bills on the second- and third-reading file, and a list of bills on the consent calendar. If a bill has no opposition expressed against it, it may be placed, at the request of the author, on the consent calendar and voted upon without debate.

Daily History.   The senate and assembly or house both produce a daily history, which shows actions taken on assembly and senate measures up to and including that day.

Weekly History.   The senate and assembly or house both produce a weekly history which contains a record of each bill's progress that week. The weekly history gives a short synopsis of the history of the bill, when it was first read, which committee it was referred to, when its writing period was over, when it was heard and in what committee, and whether it passed or failed.

Legislative Index.   The legislative index is produced several times during the legislative session. This index lists bills, constitutional amendments, concurrent resolutions, and legislative documents.

Daily Journal.   The daily journals of each house contain an accurate account of that chamber's proceedings of the preceding day. The publication includes the titles of all measures introduced, considered, or acted upon by each house.

It is important to utilize the legislative publications most accessible to you. Most of these publications can be obtained from your local congresspeople. I have also found the main branch of the public library most useful; it has a complete and current selection of legislative publications. Become familiar with the publications of your state legislature and add them to your list of valuable resources.

FEDERAL LEGISLATIVE PROCESS

The federal legislative process resembles the state process; there are, however, a few major differences.

The Senate is composed of 100 members, 2 from each state, whereas the House of Representatives is composed of 435 members elected from the 50 states, apportioned to their total population.

Congress assembles at noon on the third day of January of the year following the biennial election of members, and lasts for two years.

Choosing a President

Both houses meet in joint session on January 1, following the Presidential election, to count the electoral votes. If no candidate receives a majority of the total electoral votes, the House of Representatives chooses the President from among the three candidates having the largest number of votes, and the Senate chooses the vice president from the two candidates having the largest number of votes for that office. The Senate and the House of Representatives have equal legislative functions and powers, except that only the House of Representatives may initiate revenue bills. The chief function of the Congress is the making of laws. However, in the case of impeachment, the House of Representatives presents the charges and the Senate sits as a court to try the impeachment.

Sources of Legislation

Ideas for legislation come from a variety of sources: legislators, constituents, lobbyists, pressure groups, members of the President's Cabinet, or the President himself. A legislative counsel puts an idea into bill form, using appropriate legislative language.

From Bill to Law

As mentioned above, bills may originate in either house. An exception to this is that all bills for raising revenue must originate in the House of Representatives, but the Senate may propose or concur with amendments on these bills as on other bills. Also, appropriation bills generally originate in the House of Representatives.

In the House, any member, the resident commissioner, or the delegates may introduce a bill by placing it in the "hopper" located at the side of the clerk's desk. The Senate's procedure is more formal: the senator introducing a bill rises and states that he offers a bill for introduction, and the bill is then sent to the secretary's desk.

The bill is assigned to a committee or committees. Each committee has jurisdiction over several subject matters of legislation, and all measures affecting a particular area of the law are referred to the committee that has jurisdiction over it; therefore a bill can be heard in several committees at once.

Committee Hearings

A bill becomes the property of the committee chairman, and he may refer the bill to a subcommittee, or he may decide to hold no hearings. If the bill is of sufficient importance, however, and particularly if it is controversial, the committee will set a date for public hearings. Each committee, except the committee on rules, is required to announce to the public the date, place, and subject matter of any hearing at least one week before the commencement of that hearing, unless the committee determines that there is good cause to begin a hearing at an earlier date. Public announcements are published in the "Daily Digest" portion of the *Congressional Record,* in newspapers and periodicals.

Committee or subcommittee hearings are open to the public except when the committee or subcommittee in open session determines that all or part of the remainder of that hearing that day be closed to the public. The hearing can be closed because disclosure of testimony, evidence, or other matters being considered would endanger national security or would violate a law or rule of the House of Representatives.

At the opening of the hearing, the bill is read by the committee chairman, followed by testimony of other legislators. After all of the ranking officials have testified, private individuals can present testimony. Hearings may take weeks to complete, but once completed, the committee holds a "mark-up session" for that particular bill. During this session the views of both sides are studied in detail, and the committee amends the bill. A vote is taken to determine whether the committee will report the bill favorably, with or without amendments, or table it.

In addition to legislative functions, committees and subcommittees also have the power to conduct "oversight hearings." According to Moorhead (1978), the purpose of an oversight hearing is to analyze, appraise, and evaluate both the execution and effectiveness of laws administered by the executive branch to determine if these are areas in which additional legislation is necessary or desirable. Usually, there is less interest in oversight hearings when the executive branch and Congress are controlled by the same party.

Floor Action*

When the committees have completed their deliberation, the bill is ready for a vote by the Senate or House. There are several procedures, however, that precede the actual vote:

1. In the House, the completed committee bill is sent to the House Rules Committee (see Figure 5.2). The committee has the power to establish the length of time for debate and to determine whether floor amendments will be allowed. Except for the House Rules Committee review, procedures are the same for the House and the Senate.

---

*The sections from "Floor Action" up to the summary are reprinted with the permission of Moorehead J; in *Community Health Nursing: Patterns and Practices* ed. 2. North Scituate, Mass. Duxbury Press, 1979, p 585–589.

2. The bill is placed on a calendar and given a calendar number. In the Senate there is only one calendar, while in the House there are five.
   (a) The House Union Calendar is utilized for revenue raising or appropriations of funds.
   (b) The House Calendar is used most often for public bills and resolutions.
   (c) The House Private Calendar is for bills of a private nature, such as claims against the government.
   (d) The House Consent Calendar is for bills that are noncontroversial in nature.
   (e) The House Discharge Calendar is used to list motions to discharge bills from committees.
   Bills placed on a calendar are voted upon in numerical order, although both houses have established rules to bypass this order for quick consideration of a particular measure.
3. A bill may further be amended during floor debate. Again, because of the need to rely upon committee judgment, amendments on the floor need considerable support for favorable passage.
4. When a bill has been passed in one house, it is sent to the other house where the entire legislative process is repeated. Often, both the Senate and the House will be considering bills of a similar nature. It is unlikely that both will pass identical bills. For example, in the case of the reimbursement for nurse practitioners' bill in the 95th Congress, the Senate version preceded passage of the House version by several months. If the bills do not pass each house in identical form, then a conference committee will be arranged.

On to the President

The President has four options when a bill is sent to him. First, he can sign the bill, in which case it immediately becomes law and is sent to the General Services Administration for publication. Second, he may veto the bill within ten days (not counting Sundays) and return it to Congress. If this action is taken, the Constitution requires him to submit a statement describing his objections. Third, he may allow the bill to become law without his signature. This occurs if he takes no action for ten days while Congress is in session. His last option is the "pocket veto": if Congress adjourns before ten days have elapsed after the passage of the bill, thus preventing the President from returning the bill, the bill is "dead" or "pocket vetoed."

To override a veto takes a two-thirds majority vote in each house.

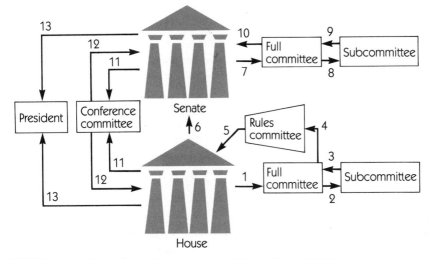

FIGURE 5.2.   Federal legislation process. (From Zinn, 1976.)

KEEPING UP WITH CONGRESS

Just as it is important for the Congress to have access to information and resources during its deliberations, it is equally important for those participating in the legislative process to know the information resources available from the federal government, and when Congress is acting or planning to act. This list provides an overview of what resources are available and how they may be obtained.

Daily Congressional Activity

Floor Debate, Scheduling, and Voting.   To determine when a bill is scheduled for floor debate, contact the Majority Whip's Office (Senate Majority Whip [202] 224-3004; House Majority Whip [202] 225-5606).

For recorded messages that are revised throughout the day on floor debate, scheduling, and voting, the Democratic and Republican Cloakrooms may be contacted:

Senate Democratic Cloakroom (202) 224-8541
Senate Republican Cloakroom (202) 224-8601
House Democratic Cloakroom (202) 225-7400
House Republican Cloakroom (202) 225-7430

Bill Status.   There are four ways to determine the status of a bill by telephone. The Bill Status Office ([202] 225-1772) can give you an update on any Senate or House bill, including date of introduction, sponsors and co-sponsors, dates of committee hearings, and current status of the bill in the legislative process. Information is current (within the preceding 24 hours) and requests should be made by bill number.

The committee or subcommittee having jurisdiction over the bill also can provide current information.

If the bill has been referred to the floor for action, the majority whip can provide current information on when it will be scheduled for a vote: Senate Majority Whip (202) 224-2158; House Majority Whip (202) 225-5606.

Future Congressional Activity

Committee Hearings and Schedules   In addition to consulting the listing of committee schedules in the *Congressional Record*, inquiries can be made directly to the committee or subcommittee staff.

Some health committees distribute periodic press releases on committee schedules or hearings (see Daily Hearings, below).

Week's Floor Schedule.   The week's floor schedule in the Senate and the House is determined by their respective majority whips. Contact their offices for specific information: Senate Majority Whip (202) 224-3004; House Majority Whip (202) 225-5606.

Additionally, both whip offices distribute weekly press releases on the upcoming week's schedule. To be placed on the mailing list, write: Senate Majority Whip, S-148; Capitol; Washington, DC 20510; and House Majority Whip, H-107; Capitol, Washington, DC 20515.

Presidential Signature.   To determine if the President of the United States has signed a bill that has passed the Congress, contact the White House Records Office ([202] 456-2226), referring to the bill by number, or the Archives, ([202] 523-5237).

Vacations, Adjournments, and Recesses.   For information about vacations, adjournments, and recesses, contact the whip's office.

Daily Hearings.   To determine what hearings are to be conducted for a given day, the following sources are helpful:

Washington Post: "Today's Activities in the Senate and House"
United Press International: "Datebook"
Associated Press: "Datebook"

The *Congressional Record* lists hearings for the next day, while the last edition of the week lists publicly announced hearings for the following week (see ordering information below).

The House Interstate and Foreign Commerce Subcommittee on Health and the Environment places interested parties on a press release mailing list, which announces public hearings in advance. Similarly, the House Ways and Means Committee distributes announcements.

Rules Covering Debate. For information on rules covering current debate, contact the Senate or House parliamentarian, respectively: Senate Parliamentarian (202) 224-6128; House Parliamentarian (202) 225-7373.

Legislative Documents of Assistance

Congressional Record. The *Congressional Record* is a verbatim transcript of the proceedings of the Senate and House. It includes a "Daily Digest" summarizing floor action, committee activities, and committee meetings scheduled for the next day. The last edition of the week (usually Thursday or Friday) lists hearings scheduled for the coming week.

Single copies may be purchased by sending 25 cents to the Congressional Record Office, H-112; Capitol; Washington, DC 20515, specifying the date of the issue requested. An annual subscription for $45 may be ordered from the Superintendent of Documents; Government Printing Office; Washington, DC 20401.

Digest of Public General Bills. This digest lists all bills, in numerical order, introduced in Congress. Enacted bills are also listed, showing subject and author. Published five or more times each session of Congress, with supplements, it is available from the Superintendent of Documents; Government Printing Office; Washington, DC 20401.

Bills, Committee Reports, Conference Reports, Public Laws. To obtain one free copy of a bill, send a self-addressed label to the Senate Document Room (for Senate items) S-325; Capitol; Washington, DC 20510; or House Document Room (for House items) H-226; Capitol; Washington, DC 20515. Request by bill number, committee report number, and so on. Materials may also be picked up in person at the same location.

Committee Prints and Hearing Records. To obtain a free copy of a committee report or hearing record, send a self-addressed label to the publications clerk of the committee from which the document was issued. Hearing records are generally available two months after the close of hearings.

General Accounting Office (GAO). GAO publishes a free monthly listing of reports. To be placed on the mailing list write: General Accounting Office; 441 G Street, NW; Washington, DC 20548.

Nonprofit organizations may obtain free copies of GAO publications by writing to the above address, marked Attention: Distribution Section, Room 4522. State the publication requested and indicate that the request is on behalf of a nonprofit organization. Others should remit a check for the specific amount to the same address.

Legislative History. One can trace the reverse chronology of a law by obtaining a copy of the law from the Senate or House Document Room or from the Government Printing Office. At the end of each law is a summary list of actions taken on the statute prior to enactment, including dates of passage.

Washington Health Newsletters. Congresspeople and their staffs in the health field also make use of newsletters, which periodically distribute summaries and analyses of what is happening in Congress and elsewhere in Washington. Many of these newsletters are available to the general public and are excellent sources of information and advice. They are produced by both commercial firms and non-profit organizations. A compilation of these newsletters, listing ordering information, is available from: Health Policy Center; The Graduate School; Georgetown University; Washington, DC 20057; telephone (202) 624-3092. Ask for the *Catalogue of Washington Health Newsletters.*

SUMMARY

Knowing the federal legislative process and the state legislative process allows you, as an individual and as a nurse, to become an effective change agent. Your input, provided at strategic times, will have an impact on this legislative process, thus changing ineffectual and harmful laws. In this way nurses can determine the future of their profession and the future of health care by challenging the laws of the land.

How do you challenge these laws? There are many ways to do this if you are aware of legislation introduced in either the state legislature or in Congress. Your input can be provided to the legislators by talking to them, by writing letters, or by presenting testimony. In your contact with these lawmakers you must emphasize the effects of the bill on health care and on nursing. Briefly state the reason for your position, so you can provide the legislator with some concrete information that will help him or her in the decision on how to vote. Most important, time your input for maximum impact. Nurses have important things to say about improving the health care of our nation and regarding the profession of nursing. Nurses must enter the political arena to become visible and to communicate to the legislators and to the public.

REFERENCES

Anderson RD: *Legal Boundaries of California Nursing Practice.* California, RD Anderson, 1978.

Archer H: From bill to law: The legislative process. *Imprint* 23:26, 1976.

Archer SE, Fleshman R: *Community Health Nursing: Patterns and Practice,* ed 2. North Scituate, Mass, Duxbury Press, 1979.

Babcock RS: *State and Local Government and Politics,* ed 2. New York, Random House, 1962.

Crane W, Watts MW: *State Legislation Systems.* Englewood Cliffs, NJ, Prentice-Hall, 1968.

Dellefield K: We can make a difference and we must. *Imprint* 23:18, 53, 1976.

Fleischacker U: Write your legislator: Some do's and don't's. *Journal of Maternal Child Nursing* 2:153–154, 1977.

Happing B: Step right up and help yourself. *Imprint* 23:46, 1976.

Jewell ME, Patterson SC: *The Legislative Process in the United States.* New York, Random House, 1966.

Keefe WJ, Ogul MS: *The American Legislative Process; Congress and the States,* ed 3. Englewood Cliffs, NJ, Prentice-Hall, 1973.

Moorhead J: Community health nurses; involvement in legislative activities, in Archer, SE, Fleshman, RP: *Community Health Nursing: Patterns and Practice,* North Scituate, Mass, Duxbury Press, 1979.

Nathanson I: Getting a bill through Congress. *The American Journal of Nursing* 75:1179–1181, 1975.

Robinson A: Want to get a message across? Write about it. *Imprint* 23:45, 1976.

Smothers F (ed.): *The Book of the States.* Chicago, Council of State Government, 1977–1978.

Quinn TA, Salzman E: *California Public Administration.* Sacramento, Calif, California Journal Press, 1978.

Zinn CJ: *How Our Laws Are Made.* Washington, DC, US Government Printing Office, 1976.

Part II

IN CHAPTER 6, lobbying, which is almost as old as the right of petition, is described as a strategy nurses can use to actively influence policy makers. Dona Cutting traces the development of the lobbying process from the Magna Carta in 1215 to the present day. Legislation has been passed in an attempt to regulate lobbying, but such laws are vague and ambiguous. The author describes how nurses can successfully use individual and collective strategies such as talking, writing, petitioning, and contributing time, energy, and money. Nurses have the right as citizens and the responsibility as professionals to influence policy decisions that affect the health of the public and the practice of their profession.

Jean M. Moorhead is the first nurse to be elected to the California State Assembly. Jean has a combination of attributes that made her an excellent candidate: professional expertise garnered from her work in community health nursing; political acumen developed during her tenure as a lobbyist for the California Nurses' Association in Sacramento; an easy and comfortable manner with people; fine public speaking skills; a supportive family; a background that can bear up under public scrutiny; the ability to accept personal criticism and lack of support; a high energy level and a commitment to working through the political process; credibility and a reputation for doing things well and fairly; and an attractive personality and appearance that makes her a media delight. In Chapter 7, she writes about her first primary and general election campaigns openly and engagingly: the organizing of campaign workers, strategies, and endless fundraising activities; the highs and lows of being a candidate; the role of her nurse colleagues in her cam-

Nurses' Roles in Political Processes

paign. Her frank discussion of her experiences should help other nurses who aspire for public office to understand better what is involved in a successful campaign. The process, as Jean explains, is full of peaks and valleys—neither of which can be appreciated without the other. In the long run, all of the effort pays off. We hope Jean's description of her campaign will serve as both an incentive and as a set of guidelines so that more nurses will follow suit.

In Chapter 8, Ruth P. Fleshman provides a real-life description of nurses' political activism at the grassroots level. She gives concrete examples of how nurses have gathered data for use by policymakers and have thus earned credibility and legitimacy for later, more creative kinds of policy-making participation. She shares her experiences, and those of nurses working with her, as a client-advocate before hearings of various policy bodies. She talks about coalition formation between providers and consumers and the strength these organizations have because of their combined membership. The local level is shown to be a place where nurses can participate effectively and gain satisfaction from seeing changes result from their political activism.

In Chapter 9, Cheryl Beversdorf describes her role as a nurse staff member of a congressional committee. She chronicles her professional development and points out how each of her educational and work experiences prepared her to obtain her position with the Senate Veterans' Affairs Committee. Finally, she provides some hints on how other nurses can prepare themselves for staff positions on congressional and state legislature committees.

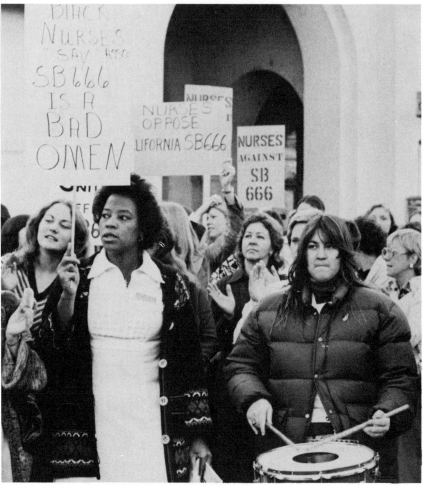

California nurses successfully defeated Senate Bill 666 through lobbying activities like this rally. *(Photo courtesy California Nurses' Association)*

CHAPTER 6

Lobbying

Dona Wilcox Cutting

CONTEMPORARY POLITICAL SCIENTISTS have interpreted the term *politics* to mean the process by which binding policies are made and carried out for society. This conception stresses the interaction between beliefs, structures, individuals, and policies (Andrain, 1974:18).

A functional part of this process is the strategy identified as lobbying. Blum describes lobbying as the active influencing of policymakers or of thoses who can and do influence them. The form chosen may vary from taking policy makers to lunch as a friendly gesture, besieging them with data, using influential people as go-betweens, or attempting to increase out-and-out pressure on policy makers through voter groups or campaign contributions (Blum, 1974:363).

HISTORY OF LOBBYING

To actively influence policy makers, or to lobby, is to exercise the constitutionally protected right to petition the government for redress of grievances (Eastman, 1978:1). The right of petition can be traced to the Magna Carta in 1215. Citizens petitioned the English parliaments regularly until government became centralized and developed separate branches and agencies. Then, citizens made fewer petitions to Parliament, but English judges continued to recognize "the birthright of the subject" (Eastman, 1978:3).

DONA WILCOX CUTTING, RN, MS, is administrative aide to Congressman Ronald Dellums in Lafayette, California.

In 1765 American colonists expressed their grievances in the resolutions of the Stamp Act Congress. They reiterated the right of British
subjects in the colonies to petition the king or either house of the Parliament. One of the basic grievances of the Declaration of Independence
was articulated as: "Our repeated Petitions have been answered only by
repeated injury." And when the Bill of Rights was adopted in 1791, the
First Amendment included these words: "The Congress shall make no
laws . . . abridging . . . the right of the people peaceably to assemble,
and to petition the Government for redress of grievances." The Supreme
Court later described the First Amendment in this manner: "The very
idea of a government, republican in form, implies a right on the part of
its citizens to meet peaceably for consultation in respect to public affairs
and to petition for redress of grievances" (Eastman, 1978:4).

Lobbying is perhaps almost as old as the right of petition. Doubtless
ever since representative assemblies began, citizens have visited them
for purposes of persuasion. Lobbying's place in our history has been so
deeply woven into the American political fabric that the history of lobbying comes close to being the history of American legislation (Eastman,
1978:4).

The participation of groups in government has its constitutional
basis in the guarantees of "freedom of speech" and the "right of citizens
to petition the government for a redress of grievances." Inordinate group
influence and corruption of elected officials by lobbyists, however, eventually led to calls for reform and regulation of lobbying (Ornstein &
Elder, 1978:95). Historically, members of Congress have been reluctant
to police the activities of fellow members. This trait, along with the First
Amendment's protections, have made reform and regulation of lobbying
difficult.

By the 1830s, the word "lobbyist" was used frequently in Washington in a derogatory way. Tales of corruption, bribery, and monumental
conflicts of interest entwined lobbying efforts by interest groups. Daniel
Webster, while a senator from Massachusetts, received $32,000 for his
efforts in the Senate on behalf of Nicholas Biddle's Bank of the United
States, which was under attack from President Andrew Jackson. Commodore Vanderbilt has been described as a frequent visitor to Washington who dined regularly at Edward Pendleton's "Palace of Fortune," a
gambling house on Pennsylvania Avenue. It was here that representatives and senators who fell into debt could be forced to vote as the
managers wished, by threats to expose the debt or by demands that the
gambling debt be paid. Commodore Vanderbilt presented a team of
horses to Pendleton after one of his visits, which happened to coincide
with a vote on the mail contracts bill. Sam Ward, the most famous
lobbyist in the 1850s, was called "King of the Lobby," and his motto
was, "The way to a man's 'Aye' is through his stomach." He threw lavish

dinner parties for members of Congress on behalf of his clients. One of Ward's clients, Hugh McCullough, an Indiana banker, paid Ward $12,-000 a year "plus dinner expenses" to "court, woo and charm congressmen, especially Democrats, prone to oppose the war" between the states (Ornstein, 1978:98). These types of activities brought periodic investigations by Congress. Their report in 1855 showed numerous abuses by lobbyists, including, for example, the payment by Samuel Colt of a $10,000 "contingent fee" to a House member to encourage him to support a bill to extend Colt's patent on revolvers (Ornstein & Elder, 1978:96).

Congressional investigations of lobbying increased late in the 19th century. Two of the most prominent inquiries involved the investigation of the 1875 "Whiskey Ring" scandal concerning federal liquor taxes, and the 1872 "Credit Mobilier" scandal surrounding the expansion of the Union Pacific railroad. Thereafter, in 1876, the House of Representatives adopted a resolution requiring all lobbyists to register with the clerk of the House. It was not renewed in the next Congress. After this turn of events, many state legislatures passed their own lobby registration laws, with Massachusetts leading the way in 1890 (Ornstein & Elder, 1978:98). In 1913 the first comprehensive congressional investigation of lobbying was undertaken by the Senate. The Senate Judiciary Committee investigated the lobbying tactics of a wide variety of groups. As a result, lobbying disclosure legislation was introduced by Senator William Kenyon of Iowa. The bill met with unexpected opposition from the farm and labor organizations whose representatives joined with other lobbyists in opposing it and succeeded in preventing it from coming to a final vote. It took 17 more sessions of Congress before a lobby disclosure bill was finally enacted in 1946. During the interim period, Congress's interest in lobby regulation and control ebbed and flowed, with investigation favored over legislation (Ornstein & Elder, 1978:99).

In 1946, the federal Regulation of Lobbying Act was passed as Title III of the landmark Legislative Reorganization Act of 1946. This act did not restrict in any way the activities, strategic or financial, of interest groups. The act required any individual who received monetary compensation from any person or group for the purposes of exerting pressure on Congress to register with the clerk of the House of Representatives and the secretary of the Senate. Lobbyists were required to identify their employers and state their general legislative objectives. Registered lobbyists, as well as lobbying organizations, also had to file quarterly reports with the House and Senate disclosing their lobbying expenses. The act specified misdemeanor criminal penalties for violation of these disclosure provisions (Ornstein & Elder, 1978:102).

The 1954 Supreme Court decision US v. Harriss involved a New York cotton broker, Robert M. Harriss, who, without registering with

Congress, had allegedly made payments to various other individuals to lobby Congress on legislation. A lower court had thrown both the indictments and the law out, holding that the 1946 Act was unconstitutional because it was too vague and indefinite to meet the requirements of due process. To the lower court, the registration and reporting requirements violated the constitutional right to petition Congress. The Supreme Court reversed the lower court and, in a 5–3 decision, upheld the constitutionality of the 1946 Act. The court's ruling provoked a storm of criticism, and a number of law-review articles suggested that the ruling only added to the problems inherent in the Act. The narrow interpretation of the 1954 Court ruling tended to increase opportunities for evading the provisions of the Act. Among the loopholes: the act left it up to the group to determine what proportion of total expenditures were required to be reported as being spent on lobbying; and, the act, in the eyes of the Supreme Court, covered only groups that solicited or collected money for influencing legislation—exempting from registration groups or individuals that spent their own money for lobbying.

The Court narrowly interpreted the act's definition of a group or individual's "principal purpose" for collecting or receiving money. To the Court, the law applied only to groups or individuals whose principal purpose was influencing legislation through direct contacts with members of Congress. Not only did this allow several large organizations to avoid registration on the grounds that they served many purposes in addition to direct lobbying, but it also allowed groups whose main efforts were geared towards stimulating public pressure on Congress— that is, grassroots lobbying—to be exempt.

The act was vague about the types of contacts with Congress that could be considered lobbying. The law permitted testimony before a congressional committee to be exempt, but other kinds of contacts were left open to different interpretations by different groups. Many groups ignored contacts with congressional staffers, and others drew a fine line between informational or social contacts and lobbying contacts.

The act covered only lobbying before Congress, not attempts to influence executive agencies, regulatory commissions, or the executive branch as a whole, and it did not designate or empower any agency to investigate or require registrations and reports, or to enforce compliance.

Most, if not all, of these criticisms of the 1946 law have been repeated with varying intensity by varying groups and individuals, up until the present (Ornstein & Elder, 1978:103).

The 1950s and 1960s

The history of lobbying legislation following the 1946 act is very similar to the pre-1946 period; it is characterized by special investigating committees, scandals, and controversy—but little in the way of new legislation (Ornstein & Elder, 1978:105).

The Senate recommended minor changes in lobbying in 1948; the House created a select committee to investigate lobbying in 1949; and the Senate held hearings on lobby legislation in 1951 and 1953, and introduced bills in 1954 and 1955 designed to tighten some of the loopholes in the 1946 act. The Senate created a special committee in 1956 to investigate corrupt practices involving lobbying and campaign contributions. A new lobby-registration bill was introduced in 1957, which would have closed several of the 1946 act's loopholes, but it died at the end of the 85th Congress (Ornstein & Elder, 1978:105).

In 1961 and 1962 the Senate Foreign Relations Committee investigated foreign lobbying because of the massive lobbying for sugar quotas in the 87th Congress. They wanted to amend the 1938 Foreign Agents Registration Act (FARA). Amendments to this FARA were finally enacted into law in 1966. This amended law reduced the previous registration requirements. The focus of this law was no longer on subversive activities but on the influence of foreign political propaganda on the regular decision-making process in Congress. In 1967 President Lyndon B. Johnson endorsed a bill to strengthen the 1946 Lobbying Act. It broadened lobby-registration requirements and required complete disclosure guidelines. This bill was passed by the Senate but died in the House of Representatives. This effort on the part of President Johnson stemmed from the Bobby Baker scandal of 1965. A top Senate aide, Bobby Baker, was accused of taking bribes from interest groups in return for influencing senators' votes (he later served time in a federal prison on related charges) (Ornstein & Elder, 1978:106).

The 1970s

The House Committee on Standards of Official Conduct held hearings on lobbying in 1970 and 1971, wherein the 1946 act was repeatedly condemned for its loopholes. The committee drafted a new bill: the Legislative Activities Disclosure Act, which was unacceptable to interest groups and as a result never reached the floor (Ornstein & Elder, 1978:106).

In 1974 and 1975, several state legislatures, led by California, passed lobbying statutes. The California law was adopted through referendum, and it imposed tough regulations on lobby disclosures and limited lobbying activities. The 94th Congress produced bills on lobby reform in both houses. The Senate overwhelmingly passed the Lobbying Disclosure Act of 1976, which caused the "public interest" lobbying ranks to split. Common Cause, the major force behind lobby reform, defended the bill, while Ralph Nader's Congress Watch and Public Citizens opposed many of the disclosure requirements. This disclosure act from the Senate made substantial alterations in the 1946 act. Lobbyists were defined in terms of an organization (individuals were not required to register); organizations needed to have at least one paid officer or employee to qualify as a lobby; and for an organization to be classified as a lobbying organization it had to do one of three things: (1) retain a law firm or person to lobby for the organization for at least $250 in compensation in a quarter year; (2) engage on its own behalf in 12 or more oral lobbying communications with Congress in a quarter year; or (3) spend $5,000 or more in a quarter year on direct expenses for a lobbying solicitation—a grassroots campaign—to persuade others to lobby Congress. Like the 1946 Act, this revision dealt only with lobbying of Congress, covered only disclosure of lobbying expenses and activities, and required quarterly reports. The registrations and reports were required to contain much more information than the 1946 act, however, including the size and nature of an organization's membership, how it determined its issue positions, and detailed data on grassroots solicitations (Ornstein & Elder, 1978:107).

During the same time the House produced two bills. The House Judiciary Committee bill defined lobbying in organizational terms. An organization qualified as a lobbyist if it: (1) spent over $1,250 in a quarter year to retain an individual or group to lobby for it; or (2) employed at least one individual who, in a particular quarter year, spent 20 percent of his or her time engaged in lobbying activities for the organization. This bill did not cover grassroots lobbying, but it did deal with lobbying of top-level executive branch officials—two major differences from the Senate bill.

The second bill came from the Committee on Standards of Official Conduct. It was very similar to the Judiciary Committee's version, but it also included a grassroots-qualification standard and tighter registration provisions. The House finally adopted a revised version of the Judiciary Committee bill. The broad differences between the House and Senate bills could not be ironed out, and time ran out in the session before any lobbying law could be passed (Ornstein & Elder, 1978:108).

The issue continued to be a source of controversy in the 95th Congress. Almost constant criticism pointed out that the 1946 measure was vague and ambiguous in its definitional standards and almost impossible to enforce (Congressional Research Service, 1979:47). Many private organizations testified on reform proposals, expressing their concern over the expensive and burdensome record-keeping requirements. Fear of infringement on the First Amendment right to petition the government for redress of grievances was also widely expressed (Congressional Research Service, 1979:47).

Bills focusing on public disclosure have also been introduced in the 96th Congress. The Public Disclosure of Lobbying Act of 1979 (House of Representatives Bill 4395, Rodino et al) was introduced in June and referred to the Judiciary Committee. The bill requires that an organization must register and file quarterly reports if it either: (1) spends more than $5,000 in a quarter year to retain an outside agent to prepare, draft, or make lobbying communications; or (2) employs one person who, on all or part of 13 days or more in a quarter year (or two or more persons each of whom on seven days or more in a quarter year), makes lobbying communications and spends more than $5,000 in the quarter year on such communications. The act does not apply to the following: (1) communications by an individual for the redress of grievances, or to express an opinion; (2) communications submitted in a report or in the public record of a congressional hearing; and (3) communications that concern only the existence of a bill, resolution, treaty, nomination, hearing, report, or investigation (Congressional Research Service, 1979:53).

Quarterly reports must consist of the following: (1) an itemized listing of each expenditure over $35 for the benefit of any federal officer or employee, and an identification of the beneficiary (when the expenditure is by an agent of the organization who is reimbursed or is treating the cost wholly or partially as a tax deduction); (2) a listing of expenditures for receptions or similar events held specifically for the benefit of one or more federal officers or employees where the cost of the event exceeds $500; (3) a description of 15 or fewer issues on which the organization spent "the most significant amount of its efforts"; (4) an identification of persons retained by the organization, and their expenditures; and (5) identification, by category, of significant contributions made to the organization for lobbying purposes (Congressional Research Service, 1979:53).

The Lobbying Disclosure Act of 1979 (Senate Bill 1564, Chiles) was introduced July 24, 1979, and was referred to the Committee on Governmental Affairs. It is similar to House of Representatives Bill 4395, with the following exceptions: an organization must register and file quarterly reports if it either (1) spends more than $500 during a quarterly filing period on (a) retaining one or more outside agents to make lobbying communications or for the expressed purpose of drafting such communications, or for (b) the benefit of a federal officer or employee, or both; or (2) employs one person who on all or part of each of 13 days or more in a quarter year (or two or more persons each of whom on all or part of seven days or more in a quarter year) makes lobbying communications and spends more than $500 during the quarter for (a) the lobbying-related portion of his or her employment, or for (b) the benefit of a federal officer or employee, or both (Congressional Research Service, 1979:53).

Quarterly reports require disclosure of "solicitations"—defined as "any communication directly urging, requesting or requiring another person or affiliate of the reporting organization to advocate a specific position on a particular issue and seek to influence a member of Congress with respect to such issue"—costing more than $500 individually, when the cost of all solicitations made by the reporting organization exceeds $2,500 in the quarter (Congressional Research Service, 1979:54).

Of the above-described two bills, The American Civil Liberties Union, a principal critic of lobby reform, endorses The Public Disclosure of Lobbying Act of 1979 (House of Representatives Bill 4395, Rodino et al). The main objection to this bill is raised by a powerful alliance of big business, church, and environment groups. They object to the provision that forces registered lobby groups to report the names of their major financial backers. Common Cause lobbyist Mike Cole says that he would rather have the less-stringent disclosure provision of the new law than the largely unenforceable provisions now on the books. This bill from the Judiciary Committee may prove to be more acceptable than legislation proposed in the past (Berlow, 1979:15).

Proposals to let the public know more about which special interests influence legislation in Congress have been prevalent since lobby reform fever hit Washington after Watergate. Two major issues need to be decided: (1) whether lobby groups will have to disclose the names of major contributors; and (2) whether the law should require disclosure of indirect or "grassroots" lobbying efforts, such as newspaper campaigns to encourage people to write letters to congressmen or actively lobby on legislation (Berlow, 1979:15).

Hearings have been held for the above-described bills; in the meantime, another decade closes without lobby-reform legislation being passed.

The Federal Election Commission

In 1975 the Federal Election Commission (FEC) was created to regulate the financing of all general elections for Congress and President. It was authorized to dispense matching funds on a one-to-one basis to candidates able to raise $5,000 in individual contributions of $250 or less in 20 states. The commission has six members, evenly divided between the major parties and appointed by the President. They are:

Robert O. Tiernan, chairman, who was appointed in 1975 when the FEC was formed. He is a former Rhode Island Democratic congressman. His term expired April 31, 1981.

Max L. Friedersdorf, vice-chairman. He is a Republican and was appointed in 1979. A former newspaper reporter, he was a White House aide in the Nixon and Ford years. His term expires April 30, 1983.

Joan D. Aikens, an original commissioner, who had been active in Pennsylvania Republican politics. Her term expired April 30, 1981.

Thomas E. Harris, the third remaining original member, was general counsel to the AFL-CIO for 22 years. He was reappointed in 1980 by President Carter to a second term ending April 30, 1985.

Frank P. Reiche, a Republican appointed in 1980, who was chairman of the New Jersey Election Law Enforcement Commission. His term expires April 30, 1985.

John W. McGarry, a Democrat and a former assistant attorney general of Massachusetts has also served as the special counsel on elections to the US House of Representatives. He was appointed in 1979 for a term ending April 30, 1983.

The agency's projected budget for 1980 is $8.6 million, with a staff of more than 250 workers. This budget comes from general tax dollars. The money given to candidates comes from a fund filled by taxpayers who check off a box on their income-tax returns saying they would like $1 of their taxes to go for the purpose of helping to finance federal elections for Congress and President. Detailed regulations, clear rules, guidance, and a new manual tell lawyers and accountants what they are expected to do. The FEC is responsible for all congressional elections and the Presidential election. Each campaign is assigned a team of auditors who work with the campaign from the beginning. Campaign audits will be completed one year after election day in 1980. The FEC is preparing a regulation that clarifies the issue of matching funds. If a candidate exceeds the spending limit in any state primary, that candidate is ineligible for matching funds in all states (Brown, 1979:B11).

The possibility of buying an election, such as the New Hampshire primary, with huge campaign spending for television and other media exposure is played down by the commissioners. They feel that buying an election is unlikely because the various participants of campaigns keep a sharp eye on each other. Violations of the spending limit really cannot be punished until after an election, however. The harshest penalty the FEC has ever handed out is a $10,000 fine to former Pennsylvania Governor Milton Shapps's 1976 campaign for falsifying information on matching fund requirements. There are provisions in the act for criminal prosecution for substantial and willful violations. Violations are to be handled by the Justice Department (Brown, 1979:B11).

Federal and State Campaign Reform Laws

This section is a guide to campaign laws explaining the rules for reporting campaign financial activities and showing who must file what, when, and where. The Federal Election Commission, created in 1975, regulates financing of all federal elections for Congress and President. The specifics of Federal Elections Act, the law sanctioning the Federal Election Commission, change frequently. Inquiries about the current regulations and oversight procedures may be addressed to the Federal Election Commission, 1325 K Street, NW, Washington, DC 20463. In addition, a manual and monthly newsletter, *Campaign Practices Reports,* can be obtained from Campaign Practices Reports, 2814 Pennsylvania Avenue, NW, Washington, DC 20007.

Common Cause, the citizens' lobby group, has undertaken a massive campaign to bring about reform in the ways money is used to influence politics in the United States (see the discussion of Political Action Committees in Chapter 4). In *How Money Talks in Congress* (1979), Common Cause outlines three important remedies to reduce the domination of special-interest groups and PACs on congressional elections:

1. Freeing congressional candidates from financial dependence on special-interest contributions by creating a system of partial public financing that matches small private contributions with public funds
2. Enforcing congressional codes of conduct with crackdowns on congressional conflicts of interest and outright acceptance of funds illegally. The 1980–81 convictions and resignations of participants in the Abscam scandal are illustrative of why such crackdowns are needed and how they can operate effectively.
3. Passing a new and much more stringent lobbying disclosure law that will ensure the public and members of Congress an accurate picture of the extent and nature of all lobbying activities.

Current information about Common Cause's campaigning for election and special interest reform can be obtained from it at 2030 M Street, NW, Washington, DC 20036.

Many states have enacted their own versions of fair political practice acts or campaign reform laws. Ask your state legislator's office for references of the status of these laws in your own state. A thorough knowledge of these regulations is essential to be sure that your lobbying efforts will be both effective and within the mandates of the law.

LOBBYING AND NURSING

At this point you may be asking yourself: what does all of this have to do with nursing? The simple fact is that nursing is becoming more and more shaped by political decisions (Kalisch & Kalisch, 1976:29). Politics pervades practically every area of nursing: its growth, its destiny, and its survival. Nurses must be politically oriented in order to give nursing care, to gain access to resources, and to work favorably with other health care providers (Leininger, 1978:9). Government bodies increasingly participate in health affairs, and therefore nurses need to become active in the elective process (Zimmerman, 1978:68).

Nurses need to increase greatly their participation in influencing policy decisions that affect the health of the public and the profession of nursing. Federal and state laws mandating programs and funding for health programs and education represent areas in which consistent input from nurses has, in the past, resulted in legislation and implementation compatible with standards and needs. An example of this is the Nurse Training Act of 1979 (PL 96-76), signed into law by President Carter on September 29, 1979. This law extends federal support to nursing schools and students through the fiscal year of 1980 at an authorization level of $103 million. The measure replaces the bill vetoed by the President in 1979 (Bauknecht, 1979:2). The American Nurse reported in September, 1979, that the American Nurses' Association had facilitated testimony at a hearing on problems in implementation of the Rural Health Clinics Services Act, and that the ANA had made recommendations that included definition of the law, development of a single reimbursement model, revision of various regulations, and establishment of outreach programs.

In order to have an impact on the policy decisions made by legislators and the implementation of these policies by administrative and regulatory agencies, nurses need to develop skills in lobbying strategies. Nurses have significant knowledge pertaining to health issues and to education. Providing information to legislators concerning pending legislation or providing the data base for original legislation increases the credibility of nurses and establishes nurses as a valuable resource. Decision makers recognize expertise, and they have the authority to appoint nurses to boards and commissions from which policy making originates. Asserting our political behavior to influence another person's decision through the lobbying process is vital in advocating for the health of the public and in controlling our own profession.

Where to Start

The ability to command facts, figures, and technical information in support of positions is a key resource in lobbying. Substantive information, to be used by legislators or bureaucrats to support their position or to persuade individuals to change their views, is at a premium in the political process (Ornstein & Elder, 1978:75).

The following areas in federal and state government represent access points where nurses collectively or as individuals may influence the decision-making process (Quinn, 1978:48):

Federal Government
Executive Branch:
  The President
  Cabinet departments
  Regulatory agencies
Legislative Branch:
  435 members in House of Representatives
  100 members in the Senate
  Committees and subcommittees
  Professional staffers
Judicial Branch:
  Judges (through direct litigation or "friend of the court" briefs)

State Government
Executive Branch:
  The governor
  Elected constitutional officers
  Independent commissions
  Education policy boards
  Business and transportation agency
  Resources agency
  Health and welfare agency
  State and consumer services agency
  Department of food and agriculture
  Department of industrial relations
Legislative Branch:
  Members of the state senate
  Members of the state assembly or house of representatives
  Committees and subcommittees
  Professional staffers
Judicial Branch:
  Judges

Organizations. Lobbying strategies may also be useful to nurses forming coalitions with community organizations and other professional organizations.

The Practice Setting. Politics in the practice setting also necessitates influencing another's views. Nursing must be politically oriented to give nursing care, to gain access to resources, and to work favorably with other health care providers (Leininger, 1978:9). For example, the availability, accessibility, and acceptability of health care are issues that involve influencing the viewpoints of others. Nursing needs to be visible and viable in advocating for the client, and the key is having the lobbying skills and the data to accomplish needed change.

Individual Strategies

In order to be involved in deciding the future of health care, whether on the agency, institutional, or governmental level, we have to identify the issues, learn the facts, and speak coherently about them (Embury, 1978:5). Political participation includes talking, writing, petitioning, and contributing time, energy, and money. As individuals we can be vocal about nursing. We must emphasize our importance as professional nurses, stressing our strengths, our contributions and our accomplishments. Friends, colleagues, and acquaintances in organizations and community groups need to know who we are and what we do. We can also speak to politicians, community leaders, and members of the business community. We can utilize media resources such as local weekly newspapers and radio or television talk shows. As individuals we can also telephone, write, or meet with our elected officals (Embury, 1978:6).

Writing, Meeting, and Testifying

The following suggestions are presented to facilitate the efforts of nurses to participate in the political process. We may act individually and/or collectively to contact our elected officals for the purposes of advocating for community health issues and for issues involving service and education in the nursing profession.

Guidelines for Writing to Elected Officials

US Senator:
The Honorable _____
United States Senate
Senate Office Building
Washington, DC 20510

Dear Senator _____
Yours very truly,

US Representative:
Honorable _____
Representative in Congress
House Post Office
Washington, DC 20515

Dear Mr, Ms _____
Yours very truly

Governor:
The Honorable _____
Governor, State of _____
Capitol Building
City and state

Dear Governor _____
Respectfully yours

State Senator:
The Honorable _____
Senator, _____ District
Capitol Building
City and state

Dear Senator _____
Yours very truly

State representative:

Honorable _____   Dear Mr (or Ms) _____

Members of the Assembly (or Member   Yours very truly

of the House of Representatives)

Capitol Building

City and state

Suggestions for Writing to Legislators

1. Letters written in longhand and/or telegrams should be used, not postcards or form letters.
2. Use your legislator's full name and spell it correctly.
3. Identify the bill or issue, using title and number. Discuss one issue or bill per letter, as letters are usually filed by subject.
4. Letters should be timely. Legislators need information while there is time to take action.
5. Give definite and concise reasons why you are for or against a certain bill. Your letter may help your legislator understand what a certain bill means to an important segment of his or her constituency.
6. Interpret your stand in terms of how it affects your community and the health of the public.
7. Suggest alternative actions that may be considered by your legislator; however, do not be dogmatic and demanding.
8. Share expert knowledge with your legislators. They are not experts in every field, and they welcome advice and counsel from constituents who are knowledgeable in a particular subject.
9. Be reasonably brief. Letters stand a better chance of being read if they are as concise as the substance of the issue will permit.
10. Express appreciation whenever your legislator does something that meets your approval.
11. Do not make threats or promises.
12. Do not berate your legislator. Give reasons for your disagreement and try to keep the dialogue open.
13. Do not pretend to speak for a vast constituency. Write as an individual.
14. Do not become a constant "pen pal." Do not nag or instruct your legislator on every subject. (National League for Nursing, *Government Relations Pamphlet* No. 2.)

Suggestions for Meeting with Legislators

1. Make an appointment by letter or telephone. Be prepared with alternative dates and times when you will be available.

2. State the purpose for the meeting: outline the issues you wish to discuss and refer to previous communications you have had with the legislator or his or her staff about these issues.
3. Plan your agenda. Limit your discussion to not more than three issues.
4. Avoid making a meeting a gripe session. Present alternative solutions to the issues you are discussing.
5. Relate the impact of the legislation to the member's own district.
6. Plan a presentation that will be succinct and can be covered in about 15 minutes.
7. Prepare a brief issue paper focusing on the most important points you wish to make for the legislator.
8. Offer to expand on the information you have covered. Ideally your communication with the legislator will motivate action on your issue or issues.
9. Do not be late for your appointment.
10. Do not be disappointed if your legislator is late.
11. Do not be disappointed if a legislative assistant meets with you in the event the legislator is unable to do so. He or she will be knowledgeable about your problem and able to exchange information about the legislator's viewpoint.
12. Do not stay beyond the time that has been set aside for you. You may wish to check your time allotment with your legislator after your brief presentation.
13. Do not present a long list of problems. Limit your concerns to not more than three issues that lend themselves to legislative resolution.
14. Do not speak solely in terms of your administrative problems. Your agency or your interest group provides services for the community, and the members of the community are the voters and the focal point of the legislator's interest (National League for Nursing, *Government Relations Pamphlet No. 1*).

Suggestions for Presenting Testimony

1. Become familiar with the domain of legislative committees, their subcommittees, and their membership.
2. Focus on bills that have the greatest consequences for programs in your area.
3. Contact the chairperson of the committee or the subcommittee and ask to be notified of the dates and times the hearings are scheduled.
4. Prepare for the hearing by learning the following: (a) the time limitation on the length of testimony, (b) the number of copies

of printed testimony, and (c) the deadline for submitting advance copies of testimony.

5. Select a witness who is knowledgeable on the subject and who will abide by the time limitations.
6. Do not guess at the answer to a question if you are not sure. Offer to provide the information after the hearing.
7. Do not fail to provide copies of oral testimony to colleagues who could help support your recommendations.
8. Do not wait for the hearing date to be announced before you prepare your data and testimony.
9. Do not testify beyond the time limits set in the "ground rules."
10. Do not fail to communicate with your elected representative about your plans to appear before the committee (National League for Nursing, *Government Relations Pamphlet No. 3*).

Analyzing a Legislative Bill

Nurses need to learn the intent and the effect of legislative bills that have the potential to become laws regulating health care services and nursing practice. The following outline will be helpful in analyzing bills:

Understanding the Anatomy of a Bill. In addition to the explanations in Figure 6.1, it is necessary to note at the top of the bill if there have been any amendments. In order to see exactly what changes are being made in present law, the latest version of the bill should be studied. When sending for a copy of the bill, list the bill by number, and request the most recent version of the bill, which shows all of the amendments. Bills can be obtained from legislators and from the state capitol.

Exploratory Study. The first study of a bill is usually exploratory. The Legislative Council's Digest (on the front page of the bill) will give the general idea and direction of the bill. It explains existing law and then how the proposed legislation would change those provisions. Do not rely completely on the digest—it sometimes contains errors. Once the digest is understood it will be easier to read the body of the bill and look for the proposed changes.

Use a marker to highlight important provisions. Keep reading steadily so that you get an overall view of the bill. Instead of getting mired in details, look for action words. When you come across language that does not seem clear, jot down your question in the margin. Likewise, make notes on any firsthand reactions you may have in your evaluation of the bill.

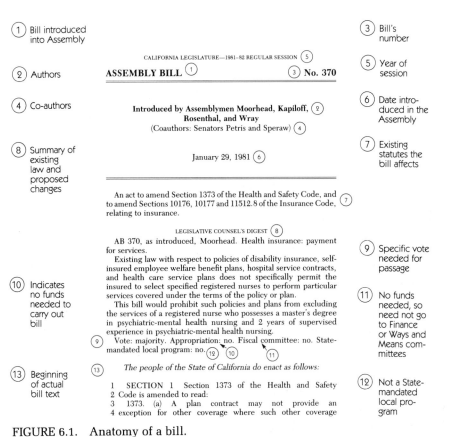

1. Bill introduced into Assembly
2. Authors
4. Co-authors
8. Summary of existing law and proposed changes
10. Indicates no funds needed to carry out bill
13. Beginning of actual bill text

3. Bill's number
5. Year of session
6. Date introduced in the Assembly
7. Existing statutes the bill affects
9. Specific vote needed for passage
11. No funds needed, so need not go to Finance or Ways and Means committees
12. Not a State-mandated local program

CALIFORNIA LEGISLATURE—1981–82 REGULAR SESSION (5)

ASSEMBLY BILL (1)   (3) **No. 370**

Introduced by Assemblymen Moorhead, Kapiloff, (2)
Rosenthal, and Wray
(Coauthors: Senators Petris and Speraw) (4)

January 29, 1981 (6)

An act to amend Section 1373 of the Health and Safety Code, and
to amend Sections 10176, 10177 and 11512.8 of the Insurance Code, (7)
relating to insurance.

LEGISLATIVE COUNSEL'S DIGEST (8)

AB 370, as introduced, Moorhead. Health insurance: payment for services.

Existing law with respect to policies of disability insurance, self-insured employee welfare benefit plans, hospital service contracts, and health care service plans does not specifically permit the insured to select specified registered nurses to perform particular services covered under the terms of the policy or plan.

This bill would prohibit such policies and plans from excluding the services of a registered nurse who possesses a master's degree in psychiatric-mental health nursing and 2 years of supervised experience in psychiatric-mental health nursing.

(9) Vote: majority. Appropriation: no. Fiscal committee: no. State-mandated local program: no. (12) (10)   (11)

(13)   The people of the State of California do enact as follows:

1   SECTION 1   Section 1373 of the Health and Safety
2 Code is amended to read:
3   1373. (a) A plan contract may not provide an
4 exception for other coverage where such other coverage

FIGURE 6.1.   Anatomy of a bill.

List under general headings the types of information you want about a bill: purpose, policies, administration, financing, and so on. Then, as you study the bill, make notes under the appropriate headings as you go along. Many bills are written so that information on a particular question, such as method of financing, is scattered through the bill. As with a jigsaw puzzle, until the related pieces have been brought together you cannot see the picture as a whole.

Varying Study Methods.   The methods to be used in further study of a bill depend upon the type of bill it is and your reasons for studying it. A bill may be: (a) an amendment to existing law. An understanding of the present law and of the changes proposed by the bill is imperative. Copies of the codes are available locally in assembly and senate field offices. (b) A multi-title or omnibus bill. These bills cover several different, though related, proposals. If you are interested in only a part or a section of a bill, it is important to understand the relationship of the subjects of your particular interest to the other provisions of the bill.

Some bills are well prepared and easy to understand; others are technical, involved, and loaded with hard-to-find provisions that run counter to a policy stated in the bill. Practice in analysis will help you understand the bill and determine the nature of action necessary to help pass or defeat it.

Determining the Origin and Motivation of a Bill. All bills have both a background and a source. Knowledge of a bill and the motives of its sponsors is a most important factor in the study of a bill. Legislators do not initiate the thousands of bills they introduce. Some proposed state legislation originates in state departments and agencies. Constituents, local governmental agencies, organizations, business, labor, and private agencies may also originate or sponsor legislation. All bills, however, must be authored and introduced in the legislature by a legislator.

Building a File of Background Information. There are several sources of materials for compiling a file of background information on a bill, and such sources also may have materials for distribution:

- the author of a bill
- the state department that will administer the bill
- organizations supporting or opposing a bill
- professional or other groups interested in the bill

Background information obtained in this way is frequently indispensable in understanding the underlying principles of a bill and the purposes that it is intended to serve. Frequently, a summary of the bill also can be obtained from these sources or the policy committee in the legislature considering the bill. However, when you know the summary was prepared by a source with a special interest, it is well to use it with caution. While helpful, none of this material is an adequate substitute for independent study and evaluation of a bill.

Cautions. Fine-sounding phrases are frequently used to conceal or confuse the real intentions of the sponsors of a bill.

Remember that when a bill contains definitions of terms, such terms must be interpreted on the basis of these definitions, regardless of their usual meanings.

A bill is a single unit, and each of its provisions must be interpreted in relation to the rest of the bill and to the rest of the code in which it will be placed (*Analyzing a Legislative Bill,* 1978:13).

Collective Strategies

With the rise of consumer groups and others dedicated to obtaining various benefits, the cornerstone of modern society is collective effort, or organized response. Legislators respond to groups that carry the greatest clout, and groups get their clout by having large memberships, well-reasoned arguments, and by convincing the legislator that their proposals are wanted by the people. With large, active memberships in nursing organizations at the local, state, and national levels, nurses will have the power they need to influence legislators (Mullane, 1976:45).

The American Nurses' Association

There are over one million employed registered nurses in the United States. Imagine the influence we could have on improving health and health care if we were united and politically active: The staff of the American Nurses' Association, for example, has nurses in every state who respond to their state nursing association's requests for follow-up lobbying with local members of Congress (Holleran, 1978:19).

Constance Holleran, former Deputy Executive Director, Government Relations Division of the American Nurses' Association, describes the role of the lobbyist as being "the eyes, ears, and at times the voice of the association." She says a good lobbyist is well informed on the issues and can communicate positions clearly and quickly. ANA lobbyists are in contact with government agencies as well as individual members of the House of Representatives and the Senate, their staffs, and their committee staffs. Interpretations of congressional intent are translated into rules and regulations in government agencies, and distortions and misreadings of congressional intent is not uncommon. Therefore the need to lobby governmental agencies is important. Holleran advises that consumer support is very important to ANA legislative efforts. Senior citizen's groups, labor organizations that negotiate for health benefits, and parents' groups must be made aware of improvements nurses can make in the health care system. They need to understand what nurses do and why nursing services are sometimes not available.

The American Nurses' Association has a membership of 200,000 compared with a membership of 1.6 million for the National Education Association (NEA). The NEA is similar in its constituency to the ANA— the NEA executive secretary calls it "a peculiar hybrid between a professional organization and a labor union." The size of such a group has an impact on its effectiveness and the availability of its revenues. The larger and better distributed an organization's membership is, the more likely it is that that organization will have political clout (Isaacs, 1978:25). (See the Yellow Pages for other lobbying groups nurses may wish to join.)

Political Action Committees

The Political Action Committee (PAC) is the dominant force in special-interest campaign contributions throughout the nation. PACs are the result of legislation in the early 1970s that limited personal contributions to federal campaigns to $1,000 but allowed political groups to contribute up to $5,000. PACs represent individual companies and associated professionals, and some are multimember associations and unions. It is predicted there will be 1,000 corporate PACs by 1980 (Quinn, 1979:96).

The Nurses' Coalition for Action in Politics (N-CAP) was established in 1974, with approval of the ANA board of directors, to act as a bipartisan, non-profit political action committee to stimulate the interest and involvement of nurses in politics. A board of trustees, some of whom are appointed by the ANA board, govern N-CAP. Registered nurses, a licensed practical nurse, and a nursing student compose the N-CAP board (Hadley, 1978:3).

In 1978 N-CAP received $98,000, three times the amount of funds accumulated prior to the 1976 election. Of the 231 candidates endorsed for the US Senate and House of Representatives, 199 were successful. In 1976 fewer than ten state PACs were in existence. This past year, state nurses' associations have organized 31 PACs. The majority of contributions came from a small segment of the nurse population in 1976. Currently many contributions fall in the $10 to $25 range, and a larger percentage of nurses are contributing in response to dues insert notices and direct-mail appeals (Curtis, 1979:5).

CONCLUSION

Legislation mandating health policy proliferates from Washington, DC, and state legislatures across the nation. We have the right as citizens and the responsibility as professional nurses to influence policy decisions that affect the health of the public and the practice of our profession. We must continue to expand our awareness of the importance of participating in the political process and of acquiring the skills necessary for that participation. Collective and individual action on the part of nursing to influence legislation and its implementation is critical to providing public health care of the highest quality. Communicating our viewpoint on health issues, and supporting it with relevant data, can provide legislators with information on which to base realistic health policy for our nation.

"Florence Nightingale, our first and still most effective lobbyist, had power. She knew who made policy, how to get to them, developed her case well, gathered her facts—presented them forcefully but tactfully and finally, through persistence, got what she needed for her cause" (Holleran, 1978:1).

REFERENCES

Analyzing a Legislative Bill, California State Teachers' Association Legislative Handbook, 1978, pp 13–14.

Andrain C: *Political Life and Social Change*, ed 2. Belmont, Calif, Duxbury Press, 1974, p 18.

Bauknecht VL: Rural clinics law reviewed. *The American Nurse* 11(8):2, 1979.

———: Carter signs NTA. *The American Nurse* 11(9):2, 1979.

Berlow A: Lobby reform bill has its best chance. *The Oakland Tribune*, November 4, 1979, p 15.

Blum HL: *Planning for Health*. New York, Human Sciences Press, 1978, p 363.

Brown PA: Election enforcers' dilemma. *The Oakland Tribune*, November 4, 1979, p 1310–1311.

Congressional Research Service: *Lobby Reform*, October 1979, pp 53–54.

Curtis B: Nurses demonstrate political awareness. *The American Nurse* 11(1):5, 1979.

Eastman H: Lobbying: Constitutionally protected right. *American Enterprise Institute Studies in Legal Policy*, 1978, pp 3–4.

Embury S: How to be involved politically. *AARN Newsletter* 34:6, April 1978.

Hadley RD: 231 N-CAP endorsements for November 7 election. *The American Nurse* 10:1,3, 1978.

Holleran C: Nursing unity—Political power. *Washington State Journal of Nursing*, Summer/Fall 1978, pp 1,19.

How Money Talks in Congress: A Common Cause Study of the Impact of Money on Congressional Decision-Making. Washington, DC. Common Cause, 1979.

Isaacs M: Nurses as a political force. *Political, Social and Educational Forces in Nursing: Input of Political Forces*, National League for Nursing Publication No. 15-1754, February 25, 1979.

Kalisch BJ, Kalisch PA: A discourse on the politics of nursing. *Journal of Nursing Administration*, March–April 1976, p 29.

Leininger M: Political nursing: Essential for health service and educational systems of tomorrow. *Nursing Administration Quarterly*, 2:9, Spring 1978.

Lobby Reform. Washington, DC, Congressional Research Service, October 1979, pp 53–54.

Mullane MK: Politics begins at work. *RN*, July 1976, p 45.

National League for Nursing: Government Relations Pamphlet No. 1, #21-1640; *No. 2*, #21-1641; *No. 3*, #21-1642, 1976.

Ornstein NJ, Elder S: *Interest Groups, Lobbying and Policymaking*. Washington, DC, Congressional Quarterly Press, 1978, pp 95–107.

Practical guide to state and national campaign reform laws. *California Journal,* 1978–1979, pp 2–12.

Quinn T A, Salzman E: The administrative agencies. *California Public Administration,* 1978, p 48.

Quinn T: Political action committees: The new campaign bankrollers. *California Journal,* March 1979, p 96.

Zimmerman A: Maintaining and expanding the nursing power base. *Nursing Administration Quarterly* 2:68, Spring 1978.

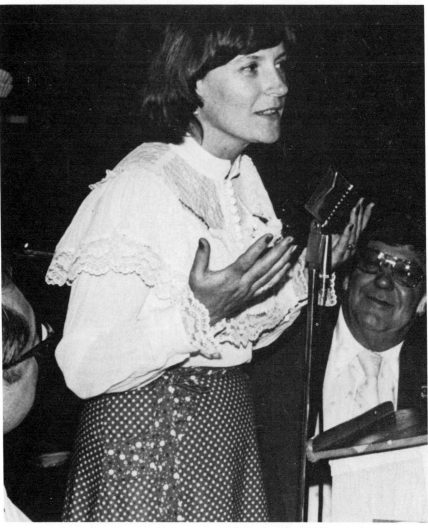

Jean Moorhead campaigning successfully for the California State
Assembly. (*Campaign photo*)

CHAPTER 7

Running for Office

Jean M. Moorhead

IT ALL STARTED in February 1978, when the assemblyman from the Fifth Assembly District in the state of California decided to run for Congress. His decision to run meant that he had to give up his assembly seat, and that the seat was open for candidates for the primary election. At first it was only with remote interest that I viewed the open seat and the candidacy. But, as the days went on, I read in the newspapers that more and more people were running for the office. And I noted that all the candidates were Democrats. I had lived in the Fifth Assembly District for almost eight years and was not so naive as to have missed the fact that most of the district was Democratic. I began to wonder, though, about what would happen to our system of free government if only one party prevailed. This thought returned each time I picked up the morning paper and read of yet another Democrat who had jumped into the Fifth Assembly District race.

One day at the California Nurses' Association office where I worked, I said, "What would you think if I ran for office?" and my boss, who was in charge of the government relations office, said, "Jean, when you are serious, come and talk to me." One of the secretaries pulled out a map of the Fifth Assembly District, and, for the first time, I saw how large it was. I looked at the map and realized that it took in a great deal of the northern part of Sacramento County, stretching up to the Placer County line on the northeast and the Sutter County line on the northwest. At home, I said to my husband, "What would you think if I ran for office?" and his response was, "I think you had better learn what that would

JEAN M. MOORHEAD, RN, MS, is Assemblywoman, Fifth District, California State Legislature, in Sacramento, California.

entail before you decide to get involved." With the purpose of educating myself, I decided to look for more data about candidacy and to gather information from the Republican State Central Committee.

I called the Republican State Central Committee and they referred me to the local committee. There was no doubt in my mind that I would run as a Republican. I have been a Republican since I was able to register to vote, and yet I am not sure at that point that I could have articulated why. I had always voted for the person not the party, but the fact that there were 11 Democrats and no Republicans running for this assembly seat stirred up my indignation.

I left phone message after phone message with the Republican County Central Committee and received no answers, so I decided to search in the legislature for more information. I took a prominent Republican assemblyman to lunch on the pretense that I was lobbying him for the nurses' association. At this point time was of the essence, because only about two weeks remained to jump into the race, and I needed a fast education. I asked him how he had won his seat in his first election 15 years before, in a district with a 62 percent Democratic registration. At the end of his story, I asked, "What would you think if I ran in the Fifth Assembly District?" Without laughing or being judgmental in any way, he said, "Well, let's get information on the district." He immediately telephoned the man who was chairperson of the Republican caucus in the state assembly and asked him to meet us in my friend's office in ten minutes.

With great speed we went back to his office in the Capitol and met the Republican caucus staff director. He showed us data on the Fifth Assembly District that indicated that the district was largely residential and had a 62 percent Democratic registration and a 31 percent Republican registration. This district was considered safe Democratic territory, so no Republican candidate who ran in the area was ever taken very seriously. However, both gentlemen treated me very kindly. The caucus chairperson asked some pointed questions including what my base would be. I did not understand the meaning of this term, so I asked him, "What do you mean, my base?" He said, "Well, where would you get $100,000 to run a campaign?" Up until then I had thought that once I was willing to be a candidate, the party would support me. So in this first part of my education, I learned that I would have to raise a lot of money. He went on to ask me if I had been active in the community, to which I replied, "No." Had I been active in school affairs? to which I replied "No." And then once again he asked what my base would be and what would be my source of funding for approximately $100,000.

Since I could not answer his question, I asked if there were someone else who might be thinking about running for office. They directed me to a man who had been an assemblyman from the area before it had been reapportioned in 1974. He was a Democrat who had turned Republican and was thinking of running again. They both suggested that I talk to him over the weekend. My colleague from the Republican caucus gave me his card and said, "If you are serious about this after the weekend, give me a call on Monday."

At that point I was almost totally committed to running for office. That weekend was a very busy time for me because I had to give a speech in San Francisco to a convention of school nurses. Had I been absolutely sure that I was going to jump into the race, I could have announced at the convention, but instead my husband and I wrestled with the question of candidacy for the entire weekend. I made an appointment to visit the former candidate and assemblyman on Saturday morning, and we met at his law office. My first impression was that the man looked to be in ill health.

We talked for some time. He, too, asked me about my base and my funding sources. He suggested that we get together with a potential third candidate, a realtor who had run unsuccessfully as a Republican in 1974. He had received only 34 percent of the vote. The attorney offered to arrange an appointment for the three of us as soon as he could. He said that a breakfast meeting would be best for him and, probably also for the other man. I agreed and left.

Early in the interview I had decided that if no other viable Republican candidate came forward, I would simply have to give running for office a try. I based this decision not on any knowledge of the political process but on a nagging and firm conviction that the voters in my district deserved a clear choice.

By Monday, I was determined to learn more. I had also promised my family that if there were another viable candidate, I would not run. The Democratic candidates were already beginning to produce buttons, brochures, bumper stickers, and so on. I realized that there was no way that I or any other Republican would be able to compete with all of them if there were competition in the Republican primary as well. California is one of the states with a partisan primary; that is, only registered Republicans may vote for Republican candidates and registered Democrats for Democratic candidates. It seemed to me that dividing the small number of Republican registered voters in the primary would weaken whatever party unity might exist and would not help the winning Republican candidate in the race for the assembly seat.

I DECIDE TO RUN

On Monday morning, I called the Republican caucus chairperson and told him that I was still serious and would like to meet with him. We set up an appointment; he would come to our home that evening at 8:00 PM. When he came that evening, I told him I had done a lot of thinking and talking with my family over the weekend and felt that people ought to have a choice in the general election. He agreed, and after talking with my husband, my children, and me, began to help me identify my base. It was he who said nursing should be my base, because of my long involvement with that profession.

I registered surprise when he suggested that I could gather together all the nurses in the state and raise almost $100,000. He pointed out that if there really were 190,000 registered nurses in the state of California and if each contributed only a dollar to my campaign, I would have more money than I would need. I pointed out that I would be lucky to get the 17,000 members who belong to the California Nurses' Association involved in the campaign. He said, "Well, if you could raise $17,000, this would attract money from other groups who would be willing to help you."

The more I thought about it, the more the idea of nursing as my political base intrigued me. I realized that if I could persuade nursing to back me, we had a real chance of getting a nurse elected to the state assembly. This had never happened in California before, and I thought: why not now and why not me?

I had to ask the former Republican assemblyman several times before getting an appointment to meet with him and the other potential candidate. When I went to the meeting, I realized that one person would leave the room as the Republican primary candidate. It was clear that we would have to decide who among us was best fit to run. I went knowing that my husband and my family were behind me, but also I had a feeling that they would be just as happy if I were not the primary candidate. I also knew in my heart that I was going to fight like mad to be that candidate.

Upon arriving at the attorney's office, I found him alone. He was unable to explain why the other man was not there. We sat down and chatted, and I felt much more in command than I had been the Saturday of our first meeting. After an hour had gone by and he was unable to reach the other man, I told him that I had decided that I was going to run and that I wouldn't take any more of his time. I left his office.

Since time was drawing near to declare candidacy, my husband and I discussed the fact that filing for candidacy would cost $256, equal to 1 percent of an assemblyperson's salary. Filing does not mean that one has to run; it is only a declaration of candidacy. After filing with the secretary of state I would have 30 days to collect signatures from 60 members of my party residing in the area in which I was going to run, in order to qualify for the ballot. One noon my husband and I went to the secretary of state's office, completed the papers that said that I wished to be a candidate for the state assembly, and wrote the check for $256. We then went back to our offices.

I am not sure what I had expected would happen then, but I can tell you that nothing happened. The press did not call, the Republican Party did not seem overwhelmed with joy, and the nurses' association did not weep with sorrow that I was leaving. My candidacy was the topic of interesting conversations at the dinner table, however. The children realized I was running for the assembly, all except three-year-old Lorna, who made a mistake and thought I was running for the "salame," but they did not really realize what it really meant because so far nothing different was happening.

The Republican County Committee chairperson did call me and expressed great interest in my running. He also informed me that I would have an opponent, a male college student. I expressed concern when I heard this, for I had come to realize I could not put together an effective primary campaign in a couple of weeks. But I was assured that my opponent was expected to put together even less of a campaign than I, since he was a college student and worked parttime in a gas station. He had been active in the Young Republicans, however, and wanted to give running a try. And so I was off and running—without fanfare.

GETTING ORGANIZED

I turned again to the Republican assembly caucus chairperson for advice. He was in somewhat of a precarious position advising me. As staff director for the Republican caucus, his job was to deal with the members of the assembly, but he loves campaigning and was willing to tutor me. So I made almost a daily pilgrimage from my office to his office in the Capitol for step-by-step instruction on how to approach the primary. The first meeting he determined we needed to call with the president of the California Nurses' Association (CNA). We decided to meet at a restaurant about halfway between the Bay Area, where she lived, and Sacramento, where we lived. We met one evening early in March to determine whether or not CNA would be interested in backing me. We outlined what was going to be needed in terms of dollars, and my advisor proposed that we go after this initial funding by a direct mailing to CNA members. He explained that such a letter needed to be written by a prominent person in the organization, preferably the president. This letter would be sent to all members, explaining the need to put a nurse in the legislature and the necessity for their help in funding such an endeavor. The president was enthusiastic and supportive and immediately told us that she would write such a letter. We just happened to have a draft of a letter with us that had been written by my advisor's staff, and with a few corrections the president willingly agreed to have it sent out.

One fact was clear all along: although CNA was willing to give me their mailing list, they obviously could not pay for the paper and the postage; the campaign would have to absorb this expense. We were very grateful to have the use of the membership list. We explained to the president that if the mailing response yielded between $10,000 to $12,000, we would be able to put that money into mailing either to other nurses on the Board of Registered Nursing list or to other groups. My advisor explained the necessity of turning whatever money we got into other fundraising appeals and events that would raise more money for the campaign. The end result would be money to print brochures, bumper stickers, buttons, billboards, and all the other things that go into a political campaign.

At about that time, I realized that Proposition 9, which had been passed by the voters in 1974, had set up some stringent guidelines for candidates to report on financial matters on a monthly basis. So the first person I needed on my campaign staff was a treasurer. I was advised to select a volunteer who could handle money and who would set up the books. It was then that I realized how few people I knew in the business world in Sacramento, since I could not come up with a single person that I felt that I could approach and ask to do that for me on a volunteer basis. I turned to a long-time friend, a health administrator with a master's degree in health education to assist me in setting up my books and to become my treasurer. We registered as a committee, calling ourselves the Committee to Elect Jean Moorhead, and received a number from the secretary of state.

Now we were officially in the business of campaigning and all contributions over $50 would be registered with the committee through the campaign treasury. My next concern was that it was getting closer and closer to the time that I needed to have those 60 Republican signatures into the secretary of state's office. I had again assumed that the Republican County Committee would help me, but I found that after a lot of asking, all that was promised was a precinct list. I realized it was going to be up to me to go from door to door in my district to try to get registered Republicans to sign the petition stating that my name would be on the ballot. There had to be 60 verified signatures, so this meant collecting more than that number, depending on how much of a risk I wanted to take. Inevitably some people sign who are not really registered as Republican, or they do not sign their name on the petition exactly as it appears on their registration, and so the secretary of state must delete their signature from the petition. At one point, I tried to get the babysitter who was then working for me on a daily basis to take my youngest daughter Lorna out for a walk in the afternoon and knock on the doors for signatures. She absolutely refused, because she did not like knocking on doors and talking to people. This was one of the functions of campaigning that was fun for me. I still do not understand why so many people find that activity so totally repugnant.

Finally, there was just one afternoon left for me to get my signatures, so my husband and I started out collecting them on a rainy Saturday in March. As we proceeded the rains became heavier, and that, coupled with the fact that my husband found more doors closed to him, as a male, than to me, led to our decision that he drive the car while I did the door-to-door work. We picked a predominantly Republican neighborhood in Sacramento, located in a country-club area. The homes were large and well groomed even on that rainy, rainy day. People opened their doors to me, invited me in, and were willing to sign. I had a very favorable reception, and, at the end of that day, we had more than enough signatures in hand. I was both encouraged and discouraged, however. I was encouraged because I had found such an overwhelmingly positive reception to a political unknown, and yet I was discouraged by the fact that this was just one neighborhood in hundreds of neighborhoods that I would have to reach between that point in March and the election in June.

My husband turned the petition in for me at the County Registrar of Voters on the following Monday. We waited to see what would happen, because if I did not have enough verified signatures I would automatically be deleted from the ballot.

Meanwhile, there were a couple of functions that I attended as a candidate. The first was put on by the Republican Women's Booster Club and was held in a beautiful mansion in Sacramento. Its purpose was to raise funds for a Republican headquarters, and all the important Republicans of Sacramento were there. When my husband and I walked in, a maid was standing by to take fur jackets upstairs to be placed in the bedroom. Not having a fur jacket, I was rather embarrassed when I took off my little string knit shawl and handed it to her. We were told to go ahead and mingle. With overwhelming impact I realized that I did not know the wealthy people of Sacramento: the people who had the potential for electing me. I was also a little frightened by their conversation, which seemed to stress a very conservative viewpoint. Although we tried to mingle, it was difficult and discouraging since no one knew me and no one realized that I was a candidate for the state assembly office. I have since come to know many of these people, of course.

Another group I was advised to contact was the Republican Federated Women's Group. I began attending their meetings after joining the organization. I have attended a handful of their meetings and have found that many of the members have been good contacts. The president of the group is a secretary at the Capitol, so I have been able to keep up with the group easily through frequent contact with her.

THE CAMPAIGN FOR THE PRIMARY

Two early formal appearances with health professionals bolstered my confidence. One was as a guest lecturer in the Legislative Processes and Strategies class at the School of Nursing, University of California at San Francisco. The graduate students and faculty were enthusiastic about my candidacy and offered their help. The second was at a California Public Health Association meeting in Oakland, where my candidacy was announced to public health people. There were many cheers and many hurrahs, and among these health people, I felt like a candidate.

During those early weeks, a long-time friend of mine, an assemblyman, set up a series of lunch meetings for me with people that he felt were key Republicans in the community in which I was running. These lunch meetings were very helpful, because when someone met me, they in turn would set up a lunch meeting with someone else they felt it was important for me to meet. I did not know it at the time, but this one-on-one approach was to become my trademark, and it seems to me I have heard it said a million times: "Jean, on a one-to-one contact you will win someone over in a very short time." So I continue to capitalize on this approach.

Prior to the public health meeting that I mentioned, we realized we were going to have to have some vehicle for soliciting money from the groups of people that I talked to. Once again, my Republican caucus mentor came through with an idea that worked very well. We printed a donation envelope that was addressed to The Committee to Elect Jean Moorhead and the post office box in Sacramento that we were using for the campaign mailing address. Inside we placed a card asking for all of the information that was required for reporting purposes under Proposition 9, the California Political Reform Act (see Chapter 7). At the bottom we added a little box that people could check if they were interested in working precincts, working in the campaign headquarters, or distributing literature for me. The first time I handed out these envelopes, I was delighted to come home with $150 in donations.

Throughout most of March and April, my campaigning was interwoven with my work for the California Nurses' Association, since I was slated to put on many courses throughout the state on a legislative process class stressing the need for nurses to have a better voice in the legislature. At the end of each course, we would declare the day officially concluded. We usually served punch and cookies for any people who wanted to stay and talk with me, and at that point I would give my campaign speech and ask people to donate to my campaign. It was apparent from the beginning that nurses would get involved in my candidacy.

One of the other links that I had to establish early was with the

Republican County Central Committee. Since Sacramento had not elected a Republican in over 24 years, there was a feeling that to get too close to the central committee was a kiss of death, and yet this committee was the link to the Republican State Central Committee and, thereby, to the Republican hierarchy. I was advised to attend one meeting and introduce myself, give my background, and find a liaison person who would be willing to provide a link between me and the committee. On March 16, I attended the Republican County Central Committee and once again was rather amazed at the polarization that took place among the members over several issues that were discussed. I decided it was politically wise to stay away from the central committee, and I did so for the remainder of the campaign.

My first actual fundraiser, a strictly social event in my honor, was held on St Patrick's Day in San Francisco by a male nurse who invited any and all nurses from the UCSF campus. He put up posters in all the prominent areas on the campus and prepared for a large crowd. When just 12 people came, he was terribly disappointed, and I was disappointed, too, though mainly for him. He had put on an elegant affair and had given me a gorgeous corsage of orchids. It was a great lesson for us both, however, because we learned that invitations have to be addressed to individuals and that they have to contain an RSVP. It was not sufficient just to post notices inviting people to come and meet the candidate. Apparently people in San Francisco in March could not have cared less about a nurse candidate from Sacramento.

As the end of March grew near, another first took place for me, the interview process. Some large organizations interview candidates and choose candidates to endorse in the primary election. The majority, however, wait until after the primary, particularly when there are so many candidates running for election. The California Teachers' Association, the Sacramento Central Labor Council and a few others, however, held interviews early.

My first interview was on a Saturday morning with the California Teachers' Association. They told me they wanted to tape the interview in order to transcribe it and sent it out to the membership, who would then vote. To be endorsed one had to receive 60 percent of the votes. My shock came when they began asking me questions. In my two years with the nurses' association, I had become very proficient in nursing areas and very conversant in all aspects of nursing concerns. Their questions, however, related to their organization, and as I knew very little about what was going on with the California Teachers' Association, I had to answer "I don't know" to many of their questions. This experience taught me what a legislator must feel like. I had always been confident of my expertise in health and wondered why legislators were so unknowledgeable in areas of health care. Now I found myself being asked to understand teachers' concerns, and I could not respond. It dawned on me that this was the reason that legislators were not knowledgeable and conversant in all areas, and that each had his or her own particular area of expertise.

By April, the newspapers were interested in doing profiles on each candidate, and I had my first experience in dealing with the press. I had decided that I would not say anything that I did not want to see in print. That is a good rule of form at any time. But I had not counted on the fact that reporters can pursue a subject until you find yourself giving an answer that perhaps you really had not intended to give. I also found that to say "No comment" was not acceptable and that, of course, the cardinal rule in dealing with the press is to realize that there is no such thing as "off the record." Any time you are talking to the press or the media, you must assume that anything you say will be heard on radio, seen on television, or printed.

Fundraisers continued to dominate my weekends. They were plagued with small attendance, and hostesses were always apologizing to me for the small numbers. Yet, there always seemed to be a reason. There were many candidates in the field. The congressional seats in Sacramento were up for election and these races emptied the pocketbook of those who had to attend congressional functions, state senate functions, supervisorial functions, city council functions and assembly functions. We decided that our most lucrative fundraisers were those following my talks to nurses. So I found myself going to nurses' groups all over the state.

The days began to get more rushed as more functions crowded closer together. Phone calls were coming from nursing groups other than those with which I was familiar. Then I found that each of the regions of the California Nurses' Association was having a spring meeting. I was close to reaching my goal of $17,000, and I needed money to put out a brochure before the election. Our one-on-one mail solicitation through CNA elicited one letter from an irate nurse who wanted an explanation of why the president of CNA was using the power of the presidency for political purposes. I responded to this one letter and so did the president. Otherwise, nurses were sending in their dollars in small amounts— not one donation was over $100. That is the way real grassroots support is demonstrated: many people giving small amounts of money. I would never have made it without this support from my nurse colleagues. This kind of support also greatly surprised and impressed the Republican Party and laid to rest their contentions that nurses would not financially support a nurse candidate.

I found that some of the people who wanted to give fundraisers for me were people I had never met. I began to experience one of the truisms that my assembly friends had told me about early in the campaign: some people you thought were your friends and avid supporters are suddenly lost to you. In their place is a whole new group of people who not only work very hard for you and your campaign but also become your very dear, long-time friends.

On Saturday, May 13, I had three different fundraisers, a full day, to say the least. I was getting to the point where I could almost predict the amount of money a 20-minute speech would raise. I decided I would like to increase my campaign funds if I could, so I asked an assembly-man friend to accompany me. He agreed and met me in San Francisco, where I made one speech, and then traveled with me to San Jose for two more. At all three appearances, my colleague gave me a tremendous boost within my own profession, since he could say things about me I could not. He also was able to speak from experience, explaining to the nurses how much they could deduct from their income tax by contrib-uting and exactly what campaigns cost. With his help, we brought home exactly double what I had expected to get that day, which put us over the top.

With the money firmly in hand, we were able to get a photographer who followed me around for one entire day snapping pictures to be used for our brochure. The caucus chairperson kept telling me that I did not need this brochure because a picture borchure called "an intro-ductory piece" would be mailed to all Republicans prior to the June 6 primary. He also pointed out that I was spending all my money for a brochure and that I did not have a campaign headquarters, a campaign secretary, a campaign manager, bumper stickers, or sign boards. By this time, mid-May, all the Democratic candidates had all these kinds of paraphernalia. I found myself in terrible conflict, wondering whether he was right. My Republican opponent had no brochures and had only appeared at a few candidates' nights, so he seemed to be no problem. When we had finished the picture taking for the brochure, the pictures and some background material were given to a public relations group that had been close to the Republican caucus. I was anxious because May was drawing to a close and the brochure was not out, and I kept saying, "We are going to be too late; we're going to be too late." I was told that timing was crucial, and that the public does not turn its atten-tion to elections until two weeks before election day. During the week before an election, people begin to look at the material coming into their home, with the realization that they are going to be expected to make a choice based on that information.

Some of the primary opponents on the Democratic side now had billboards and television spots. I was getting tremendous pressure from my colleagues in the Capitol and elsewhere, with respect to my lack of a campaign. Right after Memorial Day, the brochure came off the press. It was beautiful. It was a pictorial introduction to me and was captioned with the three words I had chosen as my ballot designation: "nurse, educator, mother," although on my brochure they added another title: "Jean Moorhead, nurse, educator, wife, and mother."

Besides interviewing candidates for the purpose of endorsement, many organizations hold a candidates' night, which is an open forum where the candidates give a 3- to 5-minute talk and the audience asks questions. Of all the aspects of campaigning, I found candidates' nights the most frightening and the least rewarding. They are frightening because you have no idea who is in the audience. You have no idea whether or not your opponent has packed the audience with people to ask you tricky or embarrassing questions, or whether these are just nice friendly homeowners who are going to ask you the usual questions that you have researched. You must perform in front of all the other candidates and your pride and integrity are caught up with trying to outdo and out perform your fellow candidates. Many times my campaign advisors suggested that I need not go to candidates' nights, particularly if the group was traditionally Democratic. They continually advised me to "work my base," which meant to educate nurses to contribute to my campaign.

The day of the primary election in California was warm and sunny. It seemed likely that I would win by a large margin in the primary since my opponent had not put out any literature and so was virtually unknown. He had marked his ballot designation as "student," which was sure to cost him votes from the older population. When I went to vote and saw my name on a ballot written in both English and Spanish, I was in awe of the whole process. Yet I had an inner confidence that I would win and that I would go on to be the Republican nominee in the general election. That night, after a dreadfully long day, my husband and I went out to dinner, and then agreed to go by the campaign headquarters of one of our friends who was running for another office. We decided we would then await the final results of the primary at home. Newspaper reporters had asked where I could be reached for a statement after the returns were in. The first return that appeared on the television set when we were at the other candidate's headquarters showed me leading with 76 percent of the vote. My opponent at that time shook my hand and wished me well and conceded that he had lost. My husband and I then went home and watched the final results. It was evident by about 11:30 PM on Tuesday, June 6, that I had become the Republican nominee for the Fifth California Assembly District. We had made it through the first test by the voters and now were really off and running!

BEGINNING THE ELECTION CAMPAIGN

With the primary out of the way, I now knew who my Democratic opponent was. I was surprised because there had been several other candidates in the primary who were more qualified than he. I had never met the man, but I knew that he had run in 1974 for the assembly and in 1976 for a county supervisorial seat. So when I was asked by a newspaper what I thought of him, I said all I knew was that he was a loser and that I hoped that he would continue the pattern.

There was a definite change in the attitude of the Republican Party toward me after June. Those who had felt they could not support one candidate over another during the primary were now ready to say that I was indeed their nominee. I received some newspaper coverage and I was always referred to as "the nurse." The label, "the nurse, Jean Moorhead," is one that I hope will stick for a long time.

Shortly after the election, I had probably one of the most bizarre fundraisers of my campaign. It was put on by a group of nurses from Stanford hospital in Palo Alto. They felt that no one had tapped the right nurses in putting on a campaign, so they proposed a marathon campaign appearance. I would have champagne with the night shift when they came off duty at eight or nine in the morning, meet with the next shift at 2 PM before they went on duty, then meet with the day shift as they came off duty, then meet with the administrators after that. It was a long, grueling day of saying the same thing over and over again to handfuls of nurses who dropped in to meet me. At the end of this exhausting day, we had received $400 for an effort that I thought was worth at least $4,000. I remember coming back to Sacramento that night and one of the people working on another campaign saying to me, "How much did you make?" When I said "$400," they said, "Oh, for a whole 12-hour day, why, that's nothing." Thanks, I thought, who needs that kind of encouragement?

One of my most important meetings, however, occurred on Monday, June 12, with a man who had once been a candidate himself. He had been involved in Republican activities for some years, although he had recently dropped out. We met on Monday, June 12, for lunch and as the meeting progressed, I could tell that he was getting more and more excited about my campaign. By the end of the lunch, I felt very definitely that I had found the perfect person to be my campaign chairman.

I had been told that immediately after the primary I must put together my "heavy-duty people": people who would to see me through the next five months of full-time campaigning to the November election. During this time I would need the back-up services of experts as well as a campaign manager to handle day-to-day matters. I wished my luncheon partner could take the job, but I knew that he could not because of other responsibilities. I also needed a campaign chairman to work for me in the district: someone who was influential in the community, someone who could get my constituents involved in my campaign. This man agreed to be that community person because he understood the things that needed to be done and he realized my feelings of inadequacy in some of these areas. He proposed to put together a luncheon meeting with a potential steering committee of 10–12 community leaders and, of course, I jumped at the opportunity.

On the following weekend, the Republican State Committee held a meeting for all the candidates. It was at this meeting that I realized I had come but a little way and still had a long, long way to go. All the candidates who had won in their primaries attended, and we spent three days listening to the different legislators talk about their different areas of concern: Proposition 13, education, crime, and so on. This was also a time to mix with the people of the Republican State Central Committee; however, it was also a shoving match because all of the candidates were competing with one another to see who was going to be among the chosen few that the Republican State Central Committee could endorse with its dollars.

It was at this time that I realized that I had done something that none of the other candidates had done. Throughout the February through June period, I had been trying to "work base," and I was grateful for the donations and support that nurses were giving me. I always felt behind, though, because we were far short of the $100,000 total goal needed for the general election campaign. What I did not realize was that my advisors had set that as an *ultimate* goal, in the hope that I would initially raise perhaps $10,000 on my own. At the Republican State Central Committee meeting I found that I was known as the nurse who had raised $17,000 of her own campaign money. Only then did I see that I had pulled off something of a miracle, not only in raising $17,000 but also in having a base of about 1,200 contributors. Most of the other candidates had between 100 to 200 contributors.

I was now in demand. A nurse and her husband flew me to Lake Shasta to attend a fundraiser and then flew me back to Sacramento. No longer was I having to beg and scramble; now nurses wanted me to attend their function because they knew that if I came, their function could be successful and money could be raised for the campaign. Again, I found myself traveling all over the state. Nurses were really getting involved! I was and still am elated about it all.

Things were beginning to change. During the first week of July my community outreach workers went with me to a caucus meeting. They were able to tell the assembled group what type of person and candidate I was. We listened to an outline of plans that would move us through the next five months to a victory in November. I was scared going into the meeting, for assembled there were people who had been at the Republican cocktail party in February. A couple of Democrats who were working on other campaigns, but who my staff people felt were important to my campaign, were also present. I told my story as I have told it here, and I am delighted to report that every single person there decided to be a part of my steering committee.

I went on vacation on July 15 with a crucial element still missing from the campaign: I still had no campaign manager. I was not yet ready to leave the California Nurses' Association and campaign full time. I needed someone to manage the day-to-day matters of the campaign. The money was beginning to come in a little bit faster, and we were planning to have more fundraisers. Each member of the steering committee had a job, and one or two people were in charge of raising finances. We had a new treasurer, because my treasurer had left the state. There were two women in charge of special events, someone was looking for a head-quarters, one woman had been assigned to be in charge of the head-quarters, and one physician was in charge of recruiting physician support. No longer could I keep juggling the calendar, answering the phone calls, writing the thank-yous, and lining up the interviews myself; it was clearly becoming more than I could do. I asked the Republican caucus staff director who might be available as a campaign manager.

Most campaign managers have been involved in politics at some time. If they're currently working in the Capitol, they take a leave of absence to become part of a candidate's organization. I got a call during my vacation that my associates felt they had found a good manager, a man who had been working as a legislative aide for an assemblyman. He had attended the Republican Party's campaign manager's school and was most interested in running a campaign. We met the end of July. I immediately liked this tall, quiet, young man who was ready to take firm command of my campaign. At that time I was tired of managing everything, tired of worrying about money, and delighted to turn the day-to-day matters over to him. I needed other people to be involved in shaping what was to come. As the campaign became more intense and I became even more busy, I knew I would have to rely increasingly on my campaign staff.

My campaign manager, community manager, and I held frequent strategy sessions. All 12 members of my campaign staff and I met every Tuesday for breakfast at 7:15 to discuss how things were going and what we needed to do next.

The campaign manager realized that the first thing he had to do was to find a campaign headquarters. One of my committee members who owns gas stations had a building in my district that we could use at a nominal rent. Originally a tire-outlet store, it was in a central location with ample parking. One of our other members, a realtor, found us a gorgeous new building in the northern area of the district, so we planned to have two headquarters. The community people went to work, and on July 31 we held our first grand opening. With a headquarters, a secretary, donated furniture, and telephones, we had a home base.

The month of August was one of the most frustrating months I have experienced. I had come back from vacation organized and ready to become a full-time candidate, only to find that the community was not holding any functions for candidates. The community was in the middle of summer vacation, and August is simply not a time that anyone is interested in coffee hours or campaign speeches. So what then does a candidate do? Well, they said, the candidate walks precincts. I was less than enthusiastic about this idea but I felt that walking precincts would give me something tangible to do, at least. I started walking precincts with my children, taking one or two with me at a time. They finally gained enough courage to talk to people on the other side of the street from me, and then we could cover twice as much territory. Walking precincts was very, very difficult in the 108° Sacramento summer, but we walked. We walked each morning and a lot of afternoons. People were very kind. They took my brochure, which was the same brochure that had been mailed to all the Republican households. I was delighted when someone would remember the brochure, and I was pleased when they would comment that I must want the position very much to be out walking in the middle of summer.

As we moved into September it was time for the grand opening of our second campaign headquarters. I was surprised by the people who came to this opening. Many of them were acquaintances of committee members, which indicated that my name was beginning to be known out in the community.

Because name identification was one of my political campaign's greatest problems, my campaign manager had me cut some radio tapes. My staff wrote the script, and I went to the radio station where I had to read it over and over to get it right. I became slightly humiliated after I had repeated my part 14 times. A professional announcer who was going to do the second of my radio ads, however, had to do his little part about 18 or 19 times. I then realized that cutting a radio spot after 14 tries was not too bad at all. During this time, the photographer that had so successfully shot the primary brochure returned to Sacramento to spend the whole day taking the slides that would be used for my television spots. This photographer felt very strongly that with so much motion on television, the most effective political spots were done with slides so that the photographer could zoom in and out. The idea was to be quiet and still, so he spent an entire day shooting pictures of me with children, with senior citizens, in the Capitol, and in my home setting in order to develop what was to become a very successful series of television spots.

About this time we received our first surprise from my opponent. This surprise arrived in the form of a process server with a summons for me to go to court. A Democrat had filed a suit against the secretary of state and me stating that my ballot designation of "Nurse, educator, mother" was misleading. The suit did not say what he thought was appropriate, but we knew that the designation he wanted to see was that of "lobbyist." This threw me into a complete panic, not because I felt that I was doing anything wrong, but because I was faced with a court case. I had no idea what sort of publicity that would yield. I also had a generalized fear of the court system because it was unknown to me. Fortunately, I had an attorney on my steering committee who took the case and handled it magnificently. The day we were to have the final verdict, the judge threw the case out on a procedural technicality. So my opponent was not able to force me to put "lobbyist" as my ballot designation, instead of "nurse, educator, mother."

Everyone but me seemed to know that after Labor Day, people began to think of fall and of political campaigns. Therefore requests for interviews by specific groups begin to multiply. Some of the same groups that had interviewed me in the primary, such as the California Teachers' Association, asked me to meet with them again. Other groups that I had not heard from also wanted to talk to me. One of these groups was the California State Employees' Association, which was well known for their usual endorsement of Democrats, an endorsement that was both written and financial. Nevertheless I met with them. I could tell that we had a rapport; I liked them, and they liked me, and the result was that they defied tradition and endorsed me. Many of the members of this group were among my most avid supporters throughout the remaining weeks of my campaign. I was also endorsed by the California School Employees' Association under similar circumstances. In order to meet with various groups of people, I held breakfast meetings, lunch meetings, and dinner meetings.

By the middle of September the campaign consumed 24 hours a day, 7 days a week. Although I was not always busy, I was always on call and never knew what to expect. Throughout this period, people constantly asked me, "How do you think you're doing?" I guess this is a question people ask because they don't know how to phrase it differently. There is probably not a candidate alive who knows exactly how he or she is doing, and obviously there is no candidate who is going to say "I'm doing horrible." You get used to saying "Well, I'm working very hard, and we're very hopeful" because you also don't want to appear overly confident. Throughout the campaign, those people who were sure that the chances of my winning were very remote because of my party designation would always speak to me in what I felt was a condescending manner. They almost patted me on the head while saying, "You poor, dumb female." Other people were much more optimistic—or unrealistic, perhaps—they said, "I hear good things about you; I think you're doing well."

I had been told by my assemblyman friend, the Republican caucus people, and my campaign manager that I would not really be able to judge how I was doing, but throughout the entire campaign from February to November I felt that I would win. I can't say why I felt this way, but late at night, or in the middle of the night if I woke up, that feeling would permeate my being. During my working hours, I was distracted by the day-to-day activities and the emotional ups and downs of the campaign, and so I didn't allow myself to feel optimistic. But if you're a candidate, no matter how you feel, you can't tell people that you think you're behind, and you can't tell people you think you're ahead, because you want to keep them interested and actively working on the campaign.

In October, when we began to get closer to the election, I began to feel a need to win because of all of the people who had helped me. By that time the campaign organization was really in full swing, and many people were walking precincts for me as individuals or as representatives of organizations. People were working in the headquarters. A marvelous camaraderie developed. I began to feel an obligation to these people and to think, "What will happen if I lose?" I mentioned this to the political experts, and the answer I got was that the people involved liked their involvement, win or lose. They got involved not knowing what the outcome of the election would be, so I should not concern myself about letting them down.

Another piece of advice I heard throughout the campaign was that I should not let myself get too emotionally high or low. I found this a most simplistic piece of advice, but it was one I tried to follow through the campaign. But when the *Sacramento Bee*, a traditionally Democratic newspaper, came out with their endorsement of me after I had been through a particularly difficult interview with them, my spirits absolutely soared, because I felt that if I could get the *Bee* endorsement at least part or perhaps half of the battle was over.

A real low occurred shortly after this, when a woman who had worked on my opponent's earlier campaigns and in the process had come to know my stepdaughter started calling and leaving threatening messages at both my husband's office and at my campaign headquarters. This had the immediate effect of throwing cold water on the emotional high that the *Bee*'s endorsement had fostered. I realized that this woman had come forward with her threats because of the publicity in the newspaper. Fortunately nothing came of them. So, although as a candidate I went through emotional ups and downs, I kept saying to myself, "Don't let the highs get too high, or the lows too low." I was able to at least temper the highs and lows, even if I was not able to prevent them from occurring.

Another important aspect of my campaign was the mail program. Our mail program during the general election was planned to begin with a letter to all registered Democrats from an angry Democrat stating that he or she could not endorse my opponent because of his poor record as a public servant. I thought it would be an easy task to find such a Democrat. However, when it came to signing their name to a letter, it was interesting to see how many people shied away. One finally stepped forward and was willing to sign the letter. We put a PS on the letter saying that we were mailing it early so that my opponent would have an opportunity to respond. No response ever came.

As the weeks went by, we prepared our second mailing to all of the registered Democrats in the district. This letter went out under the letterhead of "The Concerned Citizens' League." This group was made up of friendly Democrats who had been active in my campaign. They had documented the accusations about my opponent that had appeared in the first letter. The "Concerned Citizens' letter" described their investigation and findings. Shortly after this second letter was sent out we began to hear from my opponent's campaign group that we were involved in smear tactics and a smear campaign.

To increase my name recognition, my campaign workers placed 1,500 signs in stores, on stakes along roadways, on billboards, and anywhere else that it was possible to put them. We did this during the first week in October, and within three days they were all torn down. We were quite certain that it was my opponent's campaign group who was doing this. We became positive of this when a sheriff's officer came to our campaign headquarters and said that he had caught a man tearing down my signs in front of a large shopping center. When he questioned him, he said that he worked for my opponent and, in fact, the car he was driving was registered to my opponent's campaign manager. The police were never able to "locate" this man again and so charges were impossible to press. This was not a very satisfying ending to our 1,500 signs.

In mid-October, we had a fundraiser that was the most fun of the entire campaign. It was a Scottish *ceilidh*. A *ceilidh*, in Gaelic, means a time to sing and dance, to tell stories, and to get together with friends. We almost didn't hold it, because we were finding that since there were so many other candidates running in the Sacramento area, people were being campaigned to death and fundraisers were just not succeeding. We were having more success with small coffees and cocktail parties at which I was introduced and sat around in an informal setting, talking to people and answering their questions. Subsequently, someone from one coffee or cocktail party would host another and so they would spread. But my Scottish friends decided that we should hold the *ceilidh*, and if we made money, fine, and if we did not, fine, too. The most important thing was that we were going to have fun. As it turned out, we did make money. We sold the tickets at a very reasonable price, a friend cooked the Scottish haggis, and the whole function was a labor of love. The people who got involved cared about it, and the bagpipers played because they cared about me and the campaign. It was a marvelous, wonderful night, and we had a great time.

Throughout the month of October, I continued to walk precincts as much as possible. I also took part in formal speaking events, as well as in interviews with people who were interested in contributing but wanted to talk to me first. On Saturday, October 28, we held a nurses' precinct-walk day. This was a combination of efforts on the part of a number of nurses. One nurse, a graduate student who had done her residency with me at the California Nurses' Association, had thought of the idea early that spring and had worked through the summer to put out brochures and get people involved. We publicized the event through the California Nurses' Association's regional newsletters, and every place I went I tried to get nurses and interested others together on Oct. 28 to walk precincts. This was a massive job for the campaign people, who had to divide up the district into walkable precincts that had not yet been covered. They were choosing precincts that we considered "swing," in other words, precincts where there was a heavy Democratic registration but also a significant number of Republicans. We did not walk areas that were solidly Democratic. We planned to meet at 10 AM at the headquarters on Saturday morning. We had no idea how many people would turn up, but it turned out to be the highlight of the campaign, with nurses coming not only from Sacramento but also from Salinas, San Jose, Napa, Santa Rosa, Redding, Sonoma, San Francisco, and Stockton. As the nurses arrived, I gave them a pep talk about how nursing had been my base throughout the entire campaign. The only thing I told them about my opponent was that if people asked them whether or not he had changed his name, the answer was yes. Otherwise, we just gave them our brochure, which pointed out that I had been endorsed by the *Sacramento Bee* and the *Suburban Green Sheets*. We gave them a map and sent them on their way in teams of four.

I did not go out and walk precincts because we had enough nurses. Also, since nurses came from all over, some drifted in a little late, and I felt that I needed to be present to talk with them. Before I knew it, some of the first nurses started to come back in. As they returned, I began to hear first one and then another say, "Wow, you are winning by a landslide! Every home we went to knew of you, and they are already voting for you." As each group returned, whether they were walking the south, east or west area of the district, they all had the same thing to say. After the precinct walk, we all got together at my secretary's home for a barbecue. When I arrived, everybody clapped and cheered and said, "You're winning by a landslide!" As I mentioned earlier, I had always deep in my heart thought that I would win, but this was the first time that I dared smile and be outwardly excited about the grassroots feeling that was coming from this group of nurses. And it was especially delightful that my political base of nurses brought me the good news that the people were indeed with me and for me.

My joyful bubble, however, was about to burst, because we knew that as the last week of the campaign started my opponent would unleash a lot of mail since he had not done a mailing thus far in the campaign. We also knew that new strategies were coming, since we had read in the newspaper that the speaker of the assembly, a Democrat, had assigned another legislator to my opponent's campaign to give him a new look. They redid his hair and took away his leisure suits. We did see a lot of material mailed that week. The first brochure that went out showed that my opponent was endorsed by all the law enforcement groups, and it had a little testimonial from different people, including a woman who had almost defeated him in the primary election. Then we saw his television spots, which said that he had started to work at age 13 in a pharmacy and that he therefore would be a fiscal conservative with regard to taxes and government spending. The big shock came, however, in the middle of the week, when we got a copy of his brochure as it came off the printing press. On it was a picture of me, cut in half and entitled: "You only know half the story." Inside was their case against me: I was a lobbyist and I was being influenced in my campaign by the other 583 lobbyists. The brochure listed the amount of money I had received from organizations with lobbyists in Sacramento. The list was almost entirely false, for where I had received $500, for example, they had simply added another "0" and alleged that I had, instead, received $5,000. My campaign people, went to court and received a temporary restraining order on that piece of mail. This was served to the printing company and all of the post offices in an attempt to stop the brochure from being circulated. The court hearing was set for the next day, which brought us up to the Friday before the election. We went into court, and because that system is foreign to me, I entered with much fear and trepidation. I believed, however, that the judge would see the errors and that he would restrain the mailing. The first shock that I received was to learn that my opponent's attorney had gone to the printing company and demanded release of the brochure because they had been paid for. The printing company did not want to get involved so they released the brochures, and they had already been delivered to the post offices. The attorney for the post office made it very clear that the courts of the state of California had no jurisdication over the United States mail service, and, therefore, he was not sure whether or not they would honor an order from a California court. During the preliminary argument of the case, my opponent's attorney stated that the temporary restraining order was in violation of the First Amendment, which guarantees the freedom of speech. It is unconstitutional, he said, to restrain a piece of political mail before it is received by the people. What amazed me was that the judge pointed out that even though the brochure was a lie, it could not be restrained prior to mailing, because to do so would be to infringe on the freedom of speech. In other words, lies can be used in political mailings, and only after such material reaches the public can a restraining order be issued. The judge decided that he would wait and deliberate this case at the end of the day. At the end of the day, he lifted the restraint with no comment.

Since the brochure was already in the post office, people now began to receive it. On the Saturday before election day, which was the following Tuesday, mailboxes began to be filled with this piece of literature saying that people only knew half the story about me. I was dumbfounded that the only recourse that I had was to sue for defamation of character after the mail had reached the public. We immediately got in touch with the media and were surprised when all three of the local television stations were willing to carry the story. I was whisked from one television station to another, talking about the fact that the brochure was a lie. We also took out a full-page ad in the morning newspaper, the *Sacramento Union*. My opponent, in retaliation, asked the mayor of Sacramento to do several television spots in which he stated that no lobbyist should be elected to the assembly. The result of all this was that I received a greal deal of free publicity, and, of course, that's the name of the game. So this particular mailing backfired on my opponent. People began to telephone us stating they were shocked that someone would cut my picture in half. Many of them did not even read the brochure; when they saw the picture of me cut in half they did not wish to go any further.

The last Sunday of the campaign, my opponent and I were scheduled for a debate at a large local church. I knew he would have his people planted in the audience to ask me questions, so I filled the audience with my people, who were very upset with his latest brochure. On Sunday morning, there were about 50 people in attendance: 20 were mine, 20 were his, and perhaps 10 were members of the church. The debate started off calmly. Then one of my people started to question my opponent, who was unable to answer. A woman who had been assigned to his campaign jumped up from the audience and started screaming that I was nothing but a lobbyist. I remained very calm, but inside I felt a mixture of hatred and fear. That cold feeling was deep inside me, but I tried to give the appearance of being very calm, and I said slowly and deliberately that I was the innocent victim of a nasty onslaught of political maneuvering. After that debate, my campaign people and I went out for brunch. As we ate, there was a feeling of almost giddy hysteria, for we knew that everything that could be done was done, and that the next two days would be spent just wrapping things up. At that point, I was not sure how things were going. I knew we had a lot of publicity and that we had a lot of people on our side, but I did not know how the final vote would go.

Election day dawned bright, sunny, and clear. We had all been hoping for rain since statistics show that Republicans go to vote in the rain and Democrats do not. Election day for a candidate is the deadest day in the world because you get up early, you vote early, and then you have the entire day free until 8 PM when the polls close. There are no precincts to walk, you are not involved in a get-out-the-vote campaign, you are not involved taking people to the polls, you are supposed to just retire somewhere. I spent the day attending a parent-teacher conference at the school, returning some sweaters that I had purchased on the spur of the moment, and doing numerous errands. Finally afternoon came, and I picked up my daughter from soccer practice. Then I prepared dinner for the children. Then my husband and I went out to dinner. I made him promise that he would not talk campaign to me because if he did, I thought I would not be able to eat. We had a nice dinner and arrived at the campaign headquarters at about 9 PM, only to find an array of people already there. The campaign committee had set up refreshments and an open bar. They had also set up three television sets so we could monitor all the television stations. My campaign manager warned me, "The first returns in will show you ahead because those will be the absentee votes and most of the absentee votes are Republican. Then you will probably go behind, and then we hope you will at some point pull ahead." So when the first results came in, everybody cheered because I was leading, with 1 percent of the vote in. I was not excited, but then the next returns came in and I was still ahead. Every time we had a call from the secretary of state's office, I was still ahead, with percentages up to 60 percent. When all the votes were tallied, I had 61.8 percent of the vote in a district in which 62 percent of the voters were registered Democrats.

As that evening progressed, the media wanted me to say how I felt as a winner. Before declaring myself the winner, however, I wanted my opponent to concede the election. He never did, and I have never heard from him. I was thrilled to be a winner, but the people around me in the campaign headquarters were more thrilled, for they cheered, they yelled, they screamed, they drank, and they had a marvelous time. They had earned it. I could never have done it without them. It was busy and confusing and exciting to me, but the sense of winning was something that seemed to grow during the campaign and just reached its height that night.

The next morning, after no sleep, the media wanted to talk to me, and so it was back to the headquarters for more pictures and more stories. "How does it feel?" Of course, you are never going to say it feels tiring or crummy; you say you are delighted and thrilled. The truest statement I made was when I said, "I knew that people could discern between candidates and that people do read."

The next day, my husband and I took off for four days at the beach for a marvelous winding-down period to get away from it all. Then I was ready to return to two years as an assemblywoman for the state of California. I finally began to realize that I had won an election that no one thought I could possibly win on Dec. 4, swearing-in day, when I, with the other members of legislature, raised my hand and promised to uphold the constitution of the state of California.

EDITORS' NOTE: Since Ms Moorhead wrote this chapter, she has been elected to a second term as Assemblywoman from California's Fifth District. In March, 1981, she changed her party affiliation from Republican to Democrat. Her reasons included the increasing restriction placed on members of the Republican Caucus in the State Assembly. These restriction were interfering with her ability to serve her constituents' interests and to follow the dictates of her own conscience. The Democrats welcomed her enthusiastically. She is a respected legislator and 1981 is a reapportionment year. The long-term effects of her decision to change parties remain to be seen.

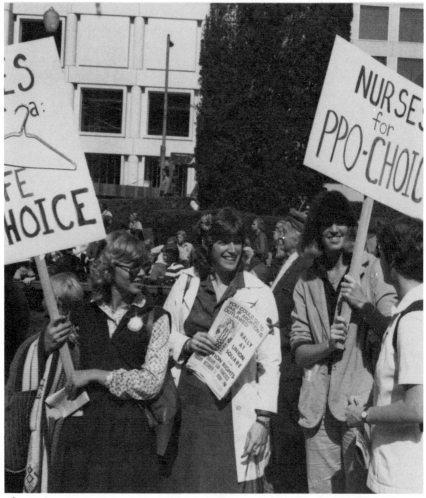

Nurses in grass roots activities to increase public awareness of health issues. *(Photo courtesy California Nurses' Association)*

CHAPTER 8

Nurses in Local Political Organizations

Ruth P. Fleshman

PARTICIPATING IN HEALTH decision making at the national level is possible for only a few nurses. It can also be difficult to have an impact on the policies and programs of the very large organizations for which many nurses work. Such feelings of ineffectiveness and frustration are probably at the root of most nurses' unwillingness to get involved in attempts to move, change, or direct health programs at any level. Practicing as an individual nurse can be such an invisible activity that neither nursing nor the health care system is affected by it. For those of us not content with only the immediate rewards of a satisfying individual professional practice, there is an alternative in working to make changes within a small arena.

Nursing Dynamics Corporation, a nonprofit organization, has provided a number of opportunities for me to practice grassroots political activities in ways not often associated with political action:

- Making changes in local systems to enhance their responsiveness to local needs
- Supporting sympathetic individuals for policy-making positions
- Forming coalitions with like-minded others, both consumers and providers
- Actually developing new and needed services

RUTH P. FLESHMAN, RN, PhD, is president of Nursing Dynamics Corporation in Mill Valley, California.

NURSES IN ACTION

When Nursing Dynamics Corporation (NDC) was founded in 1973, the two trustees, Sarah Archer and I, considered how to accomplish some of the goals the board had set for the organization (Archer & Fleshman, 1978). All of the members of the corporation had had experience working with the usual, more orthodox health agencies, as well as such experimental services as the Haight-Ashbury Free Clinic, and knew there were gaps in health services, either in relation to clients served, the methods used to deliver the services, or the kind of services being provided. We felt that existing agencies were resistant to change, which we speculated might be due to a number of factors. Often such agencies seemed to see no need to change what they had always been doing, because they saw no special value in new services. We knew that many agencies were unwilling to take any risks at all; it was easier to go along with the old services than to entertain new ideas and the possibility of failing at something new. Others simply had too much invested in the way things had always been; it is not easy, for example, to entertain the idea that specialization in children's services is no longer needed to the extent that, say, occupational health services or geriatric screening programs are.

In our early years, services for the aged were still scanty, although there were rumors that funding from a variety of sources might well become available. Since I already had experience and training in gerontology and geriatrics, I opted to limit my specialization to this population (see Fleshman & Archer, 1979:466–467 for this model of specialization). Prior to this time my work had been based in San Francisco, and my experiences there led me to realize that a few of us could not deal with that complex system. Too many diverse special interests, too many conflicting neighborhood demands, too many activists already jostling for shares of the health arena, and even too many differing elements within the aged sector were already competing within the city. Since Sarah Archer and I lived in Marin County, a suburban county just north of San Francisco, it seemed sensible to work where we need not commute—especially since gasoline had become a problem. Although the county is geographically larger than San Francisco, most of the population is located along the bay corridor on the eastern side of the county; the rural west has fewer people spread over a wide area and has a long history of few human services.

NDC's basic philosophy is to first provide services that people want, thus gaining entrée for services that you really want to provide. At a time when it was not common to do so, we began offering free blood pressure screening in community pharmacies (Fleshman & Archer, 1976). The blood pressure test was the attention-getter, but our nursing interest was in seeing if people on the street could accept the idea of health services being presented in neighborhood pharmacies by nurses prepared to offer counseling and health education on a variety of client-initiated topics. Not only did we advise about blood pressure, weight control, and smoking, but also about problems of child rearing, drugs, and home care of minor ailments, as well as making referrals for medical care. During the time that this service was offered in two Marin pharmacies, a growing bank of data was collected to reflect the characteristics and concerns of casual pharmacy patrons as well as those who returned specifically to use the counseling services.

Publicity about this program led to an invitation to provide blood pressure monitoring at the county's senior center. Clients were asked to donate a dollar for each visit, and so many signed up for each scheduled day that we felt impelled to expand the time available for the center. After observing the appeal of the counseling service, the center's director volunteered to find further funding to subsidize the program on a regular and expanded basis. This support continued until Proposition 13 resulted in curtailment of this and a number of other such community services.

Development of truly innovative services may be hampered because potential clients do not know how to value them. Also, agencies are afraid to risk either their resources or their image on an unproven idea. Thus we have found it easiest to initiate offering new services without asking for funding, either from direct consumers or from funding sources. Both are hard to convince when there has been no experience with a particular service. We find it more persuasive to simply begin a service and use the experience as documentation of both need and effectiveness. Thus the center director was finally convinced when he saw full sign-ups and a large number of individuals who had never come into his center before. In addition, my summary of the number of people served, their blood pressure status, and other health problems identified showed the scope of service more effectively than any extrapolated projections could have done. I was not so successful with the Marin pharmacy experiences, since neither of the owners would agree to subsidize the service, and the irregular client donations were too sparse to support our continuation. (One San Francisco pharmacy owner with a high sense of professional mission did pay for my counseling services for nearly a year, but could not continue during a time of economic downturn.)

RESEARCH

Although there are grounds for criticizing the pattern of gathering excesses of data before any service can be planned, we still found it disconcerting that few data were available about the health needs of elderly people living independently, that is, not in institutions. This, of course, can be understood in view of how hard it is to reach any significant number of the elderly who are not in a facility. Community-service providers, on the other hand, are often too involved in service delivery to take the time to step back for a researcher's view, and usually lack the expertise to carry out research beyond direct program evaluation. Here our academic backgrounds provided us with tools to gather data systematically, and, in her role as a university faculty member, Sarah Archer was able to get considerable mileage from designing and carrying out various survey studies focused on health services in the county. In the last years of the Comprehensive Health Planning Agencies, she was a local committee member involved in directing a number of general-service research projects, such as studying the response times of emergency ambulance services and the location of child-health programs within the county.

Sarah then went on to serve on the governing body of the Health Systems Agency. Because of NDC's focus on aging, we developed a survey tool to learn more about the health practices of aged people living in the community. Through contacts with the four-county Area Agency on Aging (AAA), we hoped to get improved access to groups of the aged by asking the leaders of existent service agencies to distribute our questionnaire. Although this was successful in Marin County, where NDC was known to be involved with service provision for the elderly, it was not true for the other three counties. Returns from these counties were negligible, and we encountered agency gatekeepers who refused us access to their aged recreation clients without ever asking the clients if they wanted this protection. At that point we decided direct contacts by those of us involved in the project could be more productive, so two of Sarah's graduate students and I began asking to make presentations of our project to organized groups. We would often be asked to make short speeches on a health topic, and we found these to be of great interest to those attending club meetings. It also served as a return payment for their participation in our survey. In that way we were able to amass 697 usable questionnaires from which we were able to learn many new things about how older people living in the community dealt with their problems of health and health care (Archer et al, 1979).

Such research projects served a number of purposes. The findings generally served as the basis for agency planning and policy development: the aging study was used by two separate AAA's, since the study provided the only health-specific data available on their clients. The graduate students learned research by participating from start-to-finish in a real-life project, and these studies earned Sarah some status points at the university. Both for other agencies and for NDC's projects, such research provides a data base for programs that are planned without local information, because such studies are generally beyond the capabilities or interests of most service providers. Program plans may present tortured extrapolations from outdated census reports or only impressionistic accounts that such programs are good things to do. Reports on such programs litter professional journals, but their anecdotal nature makes them very hard for others to apply in different localities. From a viewpoint of self-interest, I believe that utilization of research skills is the only way to keep those skills alive. Few service providers are involved in elaborate research after leaving school, and as my own curiosity needs satisfying, I find research studies worthwhile and very suited to the way I like to think.

THE AGING NETWORK

Of course, we were aware of other workers involved in services to the elderly within the county: recreation and social services workers, government planners, educators, a few other health professionals. In our early years in Marin County, there was fragmentation of health care and a lot of competition among the various providers. Finally the AAA called together all the agencies involved in all aspects of services to the aged. At this meeting a number of old battles were refought and a number of suggestions made for new ways to proceed. On the basis of that meeting, the AAA worked to develop an organization of all those in the county who were involved in or interested in services of any kind for the elderly. Although we all hoped to involve a significant number of older people, the organization, later named the Marin Section on Aging, settled down to be largely a coalition of providers. The aim was to provide a neutral territory where we could become better acquainted with one another, learn about each others' programs, and, perhaps, become less antagonistic or even positively cooperative. If nothing else, this group has provided a means of learning about a large portion of the resources available for the aged, and has occasionally served as a vehicle for concerted action around critical issues such as opposition to cutbacks of subsidies of adult education for the substantially handicapped in the day care program.

The Section meetings were only a few of the many sets of meetings that were called regarding problems in aging. Becoming known as being concerned with the health of the elderly led to invitations to Sarah and me to serve on advisory panels for training programs for new services, to join for health planning committees and other organizations, and to address existent organizations about topics related to their specific interest or on more general subjects. The number of meetings has proliferated over the years, as NDC has become more visibly involved in the service network and as services for the elderly have expanded. At times it almost seems as if there are whole days devoted to meetings with no time left to deliver services to the clients who are, after all, supposed to be the ultimate beneficiaries of the meetings. As an independent worker, I soon realized that meetings were not economically productive; only salaried bureaucrats are paid to attend them (and that contributes to why so little often gets done), and I had to become very selective about which ones to attend and how to say no to others without appearing surly. The catch, however, is that valuable information is often exchanged at such meetings, whether formally or informally. To miss them is to run the risk of losing out on vital communications. Also, meetings provide useful opportunities to see and be seen by others, both as an agency representative and as an individual. This visibility is essential, lest other people and other agencies forget one exists. Thus even though the formal content of the meeting may be dull, the value of remaining active and visible in the network may far outweigh the apparent time waste.

On occasion both Sarah and I would attend meetings but we found there were two drawbacks to this: it was a needless duplication of effort if we both went, and, since we are both fairly high-energy vocal people, some of those at the meetings were overwhelmed by the two of us. We became aware of our developing reputation among some of the network members as the "Dynamic Duo"—a slightly snide play on both our corporation's name and our energy level. Since then I have continued as the more visible one within service agencies and Sarah has specialized more with health policy aspects such as the regional Health Systems Agency. She also serves as a behind-the-scenes consultant to the executive of our day care program. (Other members of NDC's board, all of whom are nurses, have also contributed as sounding boards and consultants in the development of various service projects or by helping with knotty problems in some of the projects. We have recently added three new members to the board who are already involved in aging activities in Marin and expect to have an even greater impact on the local scene.)

Going from one meeting to another, we often joke with other agencies' staffs that "we have to stop meeting this way!" Even though there are many providers involved in the local aging network, many of the same people attend the majority of the meetings. Many of us even attend many of the same regional or national gerontology conventions, even though our particular specialties may be different. That this network is circumscribed is made clear whenever I have occasion to attend a meeting of the wider agency system—for example, when the overall county council of agencies presents a program on insurance or corporate law for non-profit organizations. Then I realize that there are many other agencies working in the county with other population groups or services and with whom I have no contact at all: the family planning agencies; the services for infants and children; the special-disease agencies that serve younger clients, such as multiple sclerosis societies, or the developmentally disabled, who seem not to live to old age. Thus I am once again reminded that I am working within a subsystem of limited size that has the potential for being comprehensible and where I can be effective.

Such concentration of effort can have a number of positive aspects. In the short run, becoming friendly with other providers gives me a chance to explain NDC and our particular perspective, and to elicit cooperation and active support in the development of our programs, and vice versa. For example, when NDC first began to work in the senior center, the center's focus was almost entirely recreational; since then the center has become much more aware of health problems and has agreed to include more health programs and to provide support services for health-related classes and activities. In long-range terms it is not always possible to predict where such contacts may help. When NDC became involved in developing day care services for the elderly, we were often surprised at the willingness of agencies to cooperate with us and to donate many of their services to help build our new program. We in turn provide services and contracts for them. The trade-offs are many and useful. Only through such continued contacts have we all been able to learn that we share similar goals of service. Now, other agencies feel comfortable about allowing us a leadership role in some activities, just as we accept their particular claims in other activities. We all hope that sometime soon it will be possible to build a coordinated system of services for the elderly, although the current economic situation suggests it may not be imminent or truly comprehensive. But many of us feel we have developed the basis for cooperation already in our county's aging-services network.

ADVOCACY

Although this term is often thought of in one-to-one relations with a needful client, we use it instead to relate to the older adult group as a whole. For NDC, advocacy takes several forms; the first I will discuss is my attempt to goad existent services to serve the elders better. One local service agency, with the perspective so many health providers have, insisted that they served everyone—everyone, that is, who actually came to them. Since the service was often regarded with suspicion by the aged, it was no surprise to me when the agency administration finally admitted that people over 65 comprised only one percent of their client population, while the county's population had between 11 and 12 percent in that age category. As of this writing, I have served for three years on the agency's annual planning task force of community members. In the first year, I had to learn a lot about the workings of the system, and I followed the lead of those members who had longer tenures in the group. When we submitted our recommendations for older-adult–service improvements to the agency board, I assumed that was the end of the task force role. However, the policy board ignored most of our advice when more vocal advocates for services to other groups demanded more for their constituents. The next year I returned to the planning task force with more knowledge and a determination to see our plans followed. I was present at the final adoption meeting of the policy board, and even though they still did not accept all we proposed, I was able to raise the issue of the absence of ongoing consultation about the aged. The board members acted as if they had never heard of the idea before (let alone annually for the past three years!) and were only too pleased to begin the procedure for appointing a standing committee of which I was subsequently elected chair. When it again became time for the annual planning task force, I was able to urge more monitoring of the entire process, and several other members attended the policy board meeting to register concerns that the aged were still not getting their proportion of the agency's services, and to urge that budget cuts not be solely directed at new services for the elderly.

Our second form of advocacy was to work for ways to support others who were willing to provide needed services outside our own particular capabilities or interests. I became aware that the older people I saw in my health counseling service desperately needed opportunities for exercise and weight control, but that individual teaching and encouragement were not enough to have a significant impact on any sizable number of those in need. The dietitian on my counseling team was interested in teaching a class on weight control, and I arranged that she work with one of Sarah's graduate students who was interested in stress management and exercise. I looked to the local high school adult education division and persuaded its principal to sponsor such a class without fee to the participants. After several sessions of this class, the student joined with a retired nurse to develop a class focused entirely on exercise and relaxation, to which most of the elderly students transferred after they had learned about nutritional factors. That exercise class, called "Remodeling Yourself," continued even when the younger nurse moved on to a different job in our aging services; the school district funded the class until Proposition 13 eliminated subsidized adult classes. (Do not let anyone tell you that tax cutting does not affect services!)

The older nurse was willing and able to continue the classes as a volunteer until her own energy began to flag. I became involved as an apprentice, even though I find it hard to imagine teaching exercise classes forever. I also could not agree to do this on a volunteer basis and sought funding from one of the local community colleges. The first one I contacted was very evasive, and I realized that this was a territorial problem, since I was proposing they pay for services given in someone else's facility. The second community college proved instantly cooperative and my colleague and I have both been paid for teaching exercise classes to community-living elderly at the senior center as well as to more handicapped elderly in the day care program.

In the early years of my own independent practice, I limited my interests to preventive services for the well elderly. On several occasions, I would be asked to turn my attention to the plight of sick old people, either those in nursing homes or those in the community who needed day care services. I kept refusing to do this on the basis of my own preference for health and a dislike of what I saw as a very depressing kind of service. Instead I kept suggesting that the inquirers should work for these ends themselves and that they should get together with like-minded others. Before long I knew several such individuals, and I advised them to make contact with each other. At last they did begin to organize a study group of service providers and community elderly. We recruited one of Sarah's graduate nursing students to, as I put it, "get in on the ground floor in developing a day care program." The student who responded was able to use the group meetings as part of her community health fieldwork, and she sparked a survey of community agencies for their estimate of the need for and probable utilization of such a service. Although all of the agencies agreed that this was an urgently needed program, none was willing to sponsor its development. When this became clear, I was authorized by my board of trustees to offer NDC as the nonprofit umbrella under which they could seek funding from the Area Agency on Aging to develop a senior day care service. I made it clear that I was not personally interested in becoming involved, and that they would have to do all the work as well as get all the satisfaction from developing the program. That lasted very briefly; both Sarah Archer and I worked with a small group in writing the proposal. I had to go before committees and the board of the funding agency to explain the concept (which I had to be taught very quickly by the graduate student); in short, I have since become far more knowledgeable about and involved in the day care program in its two-and-a-half years of expansion than I had ever intended. I continue as NDC's representative to the day care program's committee; I work with some staff members on research possibilities within parts of the program; I organized my first-ever rummage sale to benefit the program. From the start, the program has been directed by the two nurses who started with NDC as graduate students, one from the exercise classes and the other from the planning group. When the first one moved out of state, the second one assumed the executive role in a gradually diversifying set of services geared to the handicapped elderly and their aged caretakers.

Yet another form of advocacy has been in our support of cooperative directions for service provision. In general, service providers are seldom funded so well that they do not always have to look out for added funding possibilities. Such interest in self-preservation often results in a disregard for client services, the duplication of some services, and a total absence of many others. My experience with the day care program confirmed this. Because our county already had a large number of fragmented, uncoordinated services available, we developed our day care program with the intent of using diverse service elements for the benefit of a particular set of elderly day care participants. The agencies were all surprisingly willing to cooperate, especially when there were some reimbursements available for their participation. The school district supported classes that the day care director considered essential intellectual stimulation; the paratransport system contracted to pick up and deliver the handicapped participants under a very fair contract; the Title VII dining program agreed to include the day care clients at the site without charge. Having nurses in administrative roles enabled them to work knowledgeably with their clients' physicians to assess their physical status and to work for needed modifications of their medical regimes or, where that was not possible, to work with the families to get physicians more interested in elderly handicapped people. Close relations with a nearby rehabilitation hospital made it possible for some clients to have therapy for the first time in many years; some stroke patients had not been seen for a decade or more, even though they clearly benefitted from the newly instituted therapies. The experience of coordinating even these services to develop one coherent program has led us to embark this year on a far more ambitious plan to utilize extant community services for a coordinated continuum-of-care project within the county.

Cooperation of another kind has been an ongoing concern of mine within my newly adopted interest area of exercise for seniors. From talking with a few others also teaching such classes, I realized that there was a high degree of job burnout, and that many teachers dropped out because there were so many demands for exercise classes and so few people meeting the needs. In addition, it became clear that the development of some exercise classes was not related so much to the needs of the elderly as to the interests of the teacher. Thus I felt that organizing those involved in or interested in teaching exercise could start to develop peer support against burnout, provide a forum for sharing and upgrading class content, and perhaps eventually lead to a coordinated program of such classes. This was, again, one of those services that many agreed was needed, valuable, and even necessary, but which no one had the time or the energy to organize. When it became clear to me that it would require a massive energy outlay to put such a council into operation, I had to reassess my own capacities and priorities. Because of other more urgent needs, such as looking for sources of my own support as funding resources shriveled, I have put the council aside for a while. Because I have been identified as someone interested in exercise, however, I continue to get calls to provide such classes for rest homes, nursing homes, and a variety of other locations of needful elders. Each caller is urged to direct her own energies to such efforts. One recent caller knew a newly graduated sociology student with organizing energy and a desire to support herself in such an effort. I have agreed to discuss organizational shelter, even if without funds, while she develops an exercise program.

Another coalition has formed among the elderly wives of the brain-damaged men in the day care program. Once the wives' support group was strong enough to provide them with the emotional resources to deal with the ongoing stress in their uniquely difficult positions, some of the wives found released energy to begin to address larger political issues around their roles as unpaid caretakers. With my urging as well as that of the day care staff, one of the organizationally sophisticated women began to focus the group on actions they might take to publicize their problems, to promote the development of similar support groups for other women, to raise the legislature's consciousness, and to eventually develop reimbursement mechanisms for respite care for their own mental and physical health. We have urged the wives to invite all candidates for state and local offices to meet with their group. Several of the wives have appeared on videotaped public-affairs programs about the day care program, the wive's group, and the problems of being a long-term caretaker. These tapes have been presented at professional conventions, meetings of the day–health-care association, to social-work classes, and over local cable television. The wives themselves have begun to appear at hearings about local aging programs and have testified eloquently about the impact of day care on the quality of their own life. They attend candidates' appearances and are becoming quite assertive about asking for statements of political position. Most admit that without NDC's urging and on-going support, they would not have become politically active. They have begun to use their own organizational clout in some of the ways NDC does, including writing support letters for other programs, lobbying for favored candidates for local and state positions, and protesting as a group when offended by a failure of the local media to present a correct view around an issue of concern to them. Thus NDC has been able to help this group of consumers organize and function

effectively politically. In the future, we will work to develop more consumer-nurse coalitions.

A last form of advocacy that I will mention is the use of testimony
before investigative, planning, and decision-making bodies. When the
US Civil Rights Commission toured the country looking at age discrimination in access to services, I decided to present them with an
example from my own county. I learned that it was common knowledge
that a certain community-based health service was denied to persons
over 64, requiring them to use the far more expensive hospital-based
service instead. When I phoned to ask why, I was told it was a "regulation." When I asked for the specific number of the regulation, my
source could find none but assured me it was a county ruling and gave
me the name of the person at the county office who could tell me the
specifics. I phoned her and she admitted it was not a county rule, but
that she knew for certain it was a state regulation and referred me on.
The state contact person told me that it was not state policy but *county*
policy that dictated that practice. The hospital staff person to whom I
talked became very angry at my questioning. It was clear to her that
older people were likely to have many more complicating physical problems, and I was obviously frustrating her by asking why then the health
service did not establish "many more complicating physical problems"
as their basis for exclusion rather than the very secondary and, to my
view, irrelevant fact of birthdate. It was only with great difficulty that
she could finally entertain the idea that this exclusion might indeed be
discriminatory, but she ended our discussion by adding, "But you have
to draw the line somewhere!" When I so testified before the Civil Rights
Commission hearing board, I joined a number of others who demonstrated a convincing pattern of exclusion from service of the very old,
which was later published as *The Age Discrimination Study* (US Civil
Rights Commission, 1977–1978).

Local hearings are held regularly, often to provide the basis for planning new programs or assessing the impact of existent ones. The Area
Agency on Aging, for example, holds annual hearings on service needs
of the aged in specified priority areas. When a proposal was being
developed for a service for Medicaid elderly, I prepared testimony that
demonstrated the inadequate data available as to the number of eligible
clients. Without this data there could be no estimate of the feasibility
of carrying out the service with the available funds. Once again I dis-
covered a merry-go-round of information: the four departments who
gave me "firm" figures of Medicaid elderly all gave me very different
numbers, and each finally admitted that the county data system would
not permit information to be retrieved by age group. Such an incapacity
seemed impossible to all those involved but my testimony led to further

investigation that confirmed this fact. The service proposal was, obviously, not developed then, but the data system is being revised to permit information needed for rational planning to be retrieved.

In these and other presentations, I have noticed that the professional hearing officers are much impressed by a well-documented presentation, a marshalling of facts, even by statistics where available. Boards made up of laypersons are seldom as interested in such materials, which do not always make clear to them the human aspects of an issue. I had been upset by the endless anecdotes one of the other local service-providers kept presenting to a particular lay board. But when I realized that those presentations resulted in compassionate funding increases, occasionally at the expense of some program I was concerned about, I understood the value of addressing groups with materials that made sense to them. "Give them what they want" is now our motto. Thus in addresses to local service clubs, which are made up of community members whose expertise is in fields other than our own, we present stories about our clients and experiences (with personal information protected, of course). This tactic has paid off, quite literally, with an increasing number of small grants and continuing support of NDC programs by several of the service groups. In any case, presentations are always more effective if one goes into them with thoroughly prepared materials. Testimony should be brief, to-the-point, and not attempt to cover too wide a range. It is not always necessary to interpret one's testimony: my experience with the ageist community service agency, for example, stood on its own without any need on my part to include a diatribe against ageism; that emerged from the commission's hearings across the country, bolstered by repeated incidents such as my own.

BURROWING FROM WITHIN

I have mentioned several times that several of Sarah's graduate students have been involved in Marin's aging network. Our philosophy of higher education demands that students be able to test theoretical knowledge in real-life settings, and vice versa. It has been rewarding for graduate nursing students to see how they can affect service provision using NDC as a passport into Marin's service system. For some of the students, the experience has been limited to field placements for the duration of their program. Others, however, become so involved and are such impressive workers that we try to develop ways to keep them working with us after graduation. Both of the founding nurses in the day care program made a swift transition from graduate student to NDC staff. Also, as we become aware of other possible positions within the county, we try to funnel as many activist nurses as we can into these slots. One of our former master's students, Pat Goehner, worked for another agency in Marin that serves the elderly, and is an NDC trustee.

When an opening appeared on the advisory board of the service agency discussed first under "Advocacy," above, I joined with a number of others in urging that the seat be reserved for someone who could speak to issues concerning the elderly. Indirectly, I began working to promote NDC's day care executive as that person. I began to contact members of the county board of supervisors who were responsible for making the appointment. I also called friends of mine in various service agencies urging them to do likewise. In addition, I talked with several elderly people or their family members and asked them to phone the supervisors to support NDC's day care executive for the position. This lobbying paid off, and one of our own nurses became the first acknowledged advocate for the elderly on that agency's advisory board.

More recently, we began a campaign to have Sarah appointed to the board of another local planning agency. This required slightly different logistics, since she has been pursuing a deliberately less visible role in county activities, as I have noted, although she now wishes to change her role. When her name appeared with three other nominees before the supervisors, they postponed action because they knew none of the nominees well enough to make a choice. We began lobbying to make Sarah's qualifications better known. We once again mobilized local agency friends, asking them the personal favor of calling the supervisors and lobbying for Sarah for this position. I contacted a number of the elderly wives caring for brain-damaged husbands in our day care program and asked them to support Sarah as an officer and trustee of NDC. Few of them have ever met Sarah, but they were willing to support her as a reflection of their high esteem for our organization. By asking many people for these favors, Sarah was, in effect, collecting on some past favors, or calling in social credits, and putting herself in debt to others who agreed to help her. We were careful not to do too much, but to balance the extent of this effort against the fact that this is not a crucial position for either Sarah or NDC, although the long-range possibilities are good. Sarah has been appointed. Of course, when any decisions come before the board that concern NDC, Sarah will publicly declare her conflict of interest and abstain from voting. But it is clear that, with the present composition of the board, she will bring both a new perspective and some much-needed expertise in the areas of planning and evaluation. Sarah has recently been elected vice-chair.

Just as we have asked for support to accomplish our goals, we have also found it valuable to give our support to those who are in a position to accomplish goals we endorse. I have written a number of letters on NDC letterheads agreeing that some particular proposal is needed, effective, and feasible. This gives me social credit with the person submitting the proposal, and I can expect similar support letters when I seek funding for any of my needed, effective, and feasible projects. Agreeing to ask certain pertinent questions at public hearings that other providers feel they cannot ask or that staff members may not ask because of their agency position, also creates some credit against my own future needs. I will also use NDC letterheads to write letters of comment, support, or objection to issues affecting the elderly.

Because of federal, legal, and tax constraints, NDC cannot engage in any partisan political action, and we are careful not to jeopardize our position in this way; *however*, this does not preclude each of us as individual citizens from approaching candidates for office to learn their views on issues of concern to us as providers of services. We can also mobilize groups of clients to learn similar things, and we can suggest that we have roles as NDC officers that influence how we view various health issues before the legislature. We must balance this, however, with the realization that too-visible support for one candidate may bring us to the attention of his or her opponent, who may still be in a position to frustrate our organizational goals in retaliation. Thus we tend to be fairly low profile when county supervisors, for example, run for office. We are less restrained with regard to candidates for state offices who are not also local politicians with power to affect our programs. But in all cases we make it clear that we function as citizens, not as members of NDC. If we are lucky enough to support a winning candidate, the result may be slightly improved access after election time. Of course, it can also be wasted effort, as with one legislator we supported who, after election, resigned from the health committee when one of his bills aroused extreme resistance from elements of the health care industry. Our slight efforts could not offset the concerted hostility of well-funded lobbyists with major axes to grind. But one lesson of politics at all levels is that you cannot win them all. Another is that the game itself is a reward—for us as well as for those with whom and for whom we work.

TACTICS

Implicit in what I have just discussed are a number of political tactics. I will highlight some of them and describe some of the rationales for using them. Many illustrate some of the tactics introduced in Chapter 3.

Varied Approaches

Rather than trying to force all of our approaches into one format, we deliberately encourage a range of approaches. From my own position within NDC, I enjoy a gadfly role, needling agencies or making snide comments in newspaper interviews, trying to be as unsettling as possible to fixed bureaucratic ways of thinking. Meanwhile, I can rely on our day care executive to present a more soothing version of my message from within the service-agency system or as a newly appointed member of the community agency's advisory board (yes, we have infiltrated!). She can adopt the cool insider role of Nice Mrs. Marin, making her recommendations ever so much more welcome than my more extreme positions. At times even that tactic needs to be balanced by yet another approach, and so we turn to the heavy-duty credentials of Dr Archer from the university. As I have noted, until just recently, Sarah has maintained a relatively low profile in the county's activities. Thus when she does come forth, people tend to listen to her perspective since they hear from her only occasionally.

You must not think that any one of us is limited to the approaches described above. I do not go around all the time as a wild-eyed rabble rouser, even though some agency people seem to think any disagreement is the same as an attack. I have been pleased, on occasion, to find that after working with me a while, even some of the heretofore very threatened agency people will begin to agree with our goals even if they still would prefer other styles of making changes. Some of them have started to leak helpful information with the understanding that I will use these leaks effectively without revealing my sources. I have even been amazed on a couple of occasions to be offered positions within the agency systems, offers I refuse because I prefer my outsider's freedom.

Credibility

Ordinarily neither Sarah nor I use our degrees or titles, since these may intimidate other service providers and actually impede work with the elderly. We find that most people are less threatened if we identify ourselves as nurses or public health nurses whom everybody sees as harmless. But there are times when it pays to have a title, either to suggest academic authority or just to get past some physician's secretary.

Also, making it clear that we are nurses provides a ready-made access to many of the community people that we want to reach. We are building a coalition of concerned citizens and nurses who are becoming increasingly active and vocal on issues and in support of or opposition to candidates for public office. Our effectiveness in handling these kinds of coalitions is greatly aided by the fact that we have built up a good deal of credibility with the elderly community and with other service providers in our six years of involvement with and on behalf of seniors in Marin County. We guard that credibility *very* carefully.

Infiltration

Another tactic I have already mentioned is that of infiltration of other groups by members of our organization or other like-minded people. Together we are able to influence these groups to make changes or to provide services for the elderly, whose needs we have data to prove. It is often much easier for an insider to work for change in coalition with outsiders. Having other people involved also provides for a much broader base of support for issues than we could have alone. Enlisting a diverse group of people and organizations to testify at hearings or advocate at planning meetings on issues of importance to the elderly or to NDC itself also keeps me and the other members of the board from appearing to be too outspoken or even self-serving. When you are in a position to have to arrange testimony on behalf of your own organization or pet issue, remember to get a broad range of people to speak to the issue, rather than having everyone come from one point of view or one power base.

Trade-offs

As noted in Chapter 3, trade-offs are what make the world of politics run. One of the most frequent trade-off situations I find myself in is the exchange of support letters that must accompany grant proposals and planning documents. As the president of NDC, I am the one who has to give these endorsements to other agenices seeking external support or program changes. Unless I really object to what the agency is proposing to do, I quickly respond with a letter documenting the reasons why NDC supports the proposed activity. I know, as do the officers and executives of the other agencies, that it is only a matter of time before NDC too will be seeking similar documentation of their support for something we are about to undertake. I do not keep score about who owes us how many indications of support or other favors, but I do have a rough idea, and since we are a small community and all work closely together, it is easy to remember who has been asked what.

An added benefit in the trade-off business, especially since Marin County is a small community, is that most of the agencies who get support from other agencies end up by sharing whatever grants they receive through contracts for other organizations' services or personnel. Thus we all, in the long run, benefit from whatever additional resources any one group obtains. Part of this is due to the fact that cooperating agencies in our community are working together to provide comprehensive and coordinated client services rather than building up isolated empires of their own, which would result in duplications of some services and serious gaps in between.

Coalitions

As I have indicated, I have been involved in the development of several kinds of coalitions. One kind is formed between members of various consumer groups and nurses in order to bring political clout to bear on elected and appointed officials. We nurses are beginning to put our support behind candidates for various local offices in which we can be effective in shaping both policies and policy makers. We think that this kind of consumer-nurse coalition has great potential for altering a number of systems, including, of course, the health and medical care systems. Some of my colleagues and I are becoming very active in local chapters of Common Cause, the National Women's Political Caucus, the Nurses' Association, the League of Women Voters, and other politically active and effective groups. Thus we are spreading our energies and expertise around where they can have the most political effect.

Another type of coalition that is proving increasingly effective is that of service-providing organizations, for the purpose of coordinating services and stretching scarce resources. We are finding that we can give our clients better, more comprehensive, accessible, and acceptable services if we, the service providers, work cooperatively together. As mentioned earlier, we have organized a group of agencies working with the elderly into the Marin Section on Aging, of which I am an officer. This group meets regularly to discuss common goals and to share information. Thus all of us who represent agencies in this group know each other well, a situation that makes collaboration much easier to develop. I have already described the coalition of exercise instructors that I am seeking to build. I believe in the old adage that there is strength in numbers.

These are only some of the many tactics that are available and can be used to develop and provide services as well as to influence policy and policy makers on a large scale. Look carefully at your own immediate environment to see which ones you can use.

SUMMARY

I have focused in this chapter on the local political actions of Nursing Dynamics, a nonprofit corporation of which I am president. These activities are primarily concerned with the elderly population of a suburban California county and are presented in more-or-less chronological order, beginning with our first involvement in 1973. We have used our research skills to develop a data base for planning and policy making groups. We have been instrumental in the formation and maintenance of a network of agencies and providers concerned with providing services for the elderly, and we have been advocates for the needs of this population group. We have helped a group of wives who are caretakers of husbands with brain damage to become organized into a support group and to become politically active on their own behalf. We have encouraged and assisted other nurses to become members of policy making and advisory groups and other agencies as a means of influencing these groups and strengthening the elderly-care network. As individuals we have supported and opposed candidates for state and local offices. All of these activities have been local and have provided us with a great deal of satisfaction while making changes in the system.

REFERENCES

Archer SE, Fleshman RP: Doing our own thing: Community health nurses in independent practice. *Journal of Nursing Administration* 8:44–51, November 1978.

Archer SE, Fleshman RP, Carver C, Adelman L: Life-style indicators for interventions to facilitate elderly persons' independence. *Health Values* 3(3):129–135, 1979.

Fleshman RP, Archer SE: Nurse-pharmacist teams screen for hypertension. *Hospital Formulary* 11(2), 1976.

Fleshman RP, Archer SE: Nurse practitioners in community settings, in Archer SE, Fleshman RP (eds): *Community Health Nursing: Patterns and Practice*, ed 2. North Scituate, Mass, Duxbury Press, 1979, pp 455–473.

US Civil Rights Commission: *The Age Discrimination Study*, vol 1, Washington, DC, US Civil Rights Commission. December 1977, vol 2, January 1978.

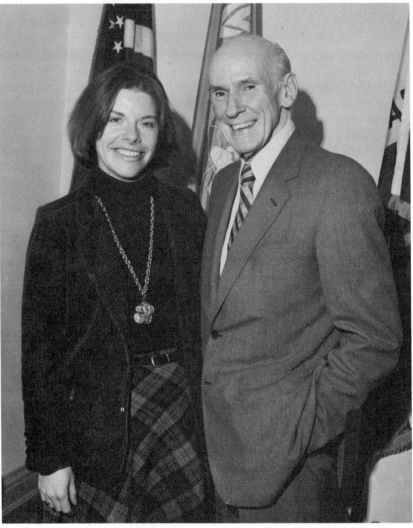

Cheryl Beversdorf and US Senator Alan Cranston while she was a member of his Senate Veterans' Affairs Committee staff. *(Photo by Congressional Photo Service)*

CHAPTER 9

The Nurse as a Member of a Congressional Committee Staff

Cheryl Beversdorf

BOTH THE NURSING profession and the diverse employment opportunities available to nurses are changing significantly and expanding rapidly. These changes have reached the point where nurses are not only being sought for positions in the more traditional hospital settings, but also in less nurse-oriented and health-related organizations such as industries, schools, corporations, professional associations, and insurance companies. In addition, the numerous and complex health issues currently coming to the attention of lawmakers and requiring action on the state, local, and national levels are increasingly calling for the expertise of health professionals. Here, too, the technical knowledge and practical experience of nurses are needed to assess appropriate action. Whether the primary interest of a health organization is returning the ill to optimal health or sustaining the good health of the well, its interest in health and health care is the fundamental factor determining its existence. This is true of the nursing profession as well.

The opportunities for nurses to mainfest their concern for the health of individuals while at the same time effecting change on a large scale are increasing, particularly in areas such as health legislation and policy. As nurses contemplate the most suitable ways to practice their profession, part of their efforts should be directed toward an active role in health policy making, in recognition of the significant impact they can make on a local or state or even national level. At present, I am a

CHERYL BEVERSDORF, RN, MScHy, is legislative assistant in the New York State Office of Federal Affairs in Washington, DC. She was a member of California US Senator Alan Cranston's staff, Veterans' Affairs Committee, United States Senate, when she wrote this chapter.

professional staff member of the US Senate Committees on Veterans' Affairs. I was hired because of my clinical nursing and administrative staff experience, my academic degrees, and, the committee's interest in my perspective as a health professional. Among the many subject areas falling under the jurisdiction of the committee, an important and complex one is veterans' hospitals and the medical care and treatment of veterans. As the only health specialist on the committee staff, it is my responsibility to provide comments, based on my technical knowledge, during committee deliberations of issues: to carry out the necessary tasks related to the committee's oversight activities; and to participate in the functions related to its legislative duties. My past educational and work experiences help me to influence important decisions that affect the health of a major segment of the nation's population.

The purpose of this chapter is threefold: first, to describe the sequence of events leading to my position as a Senate staff member; second, to explain the nature of my responsibilities on the committee staff; and, third, to give nurses a rationale to intensify their efforts toward placing themselves in positions where they will have a more direct impact on future health policy decisions.

BACKGROUND

The thought of working on the Hill in Washington, DC, occurred to me when I was doing graduate work in health planning at the School of Hygiene and Public Health at Johns Hopkins University in Baltimore, Maryland. The program led to a master's degree in health science and required two years to complete—the first year for the academic work, the second for a field placement either in a health agency, department, or institution. When assignments were being made for field placements, my advisor informed me that the Washington office of the American Optometric Association (AOA) was one of a variety of health-related organizations seeking interns. AOA's primary mission was that of increasing membership involvement in federal health programs.

As a registered nurse with an interest in health policy, I agreed that AOA would be the most appropriate placement for the year-long field assignment. During that year, I got a first-hand look at how a health profession relates to the various components of the federal government, and how health legislation and policy are subsequently influenced on the state and national level by special-interest groups. The areas to which I was assigned included health planning, health maintenance organizations (HMOs), and professional standards review organizations (PSROs). It was my responsibility to investigate innovative opportunities for the optometric profession to increase its involvement and participation in these federal health-related programs. Often the job required an update and subsequent dissemination of information regarding the current legislative status of these activities to appropriate and interested AOA members. On several occasions I had the opportunity to analyze newly enacted health legislation. After the legislation was enacted, I reviewed the federal regulations that interpreted the legislation and that specified how the law was to be implemented.

At the end of the field placement year, I was offered a full-time position with AOA. Even though the position promised a continuing opportunity to observe and participate in the operation of a health interest group, I preferred to make different use of my graduate education and background, and accepted a position as a staff liaison with the American Public Health Association (APHA). APHA is an organization whose membership is composed of public health professionals who focus on public health issues from a scientific and legislative perspective rather than from any one specific health profession viewpoint, as does AOA. As the only national public health association in the country, APHA is well know for its involvement in influencing policy on numerous and diverse public health issues. Many APHA members frequently testify on national health legislation and policy before both Senate and House committees.

As at AOA, part of my job responsibilities at APHA included the analysis and interpretation of health legislation and related federal regulations. When an issue fell within my area of responsibility, I prepared testimony for APHA members who appeared on behalf of the association at a congressional hearing. It was my job, therefore, to assure that the testimony correctly reflected APHA's position on the issue under consideration.

In order to understand the responsibilities of APHA staff liaisons, it is helpful to have a clear picture of the association's structure and how it evolved. Historically, the association welcomed the requests of most public health interest groups seeking alliance with the organization, and, as a result, staff responsibilities within the Affiliate and Section Affairs Division increased as these new units became part of the association. Each of the four liaisons, and the director, were to be responsive to a quarter of the association's 23 component sections and approximately a quarter of the 48 affiliated organizations. In addition, we responded to numerous association task forces, caucuses, boards, and special committees. Specifically, each of the liaisons provided administrative and organizational support and financial guidance to these groups and, when necessary, were available for special consultation and coordination of association-wide research projects, professional development, or special programs. During this period, APHA underwent a major reorganization, and I was appointed as the association's continuing-professional-education coordinator. For the remaining six months of my employment, I was responsible for developing the association's continuing-education program. Although the new duties were a challenge, my main interests were in health legislation and health policy. Therefore when I was offered a position as a professional staff member on the Senate Veterans' Affairs Committee, I could not turn it down. This position provided me the opportunity to participate in the complex process of writing health legislation that could become a part of the nation's policy on health.

It is important to note at this point, however, that, although experience with public health policy and legislation from a special-interest standpoint undoubtedly enhanced my eligibility for the staff position, my work and education prior to graduate school was equally significant. Before attending The Johns Hopkins University, I graduated from a diploma nursing program in Milwaukee, Wisconsin, and was a staff nurse in several civilian and army hospitals. I worked in pediatrics, obstetrics, and medical-surgical areas in the military hospital at Camp Zama, Japan, and at Walter Reed Army Medical Center in Washington, DC. Not only did the army nursing experience offer me the chance to render patient care in the military health care system, but it accorded me the veteran status that was a contributing factor to acquiring my present position.

Following discharge from the military, I attended three universities, taking various undergraduate liberal arts courses and accumulating the semester hours needed for an undergraduate degree in nursing. While in school, I worked at Group Hospitalization, Inc; the Blue Cross and Blue Shield Plans of the National Capital Area, Washington, DC; and as a medical adviser in the Blue Cross Supplemental Claims Division and the Blue Shield Regular and Special Claims Division. I was primarily responsible for reviewing and approving all cases requiring medical expertise; in addition, I participated in a special staff study that revised the Blue Shield's medical claims fee-schedule book for new surgical techniques and diagnostic procedures. This employment significantly contributed to my awareness of how a health insurance system operates and is administered. Furthermore it acquainted me with many of the problems that might require resolution if national health insurance legislation is enacted.

Thus it was the combined experience of two academic degrees and a background in civilian and military clinical nursing, health insurance administration, professional health-association management, and a veteran's status that led to my staff appointment on the Senate Veteran's Affairs Committee. The relationship between these elements was significant because they enhanced my personal and professional development. What is more important, however, they illustrate how seemingly diverse types of experiences can be combined to qualify an individual for a particular position.

THE COMMITTEE: ORGANIZATION
AND RESPONSIBILITIES

According to a Congressional Research Service memorandum on legislative developments relating to the creation of the Senate Committee on Veterans' Affairs, "Between 1946 and 1970, a number of arguments were offered and repeated in support of and in opposition to proposals to create a standing Committee on Veterans' Affairs" (December 14, 1976:6). In 1970, the 91st Congress voted to establish the committee, with the first organizational meeting taking place on February 3, 1971.

The committee in 1979 consisted of ten members, including the chairman, who, as with all congressional committees, is traditionally a member of the majority party of the Congress. Since 1977, the chairman has been Senator Alan Cranston of California. Besides Senator Cranston, the other Democratic members are Senators Herman Talmadge (Georgia), Jennings Randolph (West Virginia), Richard Stone (Florida), John Durkin (New Hampshire), and Spark Matsunaga (Hawaii).

Of the Republican members, Senator Alan Simpson (Wyoming) functions as ranking minority member, with Senators Strom Thurmond (South Carolina), Robert Stafford (Vermont), and Gordon Humphrey (New Hampshire) assigned as the other three minority members of the committee.

The committee's legislative jurisdiction is defined under the Standing Rules of the Senate. The Rules of Procedure state that the Committee on Veterans' Affairs shall consider all proposed legislation, messages, petitions, memorials, and other matters relating to the following subjects:

1. Compensation of veterans
2. Life insurance issued by the government on account of service in the armed forces
3. National cemeteries
4. Pensions of all wars of the United States, general and special
5. Readjustment of servicemen to civil life
6. Soldiers' and sailors' civil relief
7. Veterans' hospitals, medical care, and treatment of veterans
8. Veterans' measures generally
9. Vocational rehabilitation and education of veterans (Rules of Procedure, 1979, p 5)

Generally, the complex nature of most of the issues coming under the committee's jurisdiction precludes the possibility of easy or fast solutions. Matters requiring attention are resolved through extensive discussion, coordination, and deliberation among staff members who are responsible for the subject under consideration or have some knowledge or interest in the issue. The reason for collaboration and cooperation is to assure that on any issue the final action reflects committee policy. Moreover, when inquiries from interested parties are received regarding any action by the committee, all staff members must be aware of the committee's position and the reasoning for it, and be able to convey the same message.

After I began working for the committee, it became apparent that a major reason for the type of job interview I had was the need for a staff that could work closely on most issues. This requirement necessitated my return to the committee suite four separate times, for individual and small group interviews with different staff members, before the chief counsel offered me a job on the committee staff.

Of course, I welcomed the opportunity to talk with each member of the staff, particularly with those who were working on health issues and with whom I would be working most directly. Topics we discussed during most of these interviews focused primarily on the required duties of the position, but, in several conversations, my opinion on current health issues was sought, my attitude on the nursing profession was explored, and my reaction to being asked medical questions and advice should I be hired as the staff's resident health professional was queried. At the same time, the staff believed that "turnabout was fair play," and I appreciated the candor with which each of them described his or her daily workload.

Probably one of the most unusual yet enjoyable aspects of the interview was the required conversation with Senator Cranston's administrative assistant. It is important to note that, although I was applying for a position in which veterans' health care issues would be my primary concern, I would also be an employee of the chairman, which meant that my work should not conflict with his political philosophies and interests and that I would serve at his pleasure, as is typical of most staff members working for members of Congress. The interview with the administrative assistant is one of the most memorable dialogues I have ever had. Prior interviews, for this position and earlier ones, had primarily focused on the job. This interview sought instead to extract my extemporaneous comments on a range of controversial and noncontroversial issues. "How do you feel about abortion? What do you think about gun control? homosexuality? busing? On a rating scale from one to ten, if one denotes an introvert and ten an extrovert, where would you rate yourself?" (I said eight.) "Have you ever been bitten by a dog?" (Yes.) "How did you react to the dog?" (Frightened.) "How do you feel about dogs now?" (I still like them.) "Of those pictures on the wall"— he pointed to four paintings that he said were on loan from the National Collection of Fine Arts—"which do you like best?" (The earth-colored abstract.)

Needless to say, I was not prepared for this kind of rapid interrogation and felt somewhat dubious during the whole interaction. I was fearful I would give the wrong response to his queries or, even worse, be unable to utter anything at all. As the interview progressed, however, I began to relax and even enjoy the challenge of seeing how quickly I could answer his questions. What is more, it became increasingly clear that it was not so much *what* my response was—since there seemed to be no right or wrong answers—but rather that I did have answers and could give them. It seemed that he was most concerned with my reactions and my ability to analyze a situation and express myself, since that, for the most part, would be the nature of my work. It is my opinion that he wanted to be certain that I had the perception, judgment, and maturity to handle any situation that might arise should I be accepted for the job. Apparently, I convinced him that I did!

SCOPE OF COMMITTEE ACTIVITIES

Ten years ago, one of the arguments in Congress against the creation of a full committee to oversee veterans' programs was that there was insufficient legislative and oversight workload in that area to justify full committee status. That would hardly be a valid justification today, and it is fortunate for veterans that the committee became a reality.

Much of the committee work focuses on two specific veteran groups. The largest group consists of the 13 million World War II veterans who, as their median age steadily increases, are now looking to the government for health care and pension benefits. In addition, millions of Vietnam veterans have taken advantage of educational assistance and rehabilitation benefits made available by the federal government. These two groups have increased the committee workload considerably; but also, because of legislative and administrative history, the issues today are more complex and require more detailed responses than when the committee was first established. For example, in 1979 the committee held 37 days of hearings on legislative and oversight matters, executive nominations, and the recommendations of veterans' organizations; met in open executive session nine times and reported 12 bills to the Senate, 11 of which were ultimately enacted; and reviewed both the annual report of the administrator for the Veterans' Administration and the President's budget requests relating to VA programs, facilities, and agency requirements for the fiscal years 1978 and 1979. In addition, the committee reviewed reports of the General Accounting Office—the investigative and auditing agency of the Congress—concerning the operation of VA programs, as well as other reports and materials. The committee also carried on extensive correspondence with the administrator of veterans' affairs and other federal officials regarding issues of veterans' affairs.

Because each Congress passes new or revises current veterans' legislation, it is likely that the volume of the committee's work will increase in the future. What is more, as the volume increases, the amount of responsibility given to each of the committee staff members also increases. Each staff member is expected to take personal initiative with respect to the many issues assigned to him or her. Since the committee has 18 full-time staff members, the smallest on either side of Capitol Hill, high productivity is required. In order to keep up with the day-to-day activities of an executive branch agency with a budget of over $20 billion and approximately 218,000 personnel (the third largest in the federal government) whose primary mission is to provide a broad range of direct services and administer benefit programs, a great deal of responsibility rests with each staff member.

The titles of the committee staff members and their responsibilities are as follows: (1) the chief counsel, who has overall responsibility for supervising the committee staff, programs budget, and management, and for maintaining relationships with other Senate committees, Senate offices, and the public; (2) the general counsel, who is responsible for supervising the legislative staff of the committee and overseeing the legislative and congressional budgetary process; (3) three associate counsels, who have legislation and oversight responsibilities for compensation and pension matters; the VA health care system; and general government, insurance, cemeteries, burial benefits, and Vietnam-era veterans' activities; (4) two professional staff members, one of whom is responsible for the GI Bill, vocational rehabilitation, and veterans' employment issues; and a second (the position I now hold), who is responsible for special projects in the health care area and works with the associate counsel who is responsible for legislation and general oversight in the health area; (5) two research assistants, who are responsible for drafting correspondence and for performing research tasks in assigned areas; (6) one caseworker, responsible for health and hospital cases; (7) four administrative assistants; and (8) two clerks.

STAFF ACTIVITIES
AND RESPONSIBILITIES

At present I am still in the process of learning many of the legislative terms and procedures necessary in my position, and am generally striving to become versed in the committee's operational methods. Advice from colleagues, time, and on-the-job experience will undoubtedly alleviate any present problems of dealing quickly with issues under consideration.

Because of the diverse nature and the increased volume of my work, a large part of my workday is spent on keeping abreast of the committee's legislative and oversight activities. For any issue, whether health topic or policy, it may be necessary for me to analyze a report; review and comment on a publication; request information from an unlimited number of sources; draft an appropriate letter for the chairman; or investigate the nature and degree of activity in a given area by various federal agencies, health agencies, health groups, or organizations. Much of my time is spent reading a never-ending flow of newspaper clippings, articles, memoranda, circulars, publications, and correspondence that either relates directly to the VA health care system or refers to other current health issues that may have a bearing on the VA system.

Frequently, staff members must meet with Veterans' Administration employees familiar with a specific policy and discuss its present status; the potential and possibility for change or modification as needed by the VA or desired by Congress; or, in some cases, the feasibility of eliminating the policy if it is no longer contributing to the efficient operation of the system. These encounters are extremely useful in helping the staff advise the committee on the most appropriate action to take on a particular issue. In some cases, meetings with representatives of various veterans' organizations or special-interest groups provide the staff with different viewpoints and alternatives that aid in recommending suitable action.

In some instances, for certain types of technical or confidential information, I seek the assistance and advice of a colleague or a "contact" established during one of my previous positions. In Congress, federal agencies, and government-related organizations located in Washington, DC, it is not unusual for many employees to have held more than one position in a particular field of legislative and federal interest. For example, in the field of health, it is possible to have worked on matters pertaining to this area as a congressional staff member, as a civil service worker at the Department of Health and Human Services (formerly HEW) or another federal agency, or as a staff worker in the legislative office of a professional health association. I have worked for four different health-oriented organizations in the Washington area, which has given me the advantage of knowing a substantial number of health professionals who, because of their work or position, have been helpful in providing the technical information needed for my work. This "colleague network" in Washington, DC, as in all cities, is absolutely vital in developing and maintaining a perspective on how the many component agencies and support groups interact.

Since I began working for the committee, my involvement has centered on the oversight of veterans' programs rather than the committee's legislative responsibilities. Because oversight impacts and reflects legislation, however, participation in the preparation for hearings held on veterans' health legislation introduced in the Senate has been a second major area of work. Generally, the committee holds hearings to hear testimony and collect information from interested parties. With a public record established, the committee decides its view on the legislation and takes appropriate action for modifying the pending legislation before making its recommendations to the Senate.

To prepare themselves for committee hearings, members must have a clear understanding of the nature and impact of the legislation being considered; as a result, it may be necessary for a staff member, familiar with the subject area, to brief the members on the consequences of the legislation so that during the hearing they will be able to objectively assess the testimony presented by the witnesses. For example, when the committee was preparing for one of the hearings at which legislation concerning geriatric centers in VA hospitals was to be considered, they sent me to several hospitals where geriatric centers were in operation. Based on my perspective as a health professional, my responsibility was to observe the centers and report to the members the degree and caliber of activities taking place at them. In addition, I was to advise them on the appropriateness and feasibility of establishing additional centers.

For a hearing to consider legislation containing a provision to address pay and special employment benefits for VA nurses, the committee sent me to eight different VA medical facilities where the shortage of staff nurses was particularly acute. At each center I discussed recruitment and retention problems with appropriate staff members and, to the extent possible, discussed and recommended feasible short-term solutions and advised the hospital administrators of those issues that would require legislation to achieve change. In my report I focused my suggestions on what actions I thought would be necessary or most appropriate for the committee to take.

In further preparation for hearings, the staff is responsible for planning the agenda and handling the necessary logistics including scheduling the hearing date, notifying and advising witnesses, and reviewing testimony submitted by them in order to fully prepare the committee. The staff is present at the hearing to attend to any last-minute details that may arise and to provide on-the-spot advice to committee members about follow-up questions or additional questions that witnesses' responses suggest. After the hearing, the staff is responsible for securing any additional information requested of the witnesses by the committee members for inclusion in the hearing record. The staff also reviews the final hearing proceedings to assure that the record is accurate and complete.

Following the hearing, committee members consider the suggestions and testimony of the witnesses and report out the bill, including recommendations to the Senate. Depending on the action on the legislation in the House, the bill may be sent to a conference committee, which must work out the language of the final bill before it is sent to the President for his signature or veto.

CONCLUSIONS

The combination of my past experiences as a health care practitioner and patient-care administrator, and my familiarity with a methodology for accomplishing change within the system, has been extremely beneficial in assisting me to knowledgeably and professionally respond to issues and advise the committee concerning them. The fact that we as nurses can play a major role in those political areas in which the status of the nation's health care is determined is a worthwhile point to consider as we contemplate future career plans and objectives.

The number of opportunities for nurses to get involved in health legislation and policy is increasing. To effect change in the nation's health care system, more nurses must pursue those opportunities and place themselves in positions where their influence is seen and heard. At present, there are only three registered nurses working as full-time staff members on congressional committees, and each of them is actively involved in health care issues. In view of the volume of health bills introduced in Congress each year, I believe Senators and Representatives could benefit from an increase in the nursing point of view, and nurses, in turn, could gain a more diverse and comprehensive perspective on how the nation's health policies are actually formulated.

REFERENCE

Rules of Procedure, Committee on Veterans' Affairs, US Senate, 96th Congress, First sess, 1979.

Part III

Resources

IN CHAPTER 10, the Nurses' Political Yellow Pages, Sarah Ellen Archer, Patricia A. Goehner, and Ruth P. Fleshman have amassed information about a number of resources that nurses can use to become more politically active. Section 1 presents descriptions and addresses of a number of national political and professional organizations. Section 2 lists selected political resources on a state-by-state basis. Section 3 provides subscription information for a number of politically helpful periodicals and special publications. All of this is done with the intent of helping nurses gain access to information and networks.

Chapter 11 presents a comprehensive state-by-state review of bill-to-law procedures. The emphasis here is upon the structural aspects of the legislative process. This chapter is organized to afford the reader a simplified method of finding needed information and to provide a consistent format for cross referencing.

The bibliography at the end of this section provides readers with information about a number of pertinent references for nurses who seek to become more politically active.

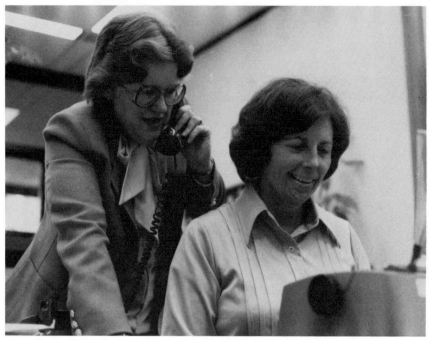

Sarah Ellen Archer and Patricia A. Goehner preparing the "Nurses' Political Yellow Pages." *(Photo by Katherine McInerney)*

CHAPTER 10

Nurses' Political
Yellow Pages

*Sarah Ellen Archer, Patricia A. Goehner,
and Ruth P. Fleshman*

THE PURPOSE OF these Yellow Pages is to provide nurses with a listing of the names and addresses of organizations that are active in political arenas. These organizations are links in a variety of information networks (see Chapter 3). The Yellow Pages can be used as a tool for active political involvement and/or as a general reference.

The chapter is divided into three sections. Section 1 contains a brief description of a number of national organizations and their central office address. Section 2 is a state-by-state listing of selected organizations that are particularly relevant to nurses seeking to become politically active on a state level. We suggest that you expand it with your experience at your state and local levels. Section 3 lists a number of publications, mainly periodicals, that we have found to be helpful in political participation.

One word of caution on the use of the Yellow Pages. Like all listings of this type, the names and addresses were current at the time the chapter was prepared. By the time you get around to using it, however, some of the contact people will have changed. Some entries—for example, the state leagues for nursing—are listed under the current president's name and address because some organizations do not have a permanent office and so must use the president's address. We have included such addresses as they were given to us on the assumption that the person who was president at the time the list was published is likely to remain an active member and therefore a viable contact person for the organization. Because of the changes that occur constantly in personnel and addresses, a listing of this kind should be updated every six months in order to be most effective. We have chosen to do the next best thing, which is to give you the most current list we can. We hope that you will find it useful.

SECTION 1: NATIONAL ORGANIZATIONS

American Civil Liberties Union

The ACLU, established in 1920, has a long history of defending individual rights through court procedures, including suits and amicus curiae briefs. Their attorneys have been involved in a wide variety of issues, with the aim of defending rights granted in the Constitution even when the exercise of those rights is not popular. In the past, they have worked on southern voter registration, freeing Japanese-Americans from internment, rights to free-association during the McCarthy era, and free speech—written or verbal—as guaranteed under the First Amendment. More recently they have been involved with issues of women's choice about abortions, and strip-searches of women traffic violators. The ACLU maintains local chapters, staffed largely with volunteer help. Members ($20 per year) receive the regular newsletter, *Civil Liberties*, as well as local bulletins covering current actions.

American Civil Liberties Union
22 E 40th St
New York, NY 10016

American Public Health Association

The APHA is the largest public health organization in the world. Its membership of over 30,000 is composed of members from all health and human services disciplines involved in health promotion and health care. The APHA has 25 sections with which members can affiliate: community health planning, dental health, environment, epidemiology, food and nutrition, gerontological health, health administration, injury control and emergency health services, international health, laboratory, maternal and child health, medical care, mental health, new professionals, occupational health and safety, podiatric health, population, public health education, public health nursing, radiological health, school health, social work, statistics, veterinary public health, and vision care. A major focus of the APHA's activities during the past several years has been in the areas of public policy and regulation. The APHA frequently gives testimony before legislative committees and regulatory bodies on issues affecting the public's health. Regular membership is $40 per year; sustaining membership is $60 per year. Members receive both *The American Journal of Public Health* and *The Nation's Health.*

American Public Health Association
1015 15th St NW
Washington, DC 20005
(202) 789-5600

Chamber of Commerce of the United States

The Chamber of Commerce is primarily a promotional organization for business and industry. Along with its other functions, however, the Chamber provides a number of publications and other types of information useful to nurse-activists. These include a series of six pamphlets entitled *Action Course in Practical Politics.* Other publications of potential interest include the Chamber's annually issued *Elections Guide* and *They Grade the Congress.*

Chamber of Commerce of the United
    States
Public Affairs Dept
1615 H St NW
Washington, DC 20006

Common Cause

When Common Cause was first established in 1970, it was designed to promote grassroots participation in government processes, especially nominations and elections to office. It has promoted broader campaign financing to reduce candidates' allegiance to major contributors, open-door meetings of government bodies, congressional codes of ethics, and a variety of other government reforms. Common Cause's staff prepares investigative studies to provide a data base for understanding government problems and suggesting remedial actions. Consistent with their grassroots policy, there are many local chapters of Common Cause that organize legislative watches and phone trees to solicit member responses to critical issues. Members receive a bimonthly magazine, *In Common,* that includes in-depth issue analyses, investigative studies, and editorial comment. Membership is $15 per year plus $5 for state Common Cause membership.

Common Cause
2030 M St NW
Washington, DC 20036
(202) 833-1200

Federation of Organizations for Professional Women

The FOPW was organized in 1972 to provide a means for women in the professions to unite around issues affecting equal opportunity in education and employment. At present, there are approximately 100 affiliated organizations, as well as individual friends supporting the federation's activities. These include involvement with the ERA, White House conferences, enforcement of Title IX, and a variety of legislation applicable to women. The federation supports two research centers and has a variety of publications, including a monthly newsletter on health-policy issues of concern to women.

Federation of Organizations for
    Professional Women
2000 P St NW, Suite 403
Washington, DC 20036
(202) 466-3547

Federation of Specialty Nursing
Organizations and ANA

The federation was formed to facilitate communication between the growing number of nursing-specialty organizations and the American Nurses' Association. The federation meets twice a year, and these meetings provide virtually the only opportunities that all nursing organizations have to meet together as equal participants in discussions about nursing. The focus of the discussions is on issues and on the sharing of information about the activities of each of the member organizations. The federation has the potential to unite the many different nursing organizations into one voice. Below is a list of the member organizations of the federation.

American Association of
    Critical-Care Nurses
PO Box C-19528
Irvine, CA 92713

American Association of Nephrology
    Nurses and Technicians
2 Talcott Rd, Suite 8
Park Ridge, IL 60068

American Association of
    Neurosurgical Nurses
625 North Michigan Ave, Suite 1519
Chicago, IL 60611

American Association of
    Nurse Anesthetists
216 Higgins Rd
Park Ridge, IL 60068

American Association of
    Occupational Health Nurses, Inc
575 Lexington Ave
New York, NY 10022

American College of Nurse Midwives
1021 14th St NW, Suite 801
Washington, DC 20005

American Nurses' Association
2420 Pershing Rd
Kansas City, MO 64108

American Public Health Association
Public Health Nursing Section
1015 15th St NW
Washington, DC 20005

American Urological Association,
   Allied
21510 S Main St
Carson, CA 90745

The Association of Operating
   Room Nurses, Inc
10170 E Mississippi Ave
Denver, CO 80231

Association of Practitioners in
   Infection Control
PO Box 546
Palatine, IL 60067

Association of Rehabilitation
   Nurses
2506 Grosse Point Rd
Evanston, IL 60201

Emergency Department Nurses'
   Association
666 N Lake Shore Dr, Suite 1729
Chicago, IL 60611

International Association for
   Enterostomal Therapy, Inc
505 N Tustin Ave, Suite 219
Santa Ana, CA 92705

National Association of Pediatric
   Nurse Associates and
   Practitioners
PO Box 56
N Woodbury Rd
Pitman, NJ 08071

National Intravenous Therapy
   Association, Inc
850 Third Ave, 11th Floor
New York, NY 10022

National Nurses' Society on
   Alcoholism
733 Third Ave
New York, NY 10017

The Nurses' Association of the
   American College of
   Obstetricians and Gynecologists
1 E Wacker Dr, Suite 2700
Chicago, IL 60601

Oncology Nursing Society
701 Washington Rd
Pittsburgh, PA 15228

Orthopedic Nurses, Inc
3165 E Shadowlaw
Atlanta, GA 30305

League of Women Voters

The LWV was founded in 1920 as an outgrowth of the National American Women's Suffrage Association. One of the LWV's first tasks was to educate US women to use their newly won right to vote effectively. Since then the LWV has expanded to serve all voters and to influence political actions and the shaping of public policy. The LWV is staunchly nonpartisan, supporting neither specific candidates nor political parties. Candidates' and issues' nights are among the LVW's activities at all levels and provide opportunities for the public to listen to and question candidates and referenda sponsors about issues. These activities are carried on through the League of Women Voters Education Fund. Contact people and addresses of state leagues are listed in Section 2 of this chapter. Dues are $25 per year.

League of Women Voters
1730 M St NW
Washington, DC 20005
(202) 296-1770

National Association for Women Deans, Administrators and Counselors

NAWDAC members are those professionally involved in or interested in the education of women and girls at all levels, public and private. With 30 state organizations, NAWDAC sponsors annual national, regional, and state conferences and workshops that are planned around specific issues or skill-building needs and provide a time for developing professional support. Members may be classified by their teaching levels: the earliest grades through early adolescence; high schools, community and junior colleges; universities; and continuing education. The association produces a quarterly journal on trends, issues, practices, and research; its quarterly bulletin deals with NAWDAC activities. Other publications include bibliographies and special-topic monographs.

National Association for Women
    Deans, Administrators and
    Counselors
1625 I St NW, Suite 624A
Washington, DC 20006
(202) 659-9330

The National League for Nursing

The NLN was formed in 1950 by combining the National League for Nursing Education, the National Organization for Public Health Nurses, and the Association of Collegiate Schools of Nursing. Membership is open to nurses, other health care providers, and members of the public who are interested in nursing. The NLN publishes many resource documents, including proceedings from NLN-sponsored conferences and data books on nursing. The organization is very active on many political issues at all levels of government. (See Section 2 for addresses of state leagues for nursing.) The NLN is composed of six councils: Associate Degree Programs, Baccalaureate and Higher Degree Programs, Diploma Programs, Home Health Agencies and Community Health Services,

Hospital and Related Institutional Nursing Services, and Practical Nursing Programs. Dues are $40 per year.

National League for Nursing
10 Columbus Circle
New York, NY 10019
(212) 582-1022

National Organization for Women

Formed in 1966, NOW has worked at consciousness-raising on a variety of levels. Involved most deeply in ratification of the Equal Rights Amendment at this time, NOW has been and continues to be concerned with women's entry into full participation in all spheres of society. This is seen in opposition to economic discrimination against working women, women seeking credit, and female pensioners. NOW was the first major feminist organization to work for women's reproductive rights, including access to contraception and abortion. NOW challenged sex discrimination in classified advertising for jobs, in academic promotions, in union hiring practices, and in many other circumstances through use of legal challenges. Various special-interest committees have addressed particular issues: the Media Reform Committee has monitored television and protested stereotyped women's roles. Recent topics of concern have been low-paid pink-collar and household workers, housewives (the unpaid workers), and violence against women. NOW successfully fought the restraint-of-trade charge brought after they persuaded many other organizations to plan no meetings or conventions in non-ERA states. NOW holds state, regional, and national conferences on current issues. There are many NOW chapters within each state; the state coordinators can direct you to the closest one to you. National NOW dues are $20.

National Organization for Women
425 13th St NW, Suite 1048
Washington, DC 20004
(202) 347-2279

National Women's Education Fund

The National Women's Education Fund was established in 1972 for the sole purpose of providing education programs and information to increase the number of women in public life. Along with other activities, the fund offers materials, consulting services, and seminars to build women's skills and motivation for involvement in political activities and to assist women already prominent in public life. The fund is a nonpartisan organization whose activities are supported by foundation grants and contributions from corporations, unions, and a variety of nonprofit groups. Contributions are tax-deductible. Among their publications is *Campaign Workbook,* an excellent step-by-step guide to campaigning for state and local offices.

The fund networks with the Public Leadership Education Network, which is composed of five institutions of higher education: Carlow College (Pittsburgh, Pa), Goucher College (Towson, Md), Spellman College (Atlanta, Ga) Stephens College (Columbia, Mo) and Wells College (Aurora, NY); and the Center for the American Woman and Politics, part of the Eagleton Institute of Politics at Rutgers University in New Brunswick, NJ. CAWP's purpose is to conduct programs to develop and disseminate information about women's political participation, and to encourage women's full and effective participation in public life. The addresses of these three network organizations are:

National Women's Education Fund
Rosalie Whelan, Executive Director
1410 Q St, NW
Washington, DC 20009
(202) 462-8606

Public Leadership Education Network
Katherine E. Kleeman, Coordinator
1410 Q St, NW
Washington, DC 20009
(202) 462-8606

Center for the American Women
 and Politics
Ruth Mandel, Director
Eagleton Institute of Politics
Rutgers University
New Brunswick, NJ 08901

National Women's Health Network

Concerned primarily about issues affecting women's health, the network has developed a series of up-to-date guides on aspects of health related to reproduction. They regularly publish news alerts on special topics; they were first to announce the risks to children of women who had been given DES. Their concern about the effects of hormonal drugs has led to alerts, testimony, pressure, and lawsuits about risks associated with the birth control pill and other invasive contraceptive methods, postmenopausal estrogens, and Depo-Provera. Other testimony has been developed on forced, uninformed sterilization and on acceptable principles for a national health plan. Fetal alcohol syndrome has received their wide attention, as have infant formula abuses and the Nestlé boycott. Wider issues the network has publicized include attempts to neutralize the Occupational Safety and Health Administration and, in support of their strong antinuclear position, they have sponsored a variety of anti-nuke events. From its start in 1975 by five feminists, the NWHN now represents over a thousand local women's health groups, projects, clinics, professionals, and consumers.

National Women's Health Network
2025 I St NW, Suite 105
Washington, DC 20006
(202) 223-6886

National Women's Political Caucus

The NWPC was founded in 1971 with the goals of getting more women into public office and increasing government's awareness of feminist issues such as the ERA. A number of NWPC members are now candidates for or are already elected to public offices. The NWPC now has over 30,000 members in all states. (See Section 2 of this chapter for the address of the NWPC in your state.) A major aim of the NWPC is to get more women appointed as judges and, eventually, to have a woman appointed to the Supreme Court. Another goal is that of increasing women's participation and power in the national political parties so that women will have greater influence on platforms and policies. The NWPC publishes *Women's Political Times* six times a year. Dues are $25 per year.

National Women's Political Caucus
1411 K St NW, Suite 1110
Washington, DC 20005
(202) 347-4456

Nurses' Coalition for Action in Politics

N-CAP is a political action committee established in 1974. N-CAP is the political-action arm of the American Nurses' Association. To comply with the laws governing organizations' political activities, N-CAP is a separate organization from the ANA and has its own board of trustees. N-CAP's purposes are to educate nurses about political activities in order to encourage their involvement, and to raise funds to support the political campaigns of candidates who have demonstrated support for nursing and health care. N-CAP functions on the national level. N-CAP's contributions to 231 candidates in 1978 amounted to $98,000; of these candidates, 199 won their elections. In the same election the American Medical Association's political action committee spent $1,562,545

(*Facts About N-CAP*, August 1979). Personal contributions should be sent directly to N-CAP, as should requests for information.

N-CAP
(Nurses Coalition for Action in
    Politics)
1030 15th St NW, Suite 408
Washington, DC 20005

State N-PACs

The N-CAP at the state level is referred to as N-PAC, political action committee. The most recent listing of state N-PACs shows that there are 34 states that have them. (See state listings.) These organizations help to politically educate nurses in their state, and collect and contribute funds to candidates for state offices who are friendly to nursing issues and support good health care.

Public Citizen

Public Citizen is perhaps better known as the advocacy organization formed by Ralph Nader. Under its aegis, study groups work on special areas of concern; a well-known example is the 1971 publication on nursing homes, *Old Age: The Last Segregation*. More recently, Public Citizen has begun a Congress Watch campaign, training local consumers to utilize their rights and to develop activism skills. Well-publicized meetings with local members of Congress have advanced the consumer viewpoint over those of special-interest lobbies to influence legislation for a stronger freedom-of-information law, a consumer cooperative bank, toxic substances laws, and greater auto safety. Public Citizen operates on a local level, and the national office should be able to give you information about Congress Watch locals near you. An annual contribution of $15 or more supports national and local efforts and brings you the *Congress Watcher*, with regular ratings of Congress members' voting records.

Public Citizen
PO Box 19404
Washington, DC 20036

Women's Action Alliance

The national center of women's programs and issues has sought since 1971 to identify program resources and connect them with individuals and groups, to provide public education on feminist issues, to coordinate other institutions' activities around identified issues, and to stimulate new programs around unaddressed issues. To these ends, the alliance maintains a library for its information services, with staff assistance weekdays from 10 AM to 5:30 PM for phone or letter requests. It also makes technical assistance available to women's groups developing or strengthening their programs. This assistance includes criticizing proposals and providing a variety of how-to publications. Women's national organizations agreeing with the tenets of the 11-point Women's Bill of Rights, developed in 1975, are eligible to join the National Women's Agenda Project to work jointly to achieve the goals of that bill of rights. The alliance staff aids by bringing together groups interested in influencing policies affecting women in both the public and private sectors, or other efforts to further women's equality. Information about the alliance and its projects can be obtained from the national office.

Women's Action Alliance, Inc
370 Lexington Ave, Room 603
New York, NY 10017
(212) 532-8374

Women's Equity Action League

As a non–tax-exempt organization, WEAL actively influences legislation on issues of concern to women, including passage of the 1974 Women's Educational Equity Act. Their suit against HEW in 1977 forced that department to begin eliminating a backlog of 3,000 sex discrimination complaints. Formed in 1968, WEAL now represents more than 2,000 members. Current issues include domestic violence, Title IX complaints, pension and welfare reform, and Fair Housing Law enforcement. This organization acts as a lobbyist and advocate in Congress testifying on laws that discriminate against women. Chapters and other divisions exist in some areas of the country; more information can be obtained from the main office.

Women's Equity Action League
805 15th St NW
Washington, DC 20005
(202) 638-4560

Other Organizations

The following list contains a number of national organizations about which we do not have additional information at the time of publication but which can be useful to nurses who seek greater political involvement. They are included for your reference.

American Association of
University Women
2401 Virginia Ave NW
Washington, DC 20006
(202) 785-7750

Association of State
Democratic Chairs
1625 Massachusetts Ave NW
Washington, DC 20036
(202) 797-5900
(Ann Fishman, Executive Director)

Educational Development Center for
Women's Educational Equity Act
Program
55 Chapel St
Newton, MA 02160

ERAmerica
1525 M St NW, No. 602
Washington, DC 20005
(Coalition since 1976 to mobilize
support for ERA)

Executive Women International
2188 Highland Dr, No. 203
Salt Lake City, UT 84106
(Contact: Mary L. Johnson,
[801] 486-3121)

Federally Employed Women
National Press Building, Suite 481
Washington, DC 20045
(202) 638-4404
(225 chapters)

International Organization of
Women Executives
1800 N 78 Ct
Elmwood Park, IL 60635
(312) 980-4366
(20 proposed chapters)

National Association of Female
Executives
160 E 56th St
New York, NY 10022
(30 state associations, 987 networks)

National Commission on Working
Women
1211 Connecticut Ave NW, Suite 400
Washington, DC 20036
(202) 466-6770

National Federation of Business and
Professional Women's Clubs
2021 Massachusetts Ave NW
Washington, DC 20036
(202) 293-1000

National Foundation for Women's
Health
3300 Henry Ave
Philadelphia, PA 19129
(215) 438-9355

National Student Nurses' Association
10 Columbus Circle
New York, NY 10019

Republican National Committee
310 First St SE
Washington, DC 20003
(202) 484-6790

Women Elected Municipal Officials
Massachusetts Municipal Association
131 Tremont St
Boston, MA 02135

Women into Public Leadership
14601 Holmes
Kansas City, MO 64145
(816) 942-3960

Women in State Government
Michigan State University
College of Communication, Arts,
and Sciences
East Lansing, MI 48824

Women in State Government
PO Box 2014
Empire State Plaza Station
Albany, NY 12220

Women USA
76 Beaver St
New York, NY 10005
(Bella Abzug, founder, 1979. Hotline
    for current information on ERA,
    child care, Social Security, and
    so on: [800] 221-4945, continental
    United States; [212] 344-2531 New
    York state.)

SECTION 2: STATE ORGANIZATIONS

Alabama

Alabama Democratic Headquarters
Jefferson Federal Building
Birmingham, AL 35203
(205) 252-4143

Health Systems Agencies

  Birmingham Regional Health
     Systems Agency, Inc
  1612 Tenth Ave S
  Birmingham, AL 35205
  (205) 933-1403

  Health Systems Agency
  PO Box 264
  Gadsden, AL 35902
  (205) 543-9451

  North Alabama Health Systems
     Agency
  Huntsville Madison County Jetport
  PO Box 6147
  Huntsville, AL 35806
  (205) 772-3492

  Southwest Alabama Health
     Planning Council
  812 Downtowner Blvd, Suite E
  Mobile, AL 36609
  (205) 343-3320

  Southeast Alabama Health
     Systems Agency
  PO Box 11292
  Montgomery, AL 36111
  (205) 263-4401

  West Alabama Health Council,
     Inc
  PO Box 1488
  Tuscaloosa, AL 35402
  (205) 345-4916

League of Women Voters of
    Alabama
1528 Valley Ave
Birmingham, AL 35209
(205) 933-6466

National Association for Women Deans,
    Administrators and Counselors
Martha Ann Cox, Director of Women's
    Programs
800 Lake Shore Dr
Birmington, AL 35209

National Organization for Women
Alabama NOW Coordinator
1524 Ninth Ave S
Birmingham, AL 35205
(205) 933-8192

National Women's Political Caucus
Jane Weeks
1636 Magnolia St
Gardendale, AL 35071

Nurses Political Action Committee
N-PAC Chairperson
Alabama Nurses' Association
360 N Hull St
Montgomery, AL 36104
(205) 262-8321

The Alabama Republican Executive
Committee
PO Box 3315
Birmingham, AL 35205
(205) 322-5773

State Health Planning and Develop-
ment Agency
Alabama State Department of
Public Health
Montgomery, AL 36104
(205) 832-5994

Alabama State League for
Nursing
Mable E. Lamb
2313 Locke Lane
Birmingham, AL 35226
(205) 853-1200

Alabama State Nurses'
Association
360 N Hull St
Montgomery, AL 36104
(205) 262-8321

Alaska

Alaska Democratic Headquarters
PO Box 1590
Nome, AK 99762
(907) 274-6435
(907) 274-6134

Health Systems Agencies

Northern Alaska Health Resources
Association, Inc
529 Fifth Ave, Suite 8
Fairbanks, AK 99701
(907) 456-2553

Southeast Alaska Health Systems
Agency
PO Box 7015
Ketchikan, AK 99901
(907) 225-9681

South Central Health Planning
and Development, Inc
1135 W Eighth Ave, Suite 1
Anchorage, AK 99501
(907) 278-3631

League of Women Voters of Alaska
Jean Neale Stassel
911 R St
Anchorage, AK 99501
(907) 277-2108

National Organization for Women
Alaska NOW Coordinator
1505 Third Ave
Fairbanks, AK 99701
(907) 456-8596 (home)
(907) 456-5968 (office)

[No Nurses Political Action
Committee]

Alaska (Pro Tem)
State League for Nursing
Clair E. Martin, PhD,
Dean, School of Nursing
University of Alaska
Anchorage, AK 99504
(907) 272-5522 (office)

Republican Party of Alaska
621 W Fifth Ave, Suite C
Anchorage, AK 99501
(907) 276-4667

State Health Planning and
  Development Agency
Department of Health and
  Social Services
Pouch H 01A
Juneau, AK 99811
(907) 465-3038

National Women's Political Caucus
Carol Derfner
c/o Anchorage Art Council
402 W Third Ave, No. 7
Sunset Plaza
Anchorage, AK 99501

Alaska State Nurses
  Association
1172 Gambell
Anchorage, AK 99501
(907) 274-0827

Arizona

Arizona Democratic Headquarters
1001 N Central No. 107
Phoenix, AZ 85004
(602) 257-9136

Health Systems Agencies

  Central Arizona Health Systems
    Agency
  124 W Thomas Rd
  Phoenix, AZ 85013
  (602) 263-5277

  Health Systems Agency of
    Southeastern Arizona
  120 W Broadway, La Placita Village
  PO Box 46
  Tucson, AZ 85702
  (602) 623-5733

  Navajo Health Systems Agency
  PO Box 604
  Navajo Tribal Council
  Window Rock, AZ 86515
  (602) 871-5513

Northern Arizona Health Systems
  Agency
PO Box 896
121 E Birch, Suite 503
Flagstaff, AZ 86002
(602) 779-0325

Western Arizona Health Systems
  Agency
Century Plaza
281 W 24th St, Rm 139
Yuma, AZ 85364
(602) 726-8300

League of Women Voters of Arizona
Becky Fossdal Moon
7930 E Pima
Tucson, AZ 85715
(602) 886-6117

National Organization for Women
Arizona NOW Coordinator
337 E 12th St
Tucson, AZ 85701
(602) 792-4336
(602) 882-5350 (office)
(602) 622-6229 (AZ NOW)

National Women's Political Caucus
Elly Anderson
6550 Camino Arturo
Tucson, AZ 85718
(602) 297-3422 (home

Nurses Political Action Committee
Jan Nusbaum, N-PAC Chairperson
550 N Bedford Dr
Tucson, AZ 85710

Arizona Republican State
  Committee
40 E Thomas, Suite 100
Phoenix, AZ 85012
(602) 248-8484

State Health Planning and
Development Agency
Division of Health Resources
Arizona Department of Health
Services
1740 W Adams St, Rm 101
Phoenix, AZ 85007
(602) 255-1091

[No State League for Nursing]

Arizona State Nurses' Association
4525 N 12th St
Phoenix, AZ 85014
(602) 277-4401

Arkansas

Arkansas Democratic Headquarters
300 Spring Bldg, Suite 720
Little Rock, AR 77201
(501) 374-2361

Health Systems Agencies

Delta Hills Health Systems
Agency, Inc
PO Box 701
Newport, AR 72112
(501) 523-8973

Central Arkansas Health Systems
Agency, Inc
PO Box 530
North Little Rock, AR 72110
(501) 372-6273

South Arkansas Health Systems,
Inc
PO Box 1917
1920 N College St
El Dorado, AR 71730
(501) 862-7951

West Arkansas Health Systems
Agencies, Inc
PO Drawer H
Russellville, AR 72801
(501) 986-2229

League of Women Voters of
Arkansas
Mary Lynn Reese
918 S 15th St
Rogers, AR 72856
(501) 636-8127

National Organization for Women
Arkansas NOW Coordinator
PO Box N
Rogers, AR 72756
(501) 925-2775

National Women's Political Caucus
Pat Youngdahl
7180 Rockwood Rd
Little Rock, AR 72207
(501) 661-5800 (office)
(501) 663-8284 (home)

[No Nurses Political Action Committee]

Republican Party of Arkansas
25 Arnold Dr
Texarkana, AR 75501
(501) 773-2005

Republican Party of Arkansas
Twin City Bank Building
1 River Front Pl, Suite 620
North Little Rock, AR 72114
(501) 372-7301

State Health Planning and
Development Agency
4815 W Marham St
Little Rock, AR 72201
(501) 661-2196

Arkansas State League for Nursing
Ercle Lee Bridwell
211 Adams St
Dumas, AR 71639
(501) 382-4867 (office)

Arkansas State Nurses' Association
117 S Cedar St
Little Rock, AR 72205
(501) 664-5853

California

California Democratic Headquarters
6022 Wilshire Blvd, Suite 201
Los Angeles, CA 90036
(213) 931-1161

Health Systems Agencies
Alameda-Contra Costa
Health Systems Agency
1322 Webster St, Rm 210
Oakland, CA 94612
(415) 652-5566

California California Health Systems
Agency
208 W Main St, Suite 9
Visalia, CA 93277
(209) 733-8676

Golden Empire Health System Agency
827 Seventh St, Fourth Floor
County Administrative Building
Sacramento, CA 95814
(916) 447-3201

Health Systems Agency of San Diego
and Imperial Counties
2831 Camino del Rio S, Suite 204
San Diego, CA 92108
(714) 297-4721

Inland Counties Health Systems
Agency
12150 Lacrosse Ave
PO Box 1237
Colton, CA 92324
(714) 825-7510

Los Angeles Health Planning and
Development Agency
Contact: Fran Frey
(213) 974-1100
[interim listing]

Mid-Coast Health Systems Agency
344 Salinas St, Suite 103
PO Box 1068
Salinas, CA 93901
(408) 757-2044

North Bay Health Systems Agency
55 Marina Dr, Suite 837
Petaluma, CA 94952
(707) 762-4591

Northern California Health Systems
Agency
813 E Fifth Ave
Chico, CA 95926
(916) 895-4461

North San Joaquin Valley
Health Systems Agency
3460 Oakdale Rd, Suite E
Oakdale Sylvan Plaza
Modesto, CA 95355
(209) 529-5080

Orange County Health Planning
Council
202 Fashion Lane, Suite 219
Tustin, CA 92680
(714) 832-1841

Santa Clara County
Health Systems Agency
825 N First St, Third Floor
San Jose, CA 95112
(408) 292-9572

Ventura-Santa Barbara
Health Systems Agency
3418 Loma Vista Rd, Suite B
PO Box 3966
Ventura, CA 93003
(805) 648-7939

West Bay Health Systems Agency, Inc
215 Market St, Seventh Floor
San Francisco, CA 94105
(415) 543-4930

League of Women Voters of California
Susan F. Rice
942 Market St, Suite 505
San Francisco, CA 94102
(415) 986-1532

California National Organization for Women
California NOW Coordinator
2525 Bourbon St, M-2
Orange, CA 92665
(714) 637-8533

National Association for Women Deans, Administrators and Counselors
Dr Anne Dolan, Vice President for Student Development
University of San Francisco
San Francisco, CA 94117

National Women's Political Caucus
Gloria Kapp
830 N Citrus
Los Angeles, CA 90038

Nurse Political Action Committee
Donna Ver Steeg
California Nurses' Association
921 11th St, Suite 902
Sacramento, CA 95814
(916) 446-5021

Republican State
Central Committee of California
730 L St
Fresno, CA 93721
(209) 268-4531

Republican State Central
Committee of California
2350 N Chestnut, Suite 102
Fresno, CA 93703
(209) 252-3781

Statewide Health Planning and Development Office
California State Department of Health
714 P St, Rm 1350
Sacramento, CA 95814
(916) 445-1945

California State League for Nursing
Ellen Polfus, Director
Woodland Memorial Hospital
1325 Cottonwood
Woodland, CA 95695
(916) 662-3961 (office)

California State Nurses' Association
790 Market St
San Francisco, CA 94102
(415) 986-2220

Colorado

Colorado Democratic Party Headquarters
1535 Race St
Denver, CO 80202
(303) 320-1000

Health Systems Agencies

Central Northeast Colorado Health Systems Agency, Inc
7290 Samuel Dr, Suite 316
Denver, CO 80221
(303) 427-8460

Southeast Colorado Health Systems Agency, Inc
130 Kiowa
PO Box 2410
Colorado Springs, CO 80910
(303) 475-9395

West Colorado Health Systems Agency
2525 N Seventh St
Grand Junction, CO 81501
(303) 245-3590

League of Women Voters of Colorado
Joyce Tavrow
1600 Race St
Denver, CO 80206
(303) 320-8493

National Organization for Women
Colorado NOW Coordinator
908 Garfield St
Ft Collins, CO 80524
(303) 221-0062 (home)

National Women's Political Caucus
Gerry Bean
2755 Julliard St
Boulder, CO 80303
(303) 629-2522 (home)
(303) 499-1688 (office)

Nurses Political Action Committee
Diane Duffy, Chairperson
7212 W Portland Ave
Littleton, CO 80123
(303) 986-8459

Republican State Central
    Committee of Colorado
3600 S Yosemite, Suite 999
Denver, CO 80237
(303) 779-1557

Republican State Central
    Committee of Colorado
1275 Tremont Pl
Denver, CO 80204
(303) 893-1776

State Health Planning and
    Development
Office of Medical Care Regulation
    and Development
Colorado Department of Health
4210 E 11th Ave
Denver, CO 80220
(303) 320-8333

Colorado State League for Nursing
Theresa Brofman
3131 E Alameda Ave
Denver, CO
(303) 777-9379 (home)

Colorado State Nurses' Association
5453 E Evans Pl
Denver, CO 30222

Connecticut

Connecticut Democratic Party
    Headquarters
634 Asylum Ave
Hartford, CT 06105
(203) 278-6080

Health Systems Agencies

Health Systems Agency of
    Eastern Connecticut, Inc
12 Case St, Suite 311
Norwich, CT 06525
(203) 886-1996

Health Systems Agency of
    North Central Connecticut
999 Asylum Ave
Hartford, CT 06105
(203) 249-7581

Health Systems Agency of
    South Central Connecticut, Inc
131 Bradley Rd
Woodbridge, CT 06525
(203) 397-5400

Northwest Connecticut
    Health Systems Agency
20 E Main St, Rm 324
Waterbury, CT 06708
(203) 757-9601

Southwest Connecticut
    Health Systems Agency
20 N Main St
South Norwalk, CT 06854
(203) 853-1501

League of Women Voters of
    Connecticut
Betsy Hedden
60 Connolly Pkwy
Hamden, CT 06514
(203) 288-7996

National Organization for Women
Connecticut NOW Coordinator
3 Round Hill Rd
Granby, CT 06035
(203) 653-3044 (home)

National Women's Political Caucus
Mary Lou Cassotto
35C Grimes Rd, Apt 24
Rocky Hill, CT 06067

Nurses Political Action Committee
Donna Vose
Connecticut Nurses' Association
1 Prestige Dr
Meriden, CT 06450
(203) 238-1208

Connecticut Republicans
1 High St
Hartford, CT 06103
(203) 249-9661

State Bureau of Health Planning
    and Development
Connecticut St͡ ͜ Department of
    Health
79 Elm St
Hartford, CT 06115
(203) 566-7886

Connecticut State League for Nursing
Dr Phyllis E Porter
605 Cascade Dr
Fairfield, CT 06430
(203) 255-5411 (office)

Connecticut State Nurses' Association
1 Prestige Dr
Meriden, CT 06450
(203) 238-1208

Delaware

Delaware Democratic Headquarters
621 Delaware Ave
Wilmington, DE 19801
(302) 655-7101

Delaware Health Council, Inc
2501 Silverside Rd, Suite 5
Wilmington, DC 19801
(302) 475-3820

League of Women Voters of Delaware
Ada Leigh Soles
11th and Washington Sts, YMCA
Wilmington, DE 19801
(302) 571-8948

Association for Women Deans,
    Administrators and Counselors
Becky Gates
1714 Paisley Blue Ct
Vienna, VA 22180

National Organization for Women
Delaware NOW Coordinator
Swanwick Gardens, 9 Varmar Dr
New Castle, DE 19720
(302) 652-0234 (home)
(302) 571-7545 (office)

National Women's Political Caucus
Vivian Houghton
9 Varmar Dr
Swanwick Gardens
New Castle, DE 19720
(302) 652-0234 (home)
(302) 571-7545 (office)

Nurses Political Action Committee
Margaret Alexander, Chairperson
18 Holt St
Newark, DE 19711

Delaware Republican State Committee
2008 Pennsylvania Ave
Wilmington, DE 19806
(302) 652-3132

State Health Planning and
    Development Agency
Bureau of Health Planning
    and Resource Development
Department of Health and
    Social Services
Jesse S. Cooper Building
Dover, DE 19901
(302) 678-4776

[No State League for Nursing]
Delaware State Nurses' Association
10003 Delaware Ave, Suite 201
Wilmington, DE 19806
(302) 655-6297

District of Columbia

District of Columbia
    Democratic Headquarters
1346 Connecticut Ave NW, Rm 719
Washington, DC 20036
(202) 347-5670

[No Health Systems Agencies]

League of Women Voters of the
    District of Columbia
1346 Connecticut Ave NW, Rm 718
Washington, DC 20036
(202) 785-2616

Association for Women Deans,
    Administrators and Counselors
Becky Gates
1714 Paisley Blue Ct
Vienna, VA 22180

National Organization for Women
District of Columbia
(NOW Co-coordinator)
2700 13th Rd S, No. 511
Arlington, VA 22204
(703) 979-9569 (home)

National Organization for Women
District of Columbia
NOW Co-coordinator
6704 Fifth St, NW
Washington, DC 20012
(202) 723-3945 (home)

National Women's Political Caucus
Jennifer Oldfield
(c/o Senator Hatfield)
463 Russell HOB
Washington, DC 20510
(202) 244-8320 (office)

National Women's Political Caucus
Anita Bonds
1446 Fourth St SW
Washington, DC 20024
(202) 727-6424 (office)

Nurses Political Action Committee
Alice Farber, Chairperson
Nurse-PUSH
602 Pershing Dr
Silver Spring, MD
(202) 625-2365

District of Columbia
    Republican Committee
1735 Connecticut Ave NW
Washington, DC 20009
(202) 667-4700

State Health Planning and
    Development Agency
Office of State Agency Affairs
Department of Human Resources
1329 E St NW, Third Floor
Washington, DC 20004
(202) 727-0477

District of Columbia
    State League for Nursing
VeNeta Masson
2451 39th Pl NW
Washington, DC 20007
(202) 234-0333 (office)

District of Columbia
    State Nurses' Association
3000 Connecticut Ave NW, Suite 136
Washington, DC 20008
(202) 234-3397

Florida

Florida Democratic Headquarters
PO Box 1758
Tallahassee, FL 32302
(904) 222-3411

Health Systems Agencies

    Florida Gulf Health Systems
        Agency, Inc
    The Byllard Executive Center
    10051 Fifth St N, Suite 253
    St Petersburg, FL 33702
    (813) 576-7772

    Florida Panhandle
        Health Systems Agency, Inc
    659 Jenks Ave, Suite A
    Panama City, FL 32401
    (904) 769-1406

    Health Planning and Development
        Council for Broward County
    1164 E Oakland Park Blvd
    Ft Lauderdale, FL 33301
    (305) 564-8777

    Health Planning Council, Inc
    4423 Westroads Dr
    West Palm Beach, FL 33407
    (305) 845-6070

    Health Systems Agency of
        East Central Florida, Inc
    1000 N Orlando Ave
    PO Box 459
    Winter Park, FL 32790
    (305) 628-1292

    Health Systems Agency of
        Northeast Florida, Area 3, Inc
    1045 Riverside Ave, Suite 260
    Jacksonville, FL 32204
    (904) 356-9731

    Health Systems Agency of
        South Florida
    3050 Biscayne Blvd, Suite 601
    Miami, FL 33137
    (305) 573-0220

    North Central Florida
        Health Planning Council, Inc
    2002 NW 13th St, Suite 103
    Gainesville, FL 32601
    (904) 377-4404

    South Central Florida
        Health Systems Council, Inc
    3801 Bee Ridge Rd
    Sarasota, FL 33582
    (813) 921-4621

League of Women Voters of Florida
Lois C. Harrison
1035S S Florida Ave
Lakeland, FL 33803
(813) 682-1636

National Association for Women Deans,
    Administrators and Counselors
Louise P. Mills, Associate Dean of
    Student Personnel
University of Miami
PO Box 248106
Coral Gables, FL 33124

National Organization for Women
Florida NOW Coordinator
7400 Powers Ave, 289
Jacksonville, FL 32217
(904) 737-7529

National Women's Political Caucus
Marilyn Whisler
822 Guthrie Ct
Winter Park, FL 32792
(305) 671-5799 (home)
(305) 275-2608 (office)

[No Nurses Political Action
   Committee]

Republican State Executive
   Committee of Florida
PO Box 311
Tallahassee, FL 32302
(904) 222-7920
                    or
PO Box 16402
Jacksonville, FL 32216
(904) 724-9744

State Health Planning
   and Development Agency
Office of Health Planning and
   Development
Florida State Department of Health
   and Rehabilitation Services
1323 Winewood,
Tallahassee, FL 32301
(904) 488-7721

Florida State League for Nursing
Joan Vogel, National Director
Medical Personnel Pool
303 SE 17th St
Ft Lauderdale, FL 33316
(305) 764-2200 (office)

Florida State Nurses' Association
PO Box 6985
Orlando, FL 32803
(305) 896-3261

Georgia

Georgia Democratic Headquarters
1627 Peachtree St NE, Suite 306
Atlanta, GA 30309
(404) 892-4788

Health Systems Agencies

Appalachian Georgia Health Systems
   Agency
PO Box 829
Cartersville, GA 30120
(404) 386-2431

East Central Georgia
   Health Systems Agency, Inc
Georgia Railroad Bank Building
699 Broad St, Suite 1114
Augusta, GA 30902
(404) 724-9927

Health Service Area 1—Interstate
[See Tennessee Area 3]

Health Systems Agency of
   Central Georgia, Inc
PO Box 2305
Kennesaw Life Building, Suite 700
Warner Robins, GA 31093
(912) 922-2215

North Central Georgia
   Health Systems Agency, Inc
Kennesaw Life Building, Suite 700
1447 Peachtree St NE
Atlanta, GA 30309
(404) 898-8600

Southwest Georgia
   Health Systems Agency, Inc
PO Box 4229
Albany, GA 31706
(912) 883-5070

Southeast Georgia
   Health Systems Agency, Inc
PO Box 1455
Brunswick, GA 31520
(912) 264-3525

League of Women Voters of Georgia
3272 Peachtree Rd NE, Suite 353
Atlanta, GA 30305
(404) 237-9294

National Organization for Women
Georgia NOW Coordinator
679 Courtenay Dr
Columbus, GA 31907
(404) 682-2483

National Women's Political Caucus
Kay Shearer Fors
360 Ponderosa Dr
Athens, GA 30605
(404) 549-0185 (home)

Nurses Political Action Committee
Georgia Nurses' Association
PAC Contact Person
269 Tenth St, NE
Atlanta, GA 30309
(404) 875-9766

National Association for Women Deans,
    Administrators and Counselors
Lynn Benson, Counselor
Armstrong State University
119 Albercorn St
Savannah, GA 31406

Georgia Republican Party
1 Park Pl, Suite 204
1900 Emery St NW
Atlanta, GA 30318
(404) 352-1150
                or
3100 Equitable Bldg
100 Peachtree St
Atlanta, GA 30303
(404) 572-6500

State Health Planning and
    Development Agency
43A Executive Park East NE
Atlanta, GA 30329
(404) 634-6342

Georgia State League for Nursing
Barbara Harvey
4860 Northland Dr
Atlanta, GA 30324
(404) 656-4913 (office)

Hawaii

Hawaii Democratic Headquarters
33 S King St, Suite 216
Honolulu, HI 96813
(808) 536-2258

[No Health Systems Agencies]

League of Women Voters of Hawaii
116 S King St, Suite 504
Honolulu, HI 96813
(808) 531-7448

National Organization for Women
Hawaii NOW Coordinator
1801 Tenth Ave
Honolulu, HI 96816
(808) 737-9254

Nurses Political Action Committee
Patricia Bilyk
94-178 Anania Dr, No. 359
Mililani, HI 96789

Republican Party of Hawaii
1136 Union Mall, Rm 203
Honolulu, HI 96813
(808) 533-6839
                or
PO Box 10375
Honolulu, HI 96816
(808) 524-1517

Hawaii State Health Planning
    and Development Agency
State Department of Health
1250 Punchbowl St
PO Box 3378
Honolulu, HI 96801
(808) 584-4050

Hawaii State League for Nursing
Barbara Ideta
700 Richards St, No. 1803
Honolulu, HI 96813
(808) 538-9011

Hawaii State Nurses' Association
677 Ala Moana Blvd, Suite 1014A
Honolulu, HI 96813
(808) 531-1628

Idaho

Idaho Democratic Headquarters
PO Box 445
Boise, ID 83701
(208) 333-1815

Idaho Health Systems Agency, Inc
512 W Idaho St
PO Box 8868
Boise, ID 83707
(208) 336-1660

League of Women Voters of Idaho
Sallee Gasser
420 S 12th
Pocatello, ID 83201
(208) 232-6285

National Organization for Women
Idaho NOW Coordinator
1417 E First St
Moscow, ID 83843
(208) 882-8852

[No Nurses Political Action
Committee]

Idaho Republication State
Central Committee
PO Box 2267
Simplot Building
Boise, ID 83701
(208) 343-6405
or
485 E St
Idaho Falls, ID 83401
(208) 523-4650

State Health Planning and
Development Agency
Idaho State Department of Health
and Welfare
State House
Boise, ID 83720
(208) 384-3272

[No State League for Nursing]

Idaho State Nurses' Association
1134 N Orchard
Boise, ID 83704
(208) 377-0226

Illinois

Illinois Democratic Headquarters
Bismarck Hotel, Rm 501
171 W Randolph
Chicago, IL 60601
(213) 372-1161

Health Systems Agencies

City of Chicago
Commission for Health Planning
and Resources Development
180 N Lasalle St, Suite 700
Chicago, IL 60601
(312) 744-5877

Comprehensive Health Planning
of Northwest Illinois, Inc
206 W State St, Suite 1008
Rockford, IL 61101
(815) 968-0720

Comprehensive Health Planning
in Southern Illinois
PO Box 3698
608 E College St
Carbondale, IL 62901
(618) 549-2161

East Central Illinois
  Health Systems Agency
302 E John St, Suite 1707
Champaign, IL 61820
(217) 333-3987

Health Systems Agency for Kane,
  Lake, and McHenry
  Counties, Inc.
188 S Northwest Hwy
Cary, IL 60013
(312) 639-0061

Illinois Central
  Health Systems Agency
PO Box 2200
East Peoria, IL 61611
(309) 694-6451

Illowa Health Systems Agency
2707 Kimberly Rd
Bettendorf, IA 52722
(319) 359-3661

Region 9 Health Systems
  Agency, Inc
1520 N Rock Run Dr, Suite 22
Crest Hill, IL 60435
(815) 744-2515

Suburban Cook/Dupage
  Health Systems Agency, Inc
1010 Lake St
Oak Park, IL 60301
(312) 524-9700

West Central Illinois
  Health Systems Agency, Inc
Ridgely Building, Rm 813
504 E Monroe
Springfield, IL 62701
(217) 544-3412

League of Women Voters of Illinois
Janet Otwell
67 E Madison St
Chicago, IL 60603
(312) 236-0315

National Association for Women Deans,
  Administrators and Counselors
E. Maxine Bloom
817 Robinhood Lane
LaGrange Park, IL 60525

National Organization for Women
Illinois NOW Coordinator
RR 2, Pilot Knob Rd
Galena, IL 61036
(815) 777-0504 (home)

National Women's Political Caucus
Marcia Gevers
417 Winnebago
Park Forest, IL 60466
(312) 747-1455 (home)

Nurses Political Action Committee
Illinois Nurses' Association
Springfield Office Building
608 Myers Building
1 W Old State Capitol Plaza
Springfield, IL 62701
(217) 523-0781

Illinois Republican State
  Central Committee
200 S Second St
Springfield, IL 62701
(217) 525-0011
            or
Cook County Office
127 N Dearborn St, Rm 828
Chicago, IL 60602
(312) 641-6400

State Health Planning and
  Development Agency
Department of Public Health
525 W Jefferson St
Springfield, IL 62761
(217) 785-2040

Illinois State League for Nursing
Carol Eady
1115 S Seminary
Park Ridge, IL 60068
(312) 751-6194 (office)

Illinois State Nurses' Association
6 N Michigan Ave
Chicago, IL 60602
(312) 236-9708

Indiana

Indiana Democratic Headquarters
311 W Washington
Indianapolis, IN 46204
(317) 635-8581

Health Systems Agencies

Central Indiana Health Systems
Agency, Inc
3901 W 86th St
Indianapolis, IN 46268
(317) 297-3990

North Indiana Health Systems
Agency, Inc
900 E Colfax Ave
South Bend, IN 46617
(219) 233-5149

Southern Indiana Health Systems
Agency, Inc
2222 W Eighth St
Bedford, IN 47421
(812) 275-5984

League of Women Voters of Indiana
Roberta Jaffe
539 Illinois Building
17 W Market St
Indianapolis, IN 46204
(317) 634-3588

National Association for Women
Deans, Administrators and
Counselors
Vicki Mech Fields,
Associate Dean of Students
Anderson College,
Anderson, IN 46011

National Organization for Women
Indiana NOW Coordinator
3530 Donald Ave
Indianapolis, IN 46224
(317) 291-8671 (home)
(317) 634-6481 (office)

National Women's Political Caucus
Molly Rucker
5722 Radnor Rd
Indianapolis, IN 46226
(317) 634-6173 (office)

[No Nurses Political Action
Committee]

Indiana Republican State
Central Committee
150 W Market St, Suite 200
Indianapolis, IN 46204
(317) 635-7561

State Health Planning
and Development Agency
Indiana State Board of Health
1330 W Michigan St
Indianapolis, IN 46206
(317) 633-8400

Indiana Citizens' State
League for Nursing
Marjorie Miller
214 S Eighth St
Vincennes, IN 47591
(812) 885-4408 (office)

Indiana State Nurses' Association
3231 N Meridian St, Suite 53
Indianapolis, IN 46208
(317) 923-5337

Iowa

Iowa Democratic Headquarters
1120 Mulberry
Des Moines, IA 50309
(515) 244-7292

Iowa Health Systems Agency
700 Fleming Building
218 Sixth Ave
Des Moines, IA 50309
(515) 247-8711

League of Women Voters of Iowa
Jane Teaford
610 Capital City Bank Building
E Fifth and Locust Sts
Des Moines, IA 50309
(515) 282-6897

National Organization for Women
Iowa NOW Coordinator
321 E Church St, Apt 2
Iowa City, IA 52240
(319) 351-6753 (home)

National Women's Political Caucus
Nancy Sweetman
9 N Georgia
Mason City, IA 50401
(515) 432-9231 (home)

[No Nurses Political
Action Committee]

Republican State
Central Committee of Iowa
1540 High St
Des Moines, IA 50309
(515) 282-8105
or
2300 Financial Center
Des Moines, IA 50309
(515) 243-2300

State Health Planning and
Development Agency
Iowa State Health Department
Lucas State Office Building
Des Moines, IA 50319
(515) 281-4340
(515) 281-4342

Iowa State League for Nursing
Buelane Daugherty
1630 First Ave NE, Apt D
Cedar Rapids, IA 52402
(319) 363-8213 (office)

Iowa State Nurses' Association
810 Walnut
Des Moines, IA 50309
(515) 282-9169

Kansas

Kansas Democratic Headquarters
PO Box 1914
Topeka, KS 66601
(913) 234-0425

Health Systems Agencies

Health Systems Agency of
Southeast Kansas, Inc
221 N Main St, Suite 231
Wichita, KS 67202
(316) 264-2861

Health Planning Association
of Western Kansas, Inc
25th and Vine
Hays, KS 67601
(913) 628-2868

League of Women Voters of Kansas
Marilyn T. Brandt
909 Topeka Blvd, Annex
Topeka, KS 66612
(913) 354-7478

National Organization for Women
Kansas NOW Coordinator
506 Paula
Wichita, KS 67209
(316) 722-4953 (home)

National Women's Political Caucus
Katie Krider
117 Woodlawn
Topeka, KS 66606
(913) 296-2063 (office)
(913) 235-3396 (home)

Nurses Political Action Committee
Kansas State Nurses' Association
820 Quincy, Rm 520
Topeka, KS 66612
(913) 233-8638

Kansas Republican State Committee
501 Jefferson, Suite 22
Topeka, KS 66607
(913) 234-3416
                    or
2500 W Sixth St
Lawrence, KS 66044
(913) 843-7114

State Health Planning and
    Development Agency
Bureau of Health Planning
Kansas Department of Health
    and Environment
6700 S Topeka Ave
Topeka, KS 66620
(913) 296-3745

Kansas State League for Nursing
W. Jean Schulte
1109-1/2 Drum
Hays, KS 67601
(913) 628-5835 (office)

Kansas State Nurses' Association
820 Quincy St
Topeka, KS 66612
(913) 233-8638

Kentucky

Kentucky Democratic Headquarters
PO Box 694
Frankfort, KY 40602
(502) 695-4828

Health Systems Agencies

East Kentucky
    Health Systems Agency, Inc
7 Carol Rd
PO Box 557
Winchester, KY 40391
(606) 744-7950

Kentucky Health Systems
    Agency West, Inc
1941 Bishop Lane, Suite 401
Louisville, KY 40218
(502) 456-6460

League of Women Voters of Kentucky
Marion Scott Kenkel
3421 Westridge Circle
Lexington, KY 40502
(606) 277-6871

National Association for Women Deans,
    Administrators and Counselors
Gloria G. Van Winkle
PO Box 2111
Berea College
Berea, KY 40404

National Organization for Women
Kentucky NOW Coordinator
2044 Georgian Way, Apt G58
Lexington, KY 40502
(606) 277-4446 (home)
(606) 252-3591 (work)

National Women's Political Caucus
Sara Creed
1381 Tyler Park Dr
Louisville, KY 40204

Nurses Political Action Committee
Diane Carlin
Chairperson, KY N-PAC
PO Box 8342, Station E
Louisville, KY 40208
(502) 459-6299

Republican Party of Kentucky
Capitol Ave at Third
Frankfort, KY 40601
(502) 875-5130

or

Route 1
Cave City, KY 42127
(502) 453-2231

State Health Planning and
    Development Agency
Center for Comprehensive Health
    Systems Development
Department of Human Resources
Health Service Building
275 E Main St
Frankfort, KY 40601
(502) 564-4860

Kentucky State League for Nursing
Paulina Fields Sloan
2841 Southview Dr
Lexington, KY 40503
(606) 622-1827 (office)

Kentucky State Nurses' Association
1400 S First St
PO Box 8342, Station E
Louisville, KY 40208
(502) 637-2546
(502) 637-2547

Louisiana

Louisiana Democratic Headquarters
5700 Florida Blvd, No. 322
Baton Rouge, LA 70806
(504) 923-1216

Health Systems Agencies

Mid-Louisiana Health Systems
    Agency
5420 Corporate Blvd, Suite 201
Baton Rouge, LA 70808
(504) 927-9740

New Orleans Area/Bayou-River
    Health Systems Agency, Inc
700 Masonic Temple Building
333 St Charles Ave
New Orleans, LA 70130
(504) 581-6821

North Louisiana
    Health Systems Agency, Inc
PO Box 3463
1600 Fairfield Ave, Rm 401
Shreveport, LA 71103
(318) 424-4441

League of Women Voters
    of Louisiana
June M. Rudd
850 N Fifth St, Apt 103
Baton Rouge, LA 70802
(504) 344-3326

National Association for Women Deans,
    Administrators and Counselors
Jo Eddie Schroeder
Ryan St
Lake Charles, LA 70609

National Organization for Women
Louisiana NOW Coordinator
5509 Coliseum St
New Orleans, LA 70115
(504) 891-2645 (home)
(504) 586-3981 (office)

National Women's Political Caucus
Louadrian Reed
4535 S Prieur
New Orleans, LA 70501

Nurses Political Action Committee
Sandy Bagley, PAC Contact
450 Cloud Dr, Apt 18
Baton Rouge, LA 70806
(504) 923-0268

The Republican Party of Louisiana
733 E Airport, Suite 102
Baton Rouge, LA 70806
(504) 924-6588
               or
202 Beck Building
Shreveport, LA 71101
(318) 221-6143

State Health Planning and
     Development Agency
Department of Health and
     Human Resources
150 Riverside Mall, Suite 410
Baton Rouge, LA 70801
(504) 389-6201

Louisiana State League for Nursing
Lillian Samardzija, Director
     of Nursing
Touro Infirmary
1401 Foucher St
New Orleans, LA 70115
(504) 897-8447 (office)

Louisiana State Nurses' Association
PO Box 837
Metairie, LA 70004
(504) 889-1030

Maine

Maine Democratic Headquarters
62 State St
Augusta, ME 04330
(207) 662-6233

Maine Health Systems Agency, Inc
2 Central Plaza
Augusta, ME 04333
(207) 623-1182

League of Women Voters of Maine
Alice A. Johnson
PO Box 216
Tuner, ME 04282
(207) 225-3647

National Organization for Women
Maine NOW Coordinator
23 March St
Bangor, ME 04401
(207) 942-2830

National Women's Political Caucus
Jane Riley
3 Chestnut St
Hallowell, ME 04347
(207) 623-9091

[No Nurses Political
     Action Committee]

Maine Republican State Committee
187 State St
Augusta, ME 04330
(207) 622-6247
               or
36 Pinewood Dr
Cumberland Center, ME 04021
(207) 829-5257

State Bureau of Health Planning
     and Development
Department of Human Services
State House
151 Capitol St
Augusta, ME 04333
(207) 289-2736

[No State League for Nursing]

Maine State Nurses' Association
83 Western Ave
Augusta, ME 04330
(207) 622-1057

Maryland

Maryland Democratic Headquarters
120 W Road St
Baltimore, MD 21201
(301) 539-1500

Health Systems Agencies

Central Maryland
    Health Systems Agency
501 St Paul Pl
Baltimore, MD 21202
(301) 752-3500

Department of Health
    Systems Planning
Montgomery County Government
611 Rockville Pike
Rockville, MD 20850
(301) 279-8366

Health Planning Council
    Eastern Shore, Inc
PO Box 776
Cambridge, MD 21613
(301) 228-8911

Southern Maryland
    Health Systems Agency
PO Box 85
Clinton, MD 20735
(301) 868-6206

Western Maryland
    Health Systems Agency
134 N Mechanic St
Cumberland, MD 21502
(301) 724-1616

National Association for Women Deans,
    Administrators and Counselors
Becky Gates
1714 Paisley Blue Ct
Vienna, VA 22180

League of Women Voters of Maryland
5 State Circle
Annapolis, MD 21401
(301) 269-0232 or (202) 261-2413

National Organization for Women
Maryland NOW Coordinator
11 S Augusta Ave
Baltimore, MD 21229
(301) 646-3336

National Women's Political Caucus
Pam Brewington
3613 Underwood
Chevy Chase, MD 20015

Nurses Political Action Committee
c/o Maryland Nurses' Association
2315-17 St Paul St
Baltimore, MD 21218
(301) 889-1485

Republican State
    Central Committee of Maryland
60 W St, Suite 201
Annapolis, MD 21401
(301) 269-0113

State Health Planning and
    Development Agency
Maryland Health Planning and
    Development Agency
O'Connor Building
201 W Preston St, Fifth Floor
Baltimore, MD 21201
(301) 383-2430

Maryland State League for Nursing
Donna M. Dorsey
6391 Scarlett Petal
Columbia, MD 21045
(301) 528-7698 (office)

Maryland State Nurses'
    Association, Inc
2315-17 St Paul St
Baltimore, MD 21218
(301) 889-1485

Massachusetts

Massachusetts Democratic
    Headquarters
11 Beacon St
Boston, MA 02108
(617) 367-4760

Health Systems Agencies

Central Massachusetts
    Health Systems Agency
El Grande Office Building
415 Boston Turnpike
Shrewsbury, MA 01545
(617) 845-1066

Health Planning Council
    for Greater Boston
294 Washington St, Suite 630
Boston, MA 02108
(617) 426-2022

Merrimack Valley
    Health Planning Council, Inc
120 Parker St
Lawrence, MA 01843
(617) 686-1621

Southeastern Massachusetts
    Health Planning and
    Development, Inc
PO Box 70
Middleboro, MA 02346
(617) 947-6300

Western Massachusetts
    Health Planning Council
59 Interstate Dr
West Springfield, MA 01089
(413) 781-2845

North Shore Health Planning
    Council
10 First Ave
Peabody, MA 01960
(617) 531-7006

League of Women Voters
    of Massachusetts
120 Boylston St
Boston, MA 02116
(617) 357-8380

National Association for Women Deans,
    Administrators and Counselors
Dr Alice Jeghelian,
    Assistant to the President
Boston College
Chestnut Hill, MA 02167

National Organization for Women
Massachusetts NOW Coordinaotr
27 Walker St
Cambridge, MA 02138
(617) 547-3336

National Women's Political Caucus
Donna Kuha
c/o Tucker Anthony Brokerage Firm
RL Day, Inc
1 Beacon St
Boston, MA 02108

Nurses Political Action Committee
Chris Janis, Chairperson, MASS-PAC
c/o Massachusetts Nurses'
    Association
141 Tremont
Boston, MA 02111
(617) 482-5465

Massachusetts Republican
    State Committee
73 Tremont St, Room 1125
Boston, MA 02108
(617) 523-7535
                    or
3 Suzanne Terrace
North Grafton, MA 01536
(617) 734-9000

State Health Planning
    and Development Agency
Massachusetts Department
    of Public Health
600 Washington St, Room 614
Boston, MA 02111
(617) 727-4164

Massachusetts State
   Nurses' Association
141 Tremont St
Boston, MA 02111
(617) 482-5465

Massachusetts-Rhode Island
   State League for Nursing
Mary Lou Lovering
PO Box 502
Shrewsbury, MA 01545
(617) 752-7700 (office)

Michigan

Michigan Democratic Headquarters
1535 E Lafayette
Detroit, MI 48207
(313) 393-2944

Health Systems Agencies

   Comprehensive Health Planning
      Council of Southeast Michigan
   1300 Book Building
   Detroit, MI 48226
   (313) 964-6950

   East Central Michigan
      Health Systems Agency
   1213 S Washington
   Saginaw, MI 48601
   (517) 754-0421

   Genesee, Lapeer and Shiawassee
      Health Systems Agency
   Walter Reuther Building, Room 325
   708 Root St
   Flint, MI 48503
   (313) 238-0650

   Michigan Mid-South
      Health Systems Agency, Inc
   528 Mason Plaza
   Mason, MI 48854
   (517) 676-4046

Northern Michigan
   Health Systems Agency
325 E Lake St
Hollywood Building
Petoskey, MI 49770
(616) 347-7772

Southeast Michigan
   Health Systems Agency, Inc
6126 Lovers Lane
Kalamazoo, MI 49002
(616) 323-3410

Upper Peninsula
   Health Systems Agency
1500 W Washington St
Marquette, MI 49855
(906) 228-7733

West Michigan
   Health Systems Agency
300 Peoples Building
Grand Rapids, MI 49502
(616) 459-1323

League of Women Voters
   of Michigan
202 Mill St
Lansing, MI 48933
(517) 484-5383

National Association for Women Deans,
   Administrators and Counselors
Dorothy Bennet
33165 Maplenut
Farmington, MI 48024

National Organization for Women
Michigan NOW Coordinator
13610 Cedargrove
Detroit, MI 48205
(313) 526-0930 (home)
(313) 226-7022 (office)

National Women's Political Caucus
Sally Ann Payton
1928 Lorraine Pl
Ann Arbor, MI 48104
(313) 994-8022
(313) 763-0220

Nurses Political Action Committee
Bill Ludwig, Contact, INPUT
Michigan Nurses' Association
120 Spartan Ave
East Lansing, MI 48823
(517) 337-1653

Michigan Republican State
    Committee
223 N Walnut St
Lansing, MI 48933
(517) 487-5413

State Health Planning and
    Development Agency
Office of Health and Medical Affairs
Lewis Cass Building
PO Box 30026
Lansing, MI 48909
(517) 373-8155

Michigan State League for Nursing
Mr. Sterling Breed
867 Dobbin Dr
Kalamazoo, MI 49007
(616) 383-1850 (office)

Michigan State Nurses' Association
120 Spartan St
East Lansing, MI 48823
(517) 337-1653

Minnesota

Minnesota Democratic Headquarters
730 E 38th St
Minneapolis, MN 55407
(612) 827-5421

Health Systems Agencies

Central Minnesota
    Health Systems Agency
113 Division St
Sauk Rapids, MN 56379
(612) 253-2930

Health Systems Area 1–Interstate
[see North Dakota, Area 2]

Health Systems of
    Western Lake Superior, Inc
202 Ordean Building
424 W Superior St
Duluth, MN 55802
(218) 727-8371

Metropolitan Council
300 Metro Square Building
Seventh and Robert Streets
St Paul, MN 55101
(612) 291-6351

Minnesota Health Systems, Agency 6
PO Box 156
Redwood Falls, MN 56283
(507) 637-3575

Southeastern Minnesota
    Health Systems Agency
303 Marquette Bank Building
South Broadway and Second St SE
Rochester, MN 55901
(507) 285-0900

League of Women Voters
    of Minnesota
555 Wabasha
St Paul, MN 55102
(612) 224-5445

National Organization for Women
Minnesota NOW Coordinator
220 Marshall Ave, No. 2
St Paul, MN 55102
(612) 226-9772 (home)
(612) 298-0999 (office)

National Women's Political Caucus
Carol Connolly
1382 Summit Ave
St Paul, MN 55105
(612) 698-0117 (home)

National Women's Political Caucus
1821 University Ave, Room S-291
St Paul, MN 55104

National Women's Political Caucus
Marilyn Bryant
17819 Maple Hill Rd
Wayzata, MN 55391
(612) 473-4808 (home)

Nurses Political Action Committee
Maureen Davis, Chairperson MINN-
PIN
7308 39th Ave N
New Hope, MN 55427
(612) 537-2462

Independent Republicans of
Minnesota
555 Wabasha St
St Paul, MN 55102
(612) 291-1286

State Health Planning
and Development Agency
Capitol Square Building
550 Cedar St
St Paul, MN 55101
(612) 296-2407

Minnesota State League for Nursing
Joan Janusz
764 Gramsie Rd
Shoreview, MN
(612) 483-3794 (home)

Minnesota State
Nurses' Association
Griggs-Midway Building, Suite 152
1821 University Ave
St Paul, MN 55104
(612) 646-4807

Mississippi

Mississippi Democratic
Headquarters
PO Box 1583
Jackson, MS 39205
(601) 969-2913

Mississippi Health
Systems Agency, Inc
Watkins Building, Suite 400
510 George St
Jackson, MS 39201
(601) 948-8905

League of Women Voters
of Mississippi
Route 2, PO Box 413-41
Meridian, MS 39301
(601) 483-1723

National Organization for Women
Mississippi NOW Coordinator
425 Second St
Gulfport, MS 39501
(601) 863-6075 (home)
(601) 864-8284 (office)

National Women's Political Caucus
Linda St Martin
PO Box 5433
University, MS 38677
(601) 234-6253

[No Nurses Political Action
Committee]

Mississippi Republican Party
PO Box 1178
518 E Capitol St
Jackson, MS 39205
(601) 948-5191   or
PO Box 4457
Greenville, MS 38701
(601) 335-7138

State Health Planning
and Development Agency
Watkins Building, Suite 100
510 George St
Jackson, MS 39201
(601) 354-7621

[No State League for Nursing]

Mississippi State
Nurses' Association
135 Bounds St, Suite 100
Jackson, MS 39206
(601) 366-1416

Missouri

Missouri Democratic Headquarters
PO Box 719
Jefferson City, MO 65102
(314) 636-5241

Health Systems Agencies

Area 11 Health Systems Agency
of Missouri, Inc
1326 S Morley St
Moberly, MO 65270
(816) 263-4343

Greater St Louis
Health Systems Agency, Inc
915 Olive St
St Louis, MO 63101
(314) 241-5810

Mid-America
Health Systems Agency
20 W Ninth St, Suite 715
Kansas City, MO 64105
(816) 421-2710

Missouri Area 5
Health Systems Agency Council
211 S Broadway
Poplar Bluff, MO 63901
(314) 785-7737

Southwest Missouri
Health Systems Agency
2835B E Division
Springfield, MO 65803
(417) 866-2727

League of Women Voters
of Missouri
2138 Woodson Rd, Suite 6
St Louis, MO 63114
(314) 429-6161

National Organization for Women
Missouri NOW Coordinator
PO Box 1521
Kansas City, MO 64141
(816) 561-6499 (home)
(913) 362-1303 (work)

National Women's Political Caucus
Erika Fox
214 W Concord
Kansas City, MO 64112
(816) 842-0800 (home)
(816) 361-3657 (office)

[No Nurses Political Action
Committee]

Missouri Republican State
Committee
PO Box 73
507 E High St
Jefferson City, MO 65102
(314) 636-3146
or
100 N Broadway
St Louis, MO 63102
(314) 231-0100

State Health Planning
and Development Agency
Division of Special Services
Department of Social Services
Broadway State Office Building
Jefferson City, MO 65101
(314) 751-2055

Missouri State League for Nursing
Emily Huber
6 Graymore Dr
Chesterfield, MO 63107
(314) 454-7000 (office)

Missouri State Nurses' Association
206 E Dunklin St
Box 325
Jefferson City, MO 65101
(314) 636-4623

Montana

Montana Democratic Party
PO Box 802
Helena, MT 59601
(406) 442-9520

Montana Health Systems Agency
324 Fuller Ave
Helena, MT 59601
(406) 443-5965

League of Women Voters of Montana
Ardelle C. Hulburt
16 Hidden Valley Rd
Harve, MT 59501
(406) 265-2663

National Organization for Women
Montana NOW Coordinator
2212 First Ave N
Great Falls, MT 59401
(406) 453-4129 (home)
(406) 452-9564 (office)

National Women's Political Caucus
Susan Selig Wallwork
120 Evans Ave
Missoula, MT 59801

Nurses Political Action Committee
N-PAC Chairperson
Madeline Samson
620 Floweree
Helena, MT 59601
or
N-PAC Chairperson
Fay Thomson
Wolf Creek, MT 59648

Montana Republican State
    Central Committee
1425 Helena Ave
Helena, MT 59601
(406) 442-6469
or
PO Box 753
Sidney, MT 59270
(406) 482-3212

State Health Planning
    and Development Agency
Bureau of Health Planning
    and Resource Development
State Department of Health
    and Environmental Sciences
Division of Hospital
    and Medical Facilities
Cogswell Building
Helena, MT 59601
(406) 449-3121

Montana State League for Nursing
Beverly J. Johnson
9 Nimitz Dr
Billings, MT 59101
(406) 657-4000 (office)

Montana State Nurses' Association
1716 Ninth Ave
Helena, MT 59601
(406) 442-6710

Nebraska

Nebraska Democratic Headquarters
2635 O St
Lincoln, NE 68510
(402) 475-4584

Health Systems Agencies

Greater Nebraska HSA, Inc
2201 N Wheeler
Grand Island, NE 68801
(308) 384-2368

Health Planning Council
   of the Midlands, Inc
7202 Jones St
Omaha, NE 68114
(402) 393-6404

Southeast Nebraska
   Health System Agency
215 Centennial Mall S, Room 417
Lincoln, NE 68508
(402) 432-4402

League of Women Voters of Nebraska
Patricia H. Stephen
1614 N St
Lincoln, NE 68508
(402) 475-1411

National Association for Women
   Deans, Administrators
   and Counselors
Karen McCammond, Dean of Women
Nebraska Wesleyan University
50th and St Paul Streets
Lincoln, NE 68504

National Organization for Women
Nebraska NOW Coordinator
PO Box 96
Bartley, NE 69020
(406) 453-4129 (home)
(406) 452-9564 (office)

National Women's Political Caucus
Virginia Zais
11518 Raleigh Dr
Omaha, NE 68164
(402) 493-3475 (home)
(402) 221-4117 (office)

Nurses Political Action Committee
N-PAC Chairperson
Mary Ann Sak
Nebraska Nurses' Association
10730 Pacific St, Suite 26
Omaha, NE 68114
(402) 391-8920

Nebraska Republican
   State Central Committee
Anderson Building, No. 212
116 N 12th St
Lincoln, NE 68598
(402) 475-2122

State Health Planning
   and Development Agency
Nebraska State Department of Health
301 Centennial Mall S
PO Box 95007
Lincoln, NE 68509
(402) 471-2337

Nebraska State League for Nursing
Kathleen Wach
PO Box 356
Sutton, NE 68979
(402) 463-2471 (office)

Nebraska State Nurses' Association
10730 Pacific St, Suite 26
Omaha, NE 68114
(402) 391-8920

Nevada

Nevada Democratic Headquarters
1111 Las Vegas Blvd S
Las Vegas, NV 89104
(702) 382-7397

Greater Nevada Health Systems
   Agency
1135 Terminal Way, Suite 106
PO Box 11795
Reno, NV 89510
(702) 323-1791

League of Women Voters of Nevada
Mary K. Forrester
2703 Natalie Ave
Las Vegas, NV 89121
(702) 457-3465

National Organization for Women
Nevada NOW Coordinator
1332 E Serape Circle, No. 2
Las Vegas, NV 89109
(702) 732-2618 (home)

National Women's Political Caucus
Jill Derby
Rt 3, Box 105
Gardnerville, NV 89410
(702) 782-3949

Nurses Political Action Committee
N-PAC
Jean K. Rambo, Chairperson
5936 S Topaz Rd
Las Vegas, NV 89120

Republican State
    Central Committee of Nevada
PO Box 1886
Reno, NV 89505
(702) 786-3146
                or
PO Box 460
Reno, NV 89504
(702) 323-8633

State Health Planning
    and Development Agency
Office of Health Planning
    and Resources
Nevada State Department
    of Human Resources
505 E King St, Room 605
Carson City, NV 89710
(702) 885-4720

Nevada State League for Nursing
Jo Deen Howe
4190 Billy Dr
Reno, NV 89502
(702) 827-3943 (office)

Nevada State Nurses' Association
3660 Baker Lane
Reno, NV 89509
(702) 825-3555

New Hampshire

New Hampshire Democratic
    Headquarters
77 N Main St
Concord, NH 03301
(603) 228-0191

United Health Systems Agency, Inc
2–1/2 Beacon St
Concord, NH 03301
(603) 228-1506

League of Women Voters
    of New Hampshire
Virginia A. Higgins
Nashua Rd
Pelham, NH 03076
(603) 225-5344

National Organization for Women
New Hampshire NOW Coordinator
PO Box 84
Concord, NH 03301
(603) 225-5277 (home)
(603) 224-7741 (office)

National Women's Political Caucus
Donna McEachern
50 Meadow Rd
Portsmouth, NH 03802
(603) 436-7966

Nurses Political Action Committee
N-PAC
Sister M. Augustine San Souci,
    Executive Director
New Hampshire Nurses' Association
48 West St
Concord, NH 03301
(602) 225-3783

New Hampshire
    Republican State Committee
134 N Main St
Concord, NH 03301
(603) 225-9341
                or
24 Samoset Dr
Salem, NH 0..79
(603) 893-1042

State Health Planning
    and Development Agency
State of New Hampshire
Health and Welfare Building
Hazen Dr
Concord, NH 03301
(603) 271-2221

New Hampshire
    State League for Nursing
Virginia B. Young
41 Oak St
Milford, NH 03055
(603) 673-3551 (office)

New Hampshire
    State Nurses' Association
48 West St
Concord, NH 03301
(603) 225-3783

New Jersey

New Jersey Democratic Headquarters
226 W State St
Trenton, NJ 08608
(609) 392-3367

Health Systems Agencies

Bergen-Passaic Health Systems
    Agency
2 University Plaza
Hackensack, NJ 07601
(201) 646-9090

Central Jersey Health
    Planning Council, Inc
Twin Rivers Mall,
    Professional Center
Route 33
Hightstown, NJ 08520
(609) 443-4232

Hudson Health Systems Agency
871 Bergen Ave
Jersey City, NJ 07306
(201) 451-5024

Regional Health Planning Council
8 Park Pl
Newark, NJ 07102
(201) 622-3280

Southern New Jersey
    Health Systems Agency
Kor-Center W, Suite 101
Interstate Industrial Park
Bellmawr, NJ 08031
(609) 933-0641

League of Women
    Voters of New Jersey
Joan A Crowley
460 Bloomfield Ave
Montclair, NJ 07042
(201) 746-1465

National Organization for Women
New Jersey NOW Coordinator
32 W Lafayette St
Trenton, NJ 08608
(201) 255-5246 (home)
(609) 393-7474 (work)

National Women's Political Caucus
Kathy Brock
41 Kent Pl Blvd
Summit, NJ 07901
(201) 273-3812 (home)
(201) 624-1815 (office)

Nurses Political Action Committee
Andrea Bretz Savits,
   Chairperson, N-CAP
42 Hartshorne Rd
Locust, NJ 07760
(201) 291-4270

New Jersey Republican
   State Committee
28 W State St, Room 612
Trenton, NJ 08608
(609) 989-7300
            or
409 Kenwood Dr
Moorestown, NJ 08057
(609) 235-8735

State Health Planning
   and Development Agency
Division of Health Planning
   and Resource Development
State Department of Health
Health/Agriculture Building
PO Box 1540
Trenton, NJ 08625
(609) 292-7837

New Jersey State League for Nursing
Doris A. Geyer
13 E Hillside Ave
Highlands, NJ 07732
(201) 291-4929 (home)

New Jersey State Nurses' Association
60 S Fullerton Ave, Room 201
Montclair, NJ 07042
(201) 783-9292

New Mexico

New Mexico Democratic
   Headquarters
4155 Montgomery NE
Albuquerque, NM 87109
(505) 884-8400

New Mexico Health Systems Agency
239–1/2 Johnson St
PO Box 1296
Santa Fe, NM 87501
(505) 988-8079

League of Women Voters
   of New Mexico
Route 1, PO Box 176
Santa Fe, NM 87501
(505) 455-2817

National Organization for Women
New Mexico NOW Coordinator
118 Princeton SE
Albuquerque, NM 87106
(505) 266-4496 (home)
(505) 766-3504 (office)

National Women's Political Caucus
Susan Thom Loubet
PO Box 657
Cedar Crest, NM 87008
(505) 281-5605

Nurses Political Action Committee
N-PAC
Carol Davis
N-PAC of New Mexico
460 Arroyo Tenorio
Santa Fe, NM 87501

Republican State Central
   Committee of New Mexico
3701 San Mateo NE, Suite F
Albuquerque, NM 87110
(505) 883-1776
            or
3701 San Mateo NE, Suite M
Albuquerque, NM 87110
(505) 881-6608

State Health Planning
   and Development Bureau
State Health and
   Environment Department
PO Box 968
Santa Fe, NM 87503
(505) 827-5671

[No State League for Nursing]

New Mexico
    State Nurses' Association
303 Washington SE
Albuquerque, NM 87108
(505) 268-7744

New York

New York Democratic Party
60 E 42nd St
New York, NY 10017
(212) 986-2955

Health Systems Agencies

Central New York
    Health Systems Agency
5795 Widewaters Pkwy
Dewitt, NY 13214
(315) 446-8334

Fingerlakes Health Systems Agency
360 East Ave
Rochester, NY 14604
(716) 325-2270

Health Systems Agency
    of New York City
111 Broadway
New York, NY 10006
(212) 577-0550

Health Systems Agency
    of Northeastern New York, Inc
75 New Scotland Ave
Albany, NY 12208
(518) 445-0511

Health Systems Agency
    of Western New York, Inc
Ellicott Square Building, Suite 405
Buffalo, NY 14203
(716) 854-4812

Hudson Valley
    Health Systems Agency
Sterling Lake Rd
PO Box 696
Tuxedo, NY 10987
(914) 351-5146

Nassau-Suffolk
    Health Systems Agency
560 Broad Hollow Rd
Melville, NY 11746
(516) 752-1700

New York-Penn
    Health Systems Agency
306 Press Building
19 Chenango St
Binghamton, NY 13901
(607) 722-3445

League of Women Voters of New York
817 Broadway
New York, NY 10003
(212) 677-5050

National Association for Women Deans,
    Administrators and Counselors
Sister Mary Berchmans Coyle,
    Associate Dean
School of Continuing Education
Pace University College
    of White Plains
White Plains, NY 10603

National Organization for Women
New York NOW Coordinator
294 Mulberry St
Rochester, NY 14620
(716) 442-0174 (home)

National Women's Political Caucus
Pearl Kurland
4 Jackson Ct
Guiderland, NY 12084
(518) 455-3684 (office)
(518) 456-0288 (home)

Nurses Political Action Committee
N-PAC
Mary Foley, Chairperson, NYS/NPA
519 E 88th St, Apt 2B
New York, NY 10028

New York Republican
State Committee
315 State St
Albany, NY 12210
(518) 462-2601

State Health Planning
and Development Agency
New York Health
Planning Commission
Tower Building, Room 1683
Empire State Plaza
Albany, NY 12237
(518) 474-6416

Genesee Region Citizen's
State League for Nursing
Jane Fessler
83 Stone Ridge Dr
Rochester, NY 14615
(716) 621-4118 (office)

New York State League for Nursing
Barbara Fallon
700 E Water St
Syracuse, NY 13210
(315) 474-2270 (office)

Southern New York
State League for Nursing
Dr Dorothy McMullan
233 E 69th St
New York, NY 10021
(212) 737-0926 (home)

New York State Nurses' Assocation
2113 Western Ave
Guiderland, NY 12084
(518) 456-9333

North Carolina

North Carolina Democratic
Headquarters
PO Box 12196
Raleigh, NC 27605
(919) 821-2777

Health Systems Agencies

Capital Health Systems Agency, Inc
3600 N Duke St
North Duke Mall
Durham, NC 27704
(919) 477-9881

Eastern Carolina
Health Systems Agency
301 S Evans St
Minges Building, Suite 405
PO Drawer 7306
Greenville, NC 27834
(919) 758-1372

Cardinal Health Agency, Inc
401 E 11th St
Lumberton, NC 28358
(919) 738-9316

Piedmont Health
Systems Agency, Inc
2120 Pinecroft Rd
Greensboro, NC 27407
(919) 294-5891

Southern Piedmont
Health Systems Agency
1 Charlottetown Center
1300 Baxter St, Suite 425
Charlotte, NC 28204
(704) 372-8494

Western North Carolina
Health Systems Agency
PO Drawer 1749
1 North Square
Morganton, NC 28655
(704) 433-1642

League of Women Voters
of North Carolina
2637 McDowell
Durham, NC 27705
(919) 493-1178

National Association for Women Deans,
Administrators, and Counselors
Dr Shirley K. Flynn
Office of Residence Life
University of North Carolina
Greensboro, NC 27412

National Organization of Women
North Carolina NOW Coordinator
313 Burlage Circle
Chapel Hill, NC 27514
(919) 929-2451 (home)

National Women's Political Caucus
Luetta Sellers
Rte 2 Bella Vista Dr
Edenton, NC 27932

Nurses Political Action Committee
Ora Strickland-Davis, Chairperson,
Nurse-PAC
PO Box 21444
Greensboro, NC 27420
(919) 379-5010

North Carolina Republican
Executive Committee
PO Box 10625
1033 Wade Ave
Raleigh, NC 27605
(919) 828-0678

State Health Planning
and Development Agency
Department of Human Resources
325 N Salisbury St
Raleigh, NC 27611
(919) 829-4130

North Carolina State
League for Nursing
Sister Kathryn Galligan,
Director, Nursing Service
Mercy Hospital
2001 Vail Ave
Charlotte, NC 27605
(704) 279-5000 (office)

North Carolina State
Nurses' Association
PO Box 12025
103 Enterprise St
Raleigh, NC 27605
(919) 821-4250

North Dakota

North Dakota Democratic
Headquarters
1902 E Divide Ave
Bismarck, ND 58501
(701) 255-0460

Health Systems Agencies

Agassiz Health Systems Agency
123 Demers Ave
East Grand Forks, MN 58721
(218) 773-2471

Minnesota-Dakota
Health Systems Agency, Inc
1721 S University Dr
Fargo, ND 58102
(701) 280-0002

Western North Dakota
Health Systems Agency, Inc
104 Third Ave NW
Mandan, ND 58554
(701) 663-0214

League of Women Voters
of North Dakota
3106 S Tenth St
Grand Forks, ND 58201
(701) 775-2687

National Organization for Women
North Dakota NOW Coordinator
1035 N First St
Fargo, ND 58102
(701) 237-0586 (home)

[No Nurses Political
    Action Committee]

North Dakota Republican
    State Committee
PO Box 1917
102–1/2 S Third St
Bismarck, ND 58501
(701) 255-0030
(701) 547-3129

State Health Planning
    and Development Agency
Missouri Building
1200 Missouri Ave, Room 102
Bismarck, ND 58505
(701) 224-2894

North Dakota Citizens'
    League for Nursing
James P. Swenson
PO Box 640
Bismarck, ND 58501
(701) 223-4700 (office)

North Dakota State
    Nurses' Association
219 N Seventh St
Bismarck, ND 58501
(701) 223-1385

Ohio

Ohio Democratic Headquarters
88 E Broad St
Columbus, OH 43215
(614) 221-6563

Health Systems Agencies

Area 6 Health Systems Agency, Inc
216 Putnam St
St Clair Building, Suite 205
Marietta, OH 45750
(614) 374-2200

Health Planning Association
    of Northwest Ohio
350 Holland Rd, Suite B
Maumee, OH 43537
(419) 893-0287

Health Planning and
    Development Council
405 W Liberty St
Wooster, OH 44691
(216) 264-9939

Health Planning and
    Resources Development
    Association of Central
Ohio River Valley
19 Garfield Pl, Suite 700
Cincinnati, OH 45202
(513) 621-2434

Metropolitan Health
    Planning Corporation
908 Standard Building
Cleveland, OH 44113
(216) 771-6814

Mid-Ohio Health
    Planning Federation
2015 W Fifth Ave
PO Box 2239
Columbus, OH 43216
(614) 461-4230

Health Systems Agency for
    Summit Portage County
411 Wolf Ledges Pkwy, Suite 310
Akron, OH 44311
(216) 762-9417

Health Systems Agency
    of Eastern Ohio
17 Colonia Dr
Youngstown, OH 44505
(216) 759-2794

Miami Valley
    Health Systems Agency
Third National Bank Building,
    Suite 1349
32 N Main St
Dayton, OH 45402
(513) 461-5495

West Central Ohio
    Health System Agency
616 S Collett, Suite 201
Lima, OH 45805
(419) 227-8361

League of Women Voters of Ohio
65 S Fourth St
Columbus, OH 43215
(614) 469-1505

National Association for Women Deans,
    Administrators and Counselors
Georgette Allison
Mayfield Middle School
1173 SAM Center Rd
Mayfield Heights, OH 44134

National Organization for Women
Ohio NOW Coordinator
2047 Barrows
Toledo, OH 43613
(419) 474-1240 (home)

National Women's Political Caucus
Nancy Cronin
13700 Cormere
Cleveland, OH 44120

Nurses Political Action Committee
ON-PAC
Marjorie Stanton
3941 Large Lane
Dayton, OH 45430

Republican State Central
    and Executive Committee of Ohio
50 W Broad St
Columbus, OH 43215
(614) 228-2481

State Health Planning
    and Development Agency
Ohio Department of Health
PO Box 118
450 E Town
Columbus, OH 43216
(614) 466-2253

Ohio State Nurses' Association
4000 E Main St
Columbus, OH 43213
(614) 237-5414

Cleveland Area Citizens'
    State League for Nursing
Lawrence Litwack
7358 Sylvan Dr
Kent, OH 44240
(216) 672-2662 (office)

Ohio State League for Nursing
Elsie B. Hayes
4276 Kenbury Pl
Columbus, OH 43220
(614) 422-6446 (office)

Oklahoma

Oklahoma Democratic Headquarters
3022 NW Expressway
May Executive Building, Suite 301
Oklahoma City, OK 73112
(405) 946-5648

Oklahoma Health Systems Agency
Quailridge Tower, Suite 303
11212 N May
Oklahoma City, OK 73120
(405) 751-6400

League of Women Voters of Oklahoma
400 NW 23rd St
Oklahoma City, OK 73103
(405) 525-7734

National Organization for Women
Oklahoma NOW Coordinator
2331 NW 20th St
Oklahoma City, OK 73107
(405) 528-0515

National Women's Political Caucus
Wanda Peltier
Masonic Building, Room 340
9th at Bell Streets
Shawnee, OK 74801

Nurses Political Action Committee
Jean Hall
President, ON-CAP
3417 NW 24th
Oklahoma City, OK 73107

Republican State
    Committee of Oklahoma
111-A NW 23rd St
Oklahoma City, OK 73103
(405) 528-3501

State Health Planning
    and Development Agency
Oklahoma Health
    Planning Commission
NE Tenth and Stonewall St
PO Box 53551
Oklahoma City, OK 73105
(405) 271-5161

Oklahoma State League for Nursing
Constance Baker
11609 Leaning Elm
Oklahoma City, OK 73120
(405) 271-2306 (office)

Oklahoma State Nurses' Association
2912 Paseo
Oklahoma City, OK 73103
(405) 528-1734

Oregon

Oregon Democratic Headquarters
PO Box 1012
Salem, OR 97308
(503) 370-8200

Health Systems Agencies

Eastern Oregon
    Health Systems Agency
PO Box 520
Redmond, OR 97756
(503) 548-5185

Northwest Oregon
    Health Systems Agency
Westridge Gardens 2, Suite 114
5201 SW Westgate Dr
Portland, OR 97221
(503) 297-2241

Western Oregon
    Health Systems Agency
99 W Tenth St, Room 337
Eugene, OR 97401
(503) 484-9311

League of Women Voters of Oregon
495 State St, Suite 215
Salem, OR 97301
(503) 581-5722

National Association for Women Deans,
    Administrators and Counselors
Jeanne Mackie, Counselor
Milwaukie High School
11300 SE 23rd St
Milwaukie, OR 97222

National Organization for Women
Oregon NOW Coordinator
2525 Portland, No. 22
Eugene, OR 97405
(503) 344-0290 (home)
(503) 686-3123 (office)

Oregon Women's Political Caucus
PO Box 5842
Portland, OR 97228

National Women's Political Caucus
Carol Kirchner
6137 SW 47th St
Portland, OR 97221

Nurses Political Action Committee
Marilyn Hogrefe, Chairperson,
Oregon N-PAC
33689 SE Melody Lane
Corvallis, OR 97330

Oregon Republican State
    Central Committee
Plaza 5 SW, Suite R
8700 SW 26th Ave
Portland, OR 97219
(503) 246-8221
                or
7195 SW 85th Ave
Tigard, OR 97223
(503) 244-4736

State Health Planning
    and Development Agency
Health Planning
    and Development Section
2111 Front St NE, Suite 108
Salem, OR 97310
(503) 378-4681

Oregon Citizens'
    State League for Nursing
Jean Hamilton
14903 NE Salmon Creek Ave
Vancouver WA 98665
(206) 573-0254 (home)

Oregon State
    Nurses' Association, Inc
620 SW Fifth Ave
Portland, OR 97204
(503) 228-2114

Pennsylvania

Pennsylvania Democratic
    Party Headquarters
510 N Third St
Harrisburg, PA 17101
(717) 238-9381

Health Systems Agencies

Central Pennsylvania
    Health Systems Agency, Inc
400 Market St, Third Floor
Lewisburg, PA 17837
(717) 524-2266

Health Resources Planning
    and Development, Inc
209 Senate Ave
PO Box 122
Camp Hill, PA 17011
(717) 761-3252

Health Systems Agency of
    Southeastern Pennsylvania
1616 Walnut St
Philadelphia, PA 19103
(215) 546-1616

Health Systems Agency of
    Southwestern Pennsylvania, Inc
650 Smithfield St, Suite 950
Pittsburgh, PA 15222
(412) 562-1811

Health Systems Agency of
    Northeastern Pennsylvania, Inc
Warm Building
Avoca, PA 18641
(717) 655-3703

Health Systems, Inc of
  Northwestern Pennsylvania
1545 W 38th St
Erie, PA 16508
(814) 868-4671

Health Systems Council of
  Eastern Pennsylvania, Inc
1503 Cedar Crest Blvd, Suite 109
Allentown, PA 18104
(215) 432-2575

Keystone Health System Agency
615 Howard Ave
Executive House
Altoona, PA 16601
(814) 946-3641

League of Women Voters
  of Pennsylvania
Margot Hunt
Strawbridge and Clothier
Eighth and Market Streets, 11th Floor
Philadelphia, PA 19105
(215) 328-9881

National Association for Women Deans,
  Administrators, and Counselors
Ellen Perrin, Dean of Student Services
Slippery Rock State College
Slippery Rock, PA 16057

National Organization for Women
Pennsylvania NOW Coordinator
834 Guenther Ave, No. 173
Yeadon, PA 19050
(215) 259-8334 (home)

National Women's Political Caucus
Virginia L. Brown
5720 Pemberton St
Philadelphia, PA 19143

Nurses Political Action Committee
Patricia Scuffle, Chairperson, PRN
7413 Schoyer Ave
Pittsburgh, PA 15218
(412) 371-1206

Republican State Committee
  of Pennsylvania
PO Box 1624
112 State St
Harrisburg, PA 17105
(717) 234-4901

State Health Planning
  and Development Agency
Office of Planning
  and Development
State Health Department
PO Box 90
Harrisburg, PA 17120
(717) 783-3865

Pennsylvania State
  League for Nursing
Sister Patricia Hardner
952 W Tenth St
Erie, PA 16505
(814) 838-1966 (office)

Pennsylvania State
  Nurses' Association
2515 N Front St
Harrisburg, PA 17110
(717) 234-7935

Rhode Island

Rhode Island Democratic
  Headquarters
10 Charles Orm Building
Providence, RI 02904
(401) 273-8700

League of Women Voters
  of Rhode Island
41 Seekonk St
Providence, RI 02906
(401) 274-5822

National Organization for Women
Rhode Island NOW Coordinator
54 Clyde St
Pawtucket, RI 02860
(401) 722-4787

National Women's Political Caucus
Susan McCalmont
248 Cypress St
Providence, RI 02906

Rhode Island Republican State
    Central Committee
169 Weybosset St, Suite 602
Providence, RI
(401) 421-2570
            or
10 Brayton St
West Warwick, RI 02893
(401) 821-6172

Rhode Island State
    Nurses' Association
134 Francis St
Providence, RI 02903
(401) 421-9703

State Health Planning
    and Development Agency
Health Planning
    and Resource Development
Rhode Island State
    Department of Health
75 Davis St
Providence, RI 02908
(401) 277-2231

[No State League for Nursing;
included in Massachusetts League]

South Carolina

Democratic Party
South Carolina Democratic
    Headquarters
PO Box 5965
Columbia, SC 29205
(803) 799-7798

Health Systems Agencies

Health Systems Agency
South Carolina Appalachian
    Health Council
211 Century Dr, Bldg D
PO Box 6709
Greenville, SC 29606
(803) 242-1895

Palmetto-Lowcountry
    Health Systems Agency, Inc
107 W Sixth North St
Summerville, SC 29483
(803) 871-0350

Pee Dee Reg Health
    Systems Agency, Inc
PO Box 5959
Florence, SC 29502
(803) 669-1347

Three Rivers
    Health Systems Agency, Inc
3325 Medical Park Rd
Columbia, SC 29203
(803) 779-6790

League of Women Voters
    of South Carolina
2838 Devine St
Columbia, SC 29205
(803) 771-0063

National Organization for Women
South Carolina NOW Coordinator
Route 1, PO Box 72
Chapin, SC 29036
(803) 345-1713 (home)

South Carolina Republican Party
PO Box 5247
616 Harden St
Columbia, SC 29250
(803) 799-1610
            or
Route 2, PO Box 166
Blackville, SC 29817
(803) 725-2242

State Health Planning
and Development Agency
South Carolina Department of Health
and Environmental Control
2600 N Bull St
Columbia, SC 29201
(803) 758-4162

South Carolina
State League for Nursing
Sylvia R. Lufkin
507 S Walker St
Columbia, SC 29205
(803) 254-1563 (home)

South Carolina State
Nurses' Association
1821 Gadsden St
Columbia, SC 29201
(803) 252-4781

South Dakota

South Dakota
Democratic Party Headquarters
PO Box 668
Pierre, SD 57501
(605) 224-8638

South Dakota
Health Systems Agency
216 E Clark St
Vermillion, SD 57069
(605) 624-4446

League of Women Voters
of South Dakota
PO Box 2091
Rapid City, SD 57709
(605) 343-4026

National Organization for Women
South Dakota NOW Coordinator
1112 N Huron
Pierre, SD 57501
(605) 224-1287 (home)

National Women's Political Caucus
Linda Lee Miller
RR 1, PO Box 122J
Rapid City, SD 55701
(605) 348-6547 (office)
(605) 341-7053 (home)

[No Nurses Political
Action Committee]

Republican Party
South Dakota Republican State
Central Committee
PO Box 1099
222 E Capitol St
Pierre, SD 57501
(605) 224-7347
or
405 Jefferson Ave
Murdo, SD 57559
(605) 669-2145

Office of State Health Planning
and Development
State Department of Health
Joe Foss Building
Pierre, SD 57501
(605) 224-3361

South Dakota
State League for Nursing
Ben T. Suga
1919 Cedar
Yankton, SD 57078
(605) 677-5251 (office)

South Dakota
State Nurses' Association, Inc
1505 S Minnesota, Suite 6
Sioux Falls, SD 57105
(605) 338-1401

Tennessee

Tennessee Democratic Headquarters
1080 Capitol Hill Building
Nashville, TN 37219
(615) 244-1336

Health Systems Agencies

Archa Health Systems Agency
PO Box 600
Johnson City, TN 37601
(615) 929-0193

East Tennessee
    Health Improvement Council,
    Inc.
Twelve Oaks Executive Park
5401 Kinston Pike, Suite 340
Knoxville, TN 37919
(615) 588-1202

Georgia-Tennessee
    Regional Health Commission
201 Zayre Building
401 W Ninth St
Chattanooga, TN 37402
(615) 266-2151

Mid-South Medical Center Council
Medical Center Towers Building
    Suite 1200
969 Madison Ave
Memphis, TN 38104
(901) 523-9565

West Tennessee Health
    Improvement Association, Inc
Watkins Towers, Suite 304
1804 Hwy 45 Bypass
Jackson, TN 38301
(901) 668-8236

Middle Tennessee
    Health Systems Agency, Inc
2 International Plaza Dr, Suite 200
Nashville, TN 37217
(615) 361-8100

League of Women Voters
    of Tennessee
1701-21st Ave S, Suite 425
Nashville, TN 37212
(615) 297-7134

National Association for Women Deans,
    Administrators, and Counselors
Dr Marion F. Emslie, Associate
    Dean for Student Development
Memphis State University
202 Scates Hall
Memphis, TN 38152

National Organization for Women
Tennessee NOW Coordinator
3707 Decatur Rd
Knoxville, TN 37920
(615) 579-0515 (home)

National Women's Political Caucus
Penny Edwards
208 Lynwood Terr
Nashville, TN 37205
(615) 383-7073

Nurses Political Action Committee
Elizabeth Smith, Chairperson, TN-PAC
PO Box 24510
East Tennessee State University
Johnson City, TN 37601
(605) 929-4262

Republican Party
Tennessee Republican
    State Executive Committee
510 Gay St, Suite 306
Nashville, TN 37219
(615) 259-4033

State Health Planning
    and Development Agency
Tennessee Health Planning
    and Resources Development
    Authority
Governor's Office
Capitol Blvd Building, Suite 211
226 Capitol Blvd
Nashville, TN 37219
(615) 741-3538

Tennessee State
    League for Nursing
Dr Norma Jean Long
370 Shady Pines
Memphis, TN 38117
(901) 528-6145 (office)

Tennessee State
    Nurses' Association
1720 West End Building, Suite 400
Nashville, TN 37203
(615) 329-2511

Texas

Democratic Party
Texas Democratic Headquarters
215 Stokes Building
11th and Guadalupe
Austin, TX 78701
(512) 478-8746

Health Systems Agencies

Camino Real Health
    Systems Agency, Inc
410 S Main St, Suite 212
San Antonio, TX 78204
(512) 225-4426

Central Texas
    Health Systems Agency, Inc
1106 Clayton Lane, Suite 210
West Twin Towers Building
Austin, TX 78723
(512) 458-9161

Health Systems Agency, Inc
Houston-Galveston Area
    Council Area Health Commission
3701 W Alabama
Houston, TX 77027
(713) 627-3200

Greater East Texas
Health Systems Agency, Inc
2900 N St, Suite 314
Beaumont, TX 77702
(713) 892-6962

Northeast Texas
    Health Systems Agency, Inc
Travis Terrace Building, Suite 201
505 E Travis St
Marshall, TX 75670
(214) 938-8331

Panhandle Health Systems Agency
PO Box 9257
Amarillo, TX 79105
(806) 372-3381

Permian Basin
    Health Systems Agency
PO Box 6391
Midland, TX 79701
(915) 563-1061

South Plains Health Systems, Inc
1217 Ave K
Lubbock, TX 79401
(806) 747-0181

South Texas
    Health Systems Agency
Texas A&M University
Station 1, PO Box 2378
Kingsville, TX 78363
(512) 595-5545

Texas Area 5
    Health Systems Agency, Inc
800 W Airport Freeway
PO Box 6084
Irving, TX 75062
(214) 251-2522

Tri-Region Health Systems Agency
2642 Post Oak Rd, Suite B
Abilene, TX 79605
(915) 698-9481

West Texas Health
    Systems Agency
303 N Oregon, Suite 700
El Paso, TX 79901
(915) 532-2910

League of Women Voters of Texas
1212 Guadalupe, No. 109
Austin, TX 78701
(512) 472-1100

National Association for Women Deans,
  Administrators and Counselors
Dr Ruby Morris
6436 Patrick Dr
Dallas, TX 75214

National Organization for Women
Texas NOW Coordinator
1105 Austin St
Denton, TX 76201
(817) 387-4735

National Women's Political Caucus
Evelyn Ireland
5007 Westview Dr
Austin, TX 78731
(512) 475-4285 (office)
(512) 458-2657 (home)

Nurses Political Action Committee
Karen A. Beard, Coordinator,
  Tex N-CAP
PO Box 15202
Austin, TX 78761

Texas Women's Political Caucus
Lena Guerrero
815 Brazos, Suite 304
Austin, TX 78701
(512) 474-1798

Republican Party of Texas
1011 Congress Ave, No. 502
Austin, TX 78701
(512) 477-9821
            or
PO Box 940
Mineral Wells, TX 76067
(817) 325-6911

State Health Planning
  and Development Agency
Texas Department of Health
1100 W 49th St
Austin, TX 78756
(512) 458-7111

Texas State League for Nursing
Betty H. Wade
2900 N Britain Rd
Irving, TX 75062
(214) 631-3713 (office)

Texas State Nurses' Association
314 Highland Mall Blvd, Suite 504
Austin, TX 78752
(512) 452-0645

Utah

Utah Democratic Headquarters
363 E Second St
Salt Lake City, UT 84111
(801) 328-0239

Utah Health Systems Agency
19 W South Temple, Eighth Floor
Salt Lake City, UT 84101
(801) 581-3476

League of Women Voters of Utah
211 E Third S, No. 200
Salt Lake City, UT 84111
(801) 328-4532

National Organization for Women
Utah NOW Co-coordinator
434 E 9800 S
Sandy, UT 84070
(801) 571-8468 (home)

National Organization for Women
Utah NOW Co-coordinator
718 E 700 S, Apt 8
Salt Lake City, UT 84102
(801) 363-3772 (home)

National Women's Political Caucus
Jan Johnson
PO Box 8745
Salt Lake City, UT 84108

Nurses Political Action Committee
Contact Person for N-PAC
c/o Utah Nurses' Association
1058 E Ninth S
Salt Lake City, UT 84105
(801) 322-3439
(801) 322-3430

Utah Republican State
    Central Committee
150 S Sixth E, Suite 2B
Ambassador Plaza
Salt Lake City, UT 84102
(801) 533-9777
              or
345 S State St, Suite 107
Salt Lake City, UT 84111
(801) 532-9767

State Health Planning
    and Development Agency
Office of Planning and Research
150 W North Temple
Salt Lake City, UT 84111
(801) 533-5525

Utah State League for Nursing
Dr Mary Jo Bulbrook
2822 Cobble Moor Lane
Sandy, UT 84070
(801) 581-8278 (office)

Utah State
    Nurses' Association
1058 E Ninth S
Salt Lake City, UT 84105
(801) 322-3439
(801) 322-3430

Vermont

Vermont Democratic Headquarters
109 S Wincoski Ave, Suite 207
Burlington, VT 05401
(802) 864-0431

Vermont Health Policy Corp
State Office Building
Waterbury State Office Complex
Montpelier, VT 05602
(802) 241-2920

League of Women Voters
    of Vermont
2 Railroad Ave
Essex Junction, VT 05452
(802) 879-3414

National Organization for Women
Vermont NOW Coordinator
26 Stirrup Circle
Williston, VT 05495
(802) 879-6288 (home)

National Women's Political Caucus
Daphne Gratiot
Otis Hill Farm
Woodstock, VT 05091
(802) 457-1088

[no N-PAC]
no Nurses Political Action Committee

Vermont Republican
    State Committee
PO Box 70
100 State St
Montpelier, VT 05602
(802) 223-3411
                        or
159 State St
Montpelier, VT 05602
(802) 223-6596

State Health Planning
and Development Agency
Vermont Department of Health
60 Main St
Burlington, VT 05401
(802) 862-5701

[No State League for Nursing]

Vermont State
Nurses' Association, Inc
72 Hungerford Terr
Burlington, VT 05401
(802) 864-9390

Virginia

Virginia Democratic Headquarters
701 E Franklin St, Suite 801
Richmond, VA 23219
(804) 644-1966

Health Systems Agencies

Central Virginia
Health Systems Agency
2015 Staples Hill Rd, Room 419
Blue Cross/Blue Shield Bldg
Richmond, VA 23230
(804) 355-5723

Eastern Virginia
Health Systems Agency
11 Koger Executive Center, Suite 203
Norfolk, VA 23502
(804) 461-1236

Health Systems Agency
for Northern Virginia, Inc
7245 Arlington Blvd, Suite 300
Falls Church, VA 22042
(703) 573-3100

Northwestern Virginia
Health Systems Agency, Inc
2015 Ivy Rd, Suite 314
Charlottesville, VA 22903
(804) 977-6010

Southwest Virginia
Health Systems Agency, Inc
Plaza 1 Office Park
200 S Country Club Dr
Blacksburg, VA 24060
(703) 951-0170

League of Women Voters
of Virginia
1800 Old Meadow Rd, Suite 115
McLean, VA 22102
(703) 356-5102

National Association for Women Deans,
Administrators, and Counselors
Becky Gates
1714 Paisley Blue Ct
Vienna, VA 22180

National Organization for Women
Virginia NOW Coordinator
5005 Tenth St, S, No. 3
Arlington, VA 22204
(703) 998-8362 (home)
(202) 833-9880 (office)

National Women's Political Caucus
Marianne Fowler
300B E Glendale
Alexandria, VA 22301

Nurses Political Action Committee
Christina Crutchley
Chairperson, VAN-CAP
9017 Denise Ln
Fairfax, VA 22031

Republican Party of Virginia
Ninth and Main Streets, 16th Floor
Fidelity Building
Richmond, VA 23219
(804) 780-0111
or
2831 Old Orange Rd
Culpepper, VA 22701
(703) 825-0104

State Health Planning
    and Development Agency
Division of Health Planning
    and Resources Development
State Department of Health
109 Governor St
Richmond, VA 23219
(804) 786-4891

Virginia State League for Nursing
Vida S. Huba, Nursing Chairman
Eastern Mennonite College
206 Old 33
Harrisonburg, VA 22801
(703) 433-2771 (office)

Virginia State
    Nurses' Association
1311 High Point Ave
Richmond, VA 23230
(804) 353-7311

Washington

Washington Democratic Headquarters
Lobby, Arctic Bldg
Third and Cherry
Seattle, WA 98104
(206) 623-6093

Health Systems Agencies

  Central Washington
      Health Systems Agency
  305 W Fourth Ave
  Moses Lake, WA 98837
  (206) 765-1767

  Eastern Washington
      Health Systems Agency
  1728 W Jackson
  Spokane, WA 99205
  (509) 456-3178

  Puget Sound
      Health Systems Agency
  601 Valley St
  Seattle, WA 98109
  (206) 464-6143

Southwest Washington
    Health Systems Agency
320 W Bay Dr, Suite 102
Olympia, WA 98502
(206) 753-8137

League of Women Voters
    of Washington
1406-18th Ave
Seattle, WA 98122
(206) 329-4646
(206) 329-7165

National Association for Women Deans,
    Administrators, and Counselors
Lois V. Schmidt, Assistant Principal
Gray Junior High School
3109 S 60th
Tacoma, WA 98409

National Organization for Women
Washington NOW Coordinator
Route 1, Lakeview Terr, No. B5
Grand Coulee, WA 99133
(509) 633-2399

National Women's Political Caucus
Jennifer Beltcher
6015 Hanson RD
Olympia, WA 98503
(206) 491-1074

Nurses Political Action Committee
Joyce Pashley, Chairperson,
    PUNCH
1606 Nob Hill N
Seattle, WA 98109
(206) 281-2233

Republican State Committee
    of Washington
1509 Queen Anne Ave N
Seattle, WA 98109
(206) 285-1980

State Health Planning
    and Development Agency
Health Services Division
Department of Social
    and Health Services
Mail Stop OB 44-J
Olympia, WA 98504
(206) 753-5818

[No State League for Nursing]

Washington State
    Nurses' Association, Inc
1109 Second Ave
Seattle, WA 98101
(206) 622-3613

West Virginia

West Virginia
    Democratic Headquarters
2106 Kanawha Blvd E
Charleston, WV 25311
(304) 342-8121

West Virginia
    Health Systems Agency, Inc
Morrison Building, Suite 212
815 Quarrier St
Charleston, WV 25301
(304) 348-0550

League of Women Voters
    of West Virginia
6128 Gideon Rd
Huntington, WV 25705
(304) 736-3287

National Association of Women Deans,
    Administrators, and Counselors
Dr Nell Bailey,
    Dean of Student Development
Salem College
Salem, WV 26426

National Organization for Women
West Virginia NOW Coordinator
1013 Mile Race Dr
Martinsburg, WV 25401
(304) 263-2756 (home)
(304) 725-9741 (office)

National Women's Political Caucus
Carolyn Snyder
PO Box 47
Charlestown, WV 25414
(304) 263-5951

[No Nurses Political
    Action Committee]

Republican State Executive
    Committee of West Virginia
PO Box 1007
Union Building, Suite 1108
Charleston, WV 25301
(304) 344-3446
              or
147 E Main St
Bridgeport, WV 26330
(304) 842-5995

State Health Planning
    and Development Agency
1800 Washington St E
Charleston, WV 25305
(304) 348-0546

West Virginia
    State Nurses' Association, Inc
47 Capitol City Building
Charleston, WV 25301
(304) 342-7978

West Virginia
    State League for Nursing
Judy Tiano
723 Bright Ridge Dr
Bridgeport, WV 26330
(304) 624-2302 (office)

Wisconsin

Wisconsin Democratic Headquarters
126 S Franklin St
Madison, WI 53703
(608) 255-5172

Health Systems Agencies

Health Planning Council, Inc
310 Price Pl, Suite 206
Madison, WI 53705
(608) 238-2641

North Central Area
    Health Planning Association
811 N First Ave, Room 27
Wausau, WI 54401
(715) 845-3107

Western Wisconsin
    Health Planning Organization
1707 Main St
PO Box 1084
Lacrosse, WI 54601
(608) 785-9352

Lake Winnebago Area
    Health Systems Agency
424 Washington Ave, Suite 201
Oshkosh, WI 54901
(414) 231-2907

Northeastern Wisconsin
    Health Systems Agency, Inc
828 Cherry St
Green Bay, WI 54301
(414) 432-5284

Southeastern Wisconsin
    Health Systems Agency, Inc
735 N Fifth St
Milwaukee, WI 53203
(414) 271-9788

League of Women Voters
    of Wisconsin
625 W Washington Ave
Madison, WI 53703
(608) 256-0827

National Organization for Women
Wisconsin NOW Coordinator
15700 Gebhardt Rd
Brookfield, WI 53005
(414) 784-1694 (home)

National Women's Political Caucus
Liesl Blockstein
4833 Tokay Blvd
Madison, WI 53711
(608) 274-0217

Nurses Political Action Committee
Contact Person, WINPAC
c/o Wisconsin Nurses' Association
206 E Olin Ave
Madison, WI 53713

Republican Party of Wisconsin
PO Box 31
303 E Wilson St
Madison, WI 53701
(608) 257-4765
                    or
Hough Manufacturing Company
1809 Adel St
Janesville, WI 53545
(608) 755-0663

State Health Planning
    and Development Agency
Division of Health
1 W Wilson St, Room 434
Madison, WI 53702
(608) 266-1511

Wisconsin State
    League for Nursing
Gregory R. Olson
3029 N 49th St
Milwaukee, WI 53210
(414) 445-8656 (office)

Wisconsin State
  Nurses' Association, Inc
Plankinton Building, Room 6012
161 W Wisconsin Ave
Milwaukee, WI 53203
(414) 272-3670

Wyoming

Wyoming Democratic Headquarters
PO Box 1964
Casper, WY 82601
(307) 234-8862

Wyoming Health Systems Agency, Inc
PO Box 106
Cheyenne, WY 82001
(307) 634-2726

League of Women Voters
    of Wyoming
PO Box 999
Rawlins, WY 82301
(307) 324-9582

National Organization for Women
Wyoming NOW Coordinator
3511 E Schubert Pl
Seattle, WA 98122
(206) 322-1990

National Women's Political Caucus
Jamie Ring
520 Parkview Dr
Casper, WY 82601
(307) 237-9604

[No Nurses Political
    Action Committee]

Wyoming Republican
    State Committee
PO Box 241
Casper, WY 82602
(307) 234-9166
                or
PO Box 2151
Cheyenne, WY 82001
(307) 632-7132

State Health Planning
    and Development Agency
Department of Health
    and Social Services
Division of Health
    and Medical Services
Hathaway Building
Cheyenne, WY 82002
(307) 777-7657

Wyoming State
    League for Nursing
Meredith Schneider
320 E First Ave
Cheyenne, WY 82001
(307) 634-3341 (office)

Wyoming State
    Nurses' Association, Inc
Seminoe Dam Route
Sinclair, WY 82334
307-043F4 (reached through
    Casper Rural Operator)

American Samoa

National Organization for Women
American Samoa NOW Coordinator
c/o Mary M. Smith
1820 S Bentley, No. 108
Los Angeles, CA 90025
(213) 479-6317 (home)

State Health Planning
    and Development Agency
Dept of Medical Services
LBJ Tropical Medical Center
Pago Pago, American Samoa 96799
633-5743 (international
    operator 160-684)

Guam

Guam Democratic Headquarters
PO Box 2729
Agana, Guam 96910

National Organization for Women
Guam NOW Coordinator
1820 S Bentley, No. 108
Los Angeles, CA 90025
(213) 479-6317 (home)

[No Nurses Political
    Action Committee]

Republican Party of Guam
PO Box 3404
Agana, Guam 96910
472-8621 (international operator)
            or
PO Box 1196
Agana, Guam 96910
734-9268 (international operator)

State Health Planning
    and Development Agency
GCIC Building, Suite 205
414 W Soledad Ave
Agana, Guam 96910
472-6831 (international
    operator 160-671)

Guam State Nurses' Association
PO Box 3134
Agana, Guam 96910

Mariana Islands

Commonwealth Health Planning
    and Development
c/o Office of Planning and Budget
Government of
    Northern Mariana Islands
PO Box 509
Saipan, Mariana Islands 96950
6361 (international
    operator 160-670)

Puerto Rico

Puerto Rico
    Democratic Headquarters
Edificio Bance de Ponce
PDA 18 Ave
Ponce de Leon
Santurce, PR 00907
(809) 725-4467

[No Health Systems Agency]

League of Women Voters
    of Puerto Rico
GPO Box 3724
San Juan, PR 00936
(809) 723-0348

National Organization for Women
Puerto Rico NOW Coordinator
5614 Temple Rd
Jacksonville, FL 32207
(904) 731-7578

[No Nurses Political
    Action Committee]

National Republican Party
    of Puerto Rico
PO Box 507 Hato Rey
San Juan, PR 00919
(809) 765-9932
(809) 765-2988
            or
GPO Box 6108
San Juan, PR 00936
(809) 764-7474

State Health Planning
    and Development Agency
Health Planning Division
Department of Health
Ponce de Leon Ave
San Juan, PR 00908
(809) 782-0120, ext 281

Puerto Rico
    State League for Nursing
Marjarita Rosa
Station 6, PO Box 131
Ponce, PR 00731
(809) 844-4150, ext 225
    or 226 (office)

Trust Territories

National Organization for Women
Trust Territories NOW
    Coordinator
[see American Samoa]

[No Nurses Political
    Action Committee]

State Health Planning
    and Development Agency
Trust Territory of
    the Pacific Islands
Office of the High Commissioner
Saipan, Mariana Islands 96950
9422/9355 (international
    operator 160-671)

Virgin Islands

League of Women Voters
    of the Virgin Islands
PO Box 638
St Thomas VI 00801
(809) 774-5763

National Organization for Women
Virgin Islands NOW
    Coordinator
[see Puerto Rico]

[No Nurses Political
    Action Committee]

[No National State
    League for Nursing]

Progressive Republican Party
    of the Virgin Islands
PO Box 2512
St Croix, VI 00820
(809) 773-2161

State Health Planning
    and Development Agency
Department of Health
PO Box 1442
St Thomas, VI 00801
(809) 774-5980

Virgin Island
    State Nurses' Association
PO Box 2866
St Thomas, VI 00801

SECTION 3: PUBLICATIONS

Below is a list of selected publications that we recommend as being particularly helpful to women and nurses who seek to become better informed on political issues. It is not a complete catalog, but a group of publications we have found useful.

AARP News Bulletin. Published by American Association of Retired Persons, 215 Long Beach Blvd, Long Beach, CA 90801. Sent to members.

American Nurse. Published by the American Nurses' Association, 2420 Pershing Rd, Kansas City, MO 64108. Sent to members.

Congress and Health: An Introduction to the Legislative Process and Its Key Participants, ed 3, 96th Congress. Published by National Health Council, 1740 Broadway, New York, NY 10019. Issue $6; prepared for each new Congress.

Congress in Print. Published by the *Washington Monitor,* Inc, 499 National Press Building, Washington, DC 20045. Subscription $55 per year; weekly publication.

Congressional Insight. Published at Congressional Quarterly, Inc, 1414 22nd St NW, Washington, DC 20037. Subscription $96 per year; weekly publication.

The Congressional Monitor. Published by the *Washington Monitor,* Inc, 499 National Press Building, Washington, DC 20045. Three-month trial subscription for $95, or $400 per year; daily publication while Congress is in session.

First Monday. Published by the Republican National Committee, 310 First St SE, Washington, DC 20003. Monthly publication sent to all contributors of $15 or more to the Republican National Committee.

Health Advocate. Published by the National Health Law Program, 2639 S La Cienega Blvd, Los Angeles, CA 90034. Telephone (213) 204-6010. Free upon request.

Higher Education and National Affairs. Published by the American Council on Education, 1 Dupont Circle NW, Suite 800, Washington, DC 20036. Subscription $30 per year; weekly publication on Washington activities affecting education.

Mother Jones. Published by the Foundation for National Progress, 625 Third St, San Francisco, CA 94107. Subscription $12 per year.

Ms. Published by Ms. Magazine Corporation, 370 Lexington Ave, New York, NY 10017. Subscription $10 per year.

Newsweek. The Newsweek Building, Livingston, NJ 07039. Subscription $32 per year; some special offers less.

Politics Today. Published by *Politics Today,* Inc, Presidio Plaza, Santa Barbara, CA 93101. Subscription $8.95 per year (six issues).

Savvy. Published by the Savvy Company, 111 Eighth Ave, New York, NY 10011. Subscription $18 per year.

Time. Published by Time-Life, Inc, Time-Life Building, Chicago, IL 60611. Weekly publication; subscription offers vary.

Wall Street Journal. Published by Dow Jones & Co, Inc, 22 Cortlandt St, New York, NY 10007. Subscription $63 per year.

Washington Health Record. Published by McGraw-Hill, Inc in conjunction with *Medicine and Health*, 457 National Press Building, Washington, DC 20045. Subscription $137 per year. Weekly publication on regulations and notices, legislative activity, meetings and conferences, and publications.

The Washington Journalism Review, 3122 M St NW, Washington, DC 20007. Ten issues for $16.

Washington Newsletter. Published by the American Public Health Association, Inc, 1015-15th St NW, Washington, DC 20005. Subscription $40 per year; monthly publication.

Washington Report on Medicine and Health. Published by McGraw-Hill, Inc, 457 National Press Building, Washington, DC 20045. Subscription $137 per year; published on Monday, 50 times a year.

Working Mother. Published by McCall's, PO Box 10608, Des Moines, IA 50381. Subscription $9 per year; published bimonthly.

Working Woman. Published by Hal Publications, Inc, 600 Madison Ave, New York, NY 10022. Subscription $14 per year.

US News and World Report, 2300 N St NW, Washington, DC 20037. A 35-week subscription for $17.50.

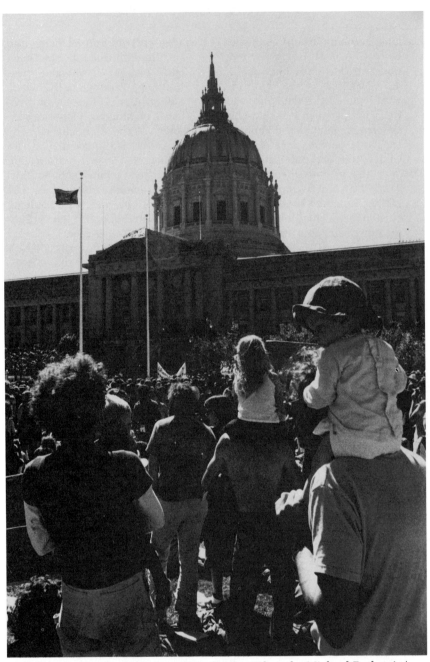

Political rally, San Francisco Civic Center. (Photo by Michael Rothstein/ Jeroboam)

States and American Samoa, Guam,
and Puerto Rico

CHAPTER 11

State-by-State
Bill-to-Law Procedures

Patricia A. Goehner

IN THE following pages are listed the specific bill-to-law procedures of all of the states and territories in the United States. Naturally, you will be most interested in the process that takes place in your own state. At some point, I suggest that you read through the other states' also, to get a feel for the variations in procedure that occur. To facilitate cross-state comparisons and contrasts, I have followed a uniform format for each state:

A. Official names of the branches of legislature
B. Convening place
C. Number of legislators
D. Terms of office
E. Legislative officers and leaders
F. Regular legislative session
G. Special legislative session
H. Bill introduction
I. Standing committees
J. Bill-to-law process
    1. By whom referred to committee
    2. Number of required readings
    3. Formal floor debate
    4. How final votes are recorded
    5. Votes required to pass a bill
    6. Fate of a passed bill before adjournment
    7. Fate of a passed bill after adjournment
    8. Passage of a bill over the governor's veto

Alabama

A. Official Names
   1. Both houses: Legislature.
   2. Upper house: Senate.
   3. Lower house: House of representatives.
B. Convening Place: State Capitol, Montgomery, AL 36104.
C. Number of Legislators
   1. Senators: 35.
   2. House of Representatives: 105.
D. Terms of Office
   1. Governor: 4 years.
   2. Senators: 4 years.
   3. Representatives: 4 years.
E. Legislative Officers and Leaders: Elected by all members of their respective chambers, except lieutenant governor, who is appointed president of the senate by the governor.
   1. Senate
      a. President: The lieutenant governor, who serves ex officio.
      b. President pro tem.
   2. House
      a. Speaker of the house.
      b. Speaker of the house pro tem.
F. Regular Legislative Session
   1. Convenes: Annually on the first Tuesday in February except during the quadrennial election year, when sessions convene on the second Tuesday in January after the quadrennial election. Legislature meets in organizational session on the second Tuesday in January after the quadrennial election.
   2. Length of Session: Session is limited to 30 legislative days in 105 calendar days.
G. Special Legislative Session
   1. Convenes: When called by the governor.
   2. Length of Session: Special session is limited to 12 legislative days within 30 calendar days.
   3. Subjects To Be Considered: May consider subjects specified in governor's proclamation convening the legislature, or legislature may determine the subject by a two-thirds vote of each house.
H. Bill Introduction
   1. Time Limitation: Legislation must be introduced by the 20th legislative day. Pre-session bill filing is allowed by both chambers in both the first and second session.
   2. Exceptions to Time Limitations: Exceptions are permitted by a special vote.
      a. Senate: Unanimous vote.
      b. House: Four-fifths of the vote of both the senate and house quorum present and voting.

I. Standing Committees
   1. Average Number in 1977
      a. Senate: 16.
      b. House: 21.
   2. Committee hearings Open to the Public
      a. Senate.
      b. House.
J. Bill-to-Law Process
   1. By Whom Referred to Committee
      a. Senate: President of the senate.
      b. House: Speaker of the house.
   2. Required Readings: Three readings of a bill are required before a final vote can take place and these readings must occur on separate days.
   3. Formal Floor Debate: Occurs after the second reading, and bills are frequently amended from the floor during this debate.
   4. Recorded Vote on Final Passage
      a. Senate: Votes are recorded manually.
      b. House: Votes are recorded by electronic vote tabulation.
   5. Passage of a Bill: Minimum vote required to pass a bill in each house is a majority of those members present.
   6. Fate of a Passed Bill Before Adjournment: The governor either signs the bill into law or vetoes it. If the governor neither signs nor vetoes the bill within six days (Sundays included), it becomes law.
   7. Fate of a Passed Bill After Adjournment: The governor either signs the bill into law or vetoes it. If the governor does neither one within ten days (Sundays included), the bill dies.
   8. Passage of a Bill Over the Governor's Veto: Requires a majority vote of the elected members of both houses.

Alaska

A. Official Names
   1. Both Houses: Legislature.
   2. Upper House: Senate.
   3. Lower House: House of representatives.
B. Convening Place: State Capitol, Juneau, AK 98824.
C. Number of Legislators
   1. Senators: 20.
   2. Representatives: 40.
D. Term of Office
   1. Governor: 4 years.
   2. Senators: 4 years.
   3. Representatives: 2 years.
E. Legislative Officers and Leaders: Elected by all members of their respective chambers.
   1. Senate: President of the senate.
   2. House: Speaker of the house.

F. Regular Legislative Session
1. Convenes: Annually on the second Monday in January, except in the January immediately following the quadrennial general election, when the first regular session convenes on the third Monday in January.
2. Length of Session: No limit on length of session.

G. Special Legislative Session
1. Convenes: When called by the governor or by a two-thirds vote of the membership.
2. Length of Session: Special session is limited to 30 calendar days.
3. Subject(s) To Be Considered: May consider subject(s) specified in the governor's proclamation convening the legislature. Only if the legislature convenes itself may it determine the subject(s) to be considered.

H. Bill Introduction
1. Time Limitations: No limit exists on the introduction of bills during the first session. Bills must be introduced by the 36th calendar day during the second session.
2. Exception to Time Limitations: Exceptions are permitted by a two-thirds vote of the membership. The governor's legislation is introduced through the Rules Committee.

I. Standing Committees
1. Average Number
   a. Senate: 9.
   b. House: 9.
2. Committee Hearings Open to Public
   a. Senate.
   b. House.

J. Bill-to-Law Process
1. By Whom Referred to Committee
   a. Senate: President of the senate.
   b. House: Speaker of the house.
2. Required Readings: Three readings of a bill are required before a final vote can take place, except by a three-fourths vote. The second and third readings occur on the same day.
3. Formal Floor Debate: Occurs after the second reading, and bills are frequently amended from the floor during this debate.
4. Recorded Votes on Final Passage: Votes are recorded by electronic vote tabulation.
5. Passage of a Bill: Minimum vote required to pass a bill in each house is a majority of the membership.
6. Fate of a Passed Bill Before Adjournment: The governor either signs the bill into law or vetoes it. If the governor does neither within 15 days (Sundays included), the bill becomes law.
7. Fate of a Passed Bill After Adjournment: The governor either signs the bill into law or vetoes it. If the governor does neither within 20 days (Sundays included), the bill becomes law.
8. Passage of a Bill Over the Governor's Veto: Requires a three-fourths vote of the members of both houses.

Arizona

A. Official Names
   1. Both houses: Legislature.
   2. Upper house: Senate.
   3. Lower house: House of representatives.
B. Convening Place: State Capitol, Phoenix, AZ 85007.
C. Number of Legislators
   1. Senators: 30.
   2. Representatives: 60.
D. Terms of Office
   1. Governor: 4 years.
   2. Senators: 2 years.
   3. Representatives: 2 years.
E. Legislative Officers and Leaders: Elected by all members of their respective chambers except for the lieutenant governor, who is elected by a statewide vote.
   1. Senate
      a. President.
      b. President pro tempore.
      c. Majority leader.
      d. Minority whip.
   2. House
      a. Speaker of the house.
      b. Speaker pro tempore.
      c. Majority leader.
      d. Minority whip.
F. Regular Legislative Session
   1. Convenes: Second Monday in January of each year.
   2. Length of Session: No limit on length of session.
G. Special Legislative Session
   1. Convenes: By a petition of two-thirds of the members of each house.
   2. Length of Session: No limit.
   3. Subject(s) To Be Considered: Special sessions are unlimited in scope.
H. Bill Introduction
   1. Time Limitation: Bills must be introduced by the 36th day of the first session, by the 29th day of the second session, and by the 10th day of a special session.
   2. Exceptions to Time Limitation: Exceptions are permitted by a two-thirds vote of a quorum or by permission of the Rules Committee.
I. Standing Committees
   1. Average Number
      a. Senate:10.
      b. House: 14.
   2. Committee Hearings Open to Public
      a. Senate.
      b. House.

J. Bill-to-Law Process
    1. By Whom Referred to Committee
        a. Senate: President of the senate.
        b. House: Speaker of the house.
    2. Required Readings: Three readings of a bill are required before a final vote can take place. These readings must occur on separate days.
    3. Formal Floor Debate: This debate takes place during the meeting of the Committee of the Whole, and bills are frequently amended from the floor during this debate.
    4. Recorded Votes on Final Passage
        a. Senate: Votes are recorded manually.
        b. House: Votes recorded by electronic vote tabulation.
    5. Passage of Bill: Minimum vote required to pass a bill in each house is a majority of the elected membership.
    6. Fate of a Passed Bill Before Adjournment: The governor either signs the bill into law or vetoes it. If the governor does neither within five days (Sundays included), the bill becomes law.
    7. Fate of a Passed Bill After Adjournment: The governor either signs the bill or vetoes it. If the governor does neither within ten days (Sundays included), the bill becomes law.
    8. Passage of a Bill Over a Governor's Veto: Requires a two-thirds vote of the elected members of both houses.

Arkansas

A. Official Names
    1. Both Houses: General assembly.
    2. Upper House: Senate.
    3. Lower House: House of representatives.
B. Convening Place: State Capitol, Little Rock, AR 72201.
C. Number of Legislators
    1. Senators: 35.
    2. Representatives: 100.
D. Terms of Office
    1. Governor: 2 years.
    2. Senators: 4 years.
    3. Representatives: 2 years.
E. Legislative Officers and Leaders: Elected by all members of their respective chamber, except the lieutenant governor, who is appointed president of the senate by the governor.
    1. Senate:
        a. President is lieutenant governor, who serves as ex officio.
        b. President pro tem.
    2. House:
        a. Speaker of the house.
        b. Speaker pro tem.

F. Regular Legislative Session
1. Convenes: Second Monday in January of odd-numbered years. Sessions may be held in even-numbered years by a two-thirds vote of members in both houses.
2. Length of Session: Session is limited to 60 calendar days; however, session may be extended for an indefinite period of time by a two-thirds vote of members in both houses.

G. Special Legislative Session
1. Convenes: When called by the governor.
2. Length of Session: No limitation on the length of session when considering subject(s) in the governor's call. After the legislature has disposed of the subject(s) in the governor's call, however, it may by a two-thirds vote of the members of both houses take up subject(s) of its own choosing in a session of up to 15 days.
3. Subject(s) To Be Considered: The legislature may determine subject(s) to be considered only after they have disposed of subject(s) in the governor's call. This can be done by a two-thirds vote of the members of both houses.

H. Bill Introduction
1. Time Limitations: General bills must be introduced by the 55th day; however, all appropriation bills must be introduced by the 50th day.
2. Exception to Time Limitations: Exceptions are permitted by a two-thirds vote of the membership.

I. Standing Committees
1. Average Number
    a. Senate: 10.
    b. House: 10.
    c. Joint: 2.
2. Committee Hearings Open to Public
    a. Senate.
    b. House.

J. Bill-to-Law Process
1. By Whom Referred to Committee
    a. Senate: Rules Committee.
    b. House: Speaker of the house.
2. Required Readings: Three readings of a bill are required before a final vote can take place, and these readings must occur on separate days except by a two-thirds vote.
3. Formal Floor Debate: Occurs after the third reading, and bills are frequently amended from the floor during this debate.
4. Recorded Vote on Final Passage
    a. Senate: Votes are recorded manually.
    b. House: Votes are recorded by electronic vote tabulation.
5. Passage of a Bill: Minimum vote required to pass a bill in each house is a majority of the elected members.
6. Fate of a Passed Bill Before Adjournment: The governor either signs the bill into law or vetoes it. If the governor does neither within five days (Sundays excluded), the bill becomes law.

7. Fate of a Passed Bill After Adjournment: The governor either signs the bill into law or vetoes it. If the governor does neither within 20 days (Sundays included), the bill becomes law.
8. Passage of a Bill Over the Governor's Veto: Requires a majority vote of the elected members of both houses.

California

A. Official Names
   1. Both Houses: Legislature.
   2. Upper House: Senate.
   3. Lower House: Assembly.
B. Convening Place: State Capitol, 10th at L Street, Sacramento, CA 95814.
C. Number of Legislators
   1. Senators: 40.
   2. Assemblypersons: 80.
D. Term of Office
   1. Governor: 4 years.
   2. Senators: 4 years.
   3. Assemblypersons: 2 years.
E. Legislative Officers and Leaders: Elected by all members of their respective chambers, except the president of the senate, the lieutenant governor, who is appointed by the governor.
   1. Senate
      a. President: The lieutenant governor, who serves ex officio.
      b. President pro tem.
   2. Assembly
      a. Speaker of the assembly.
      b. Speaker pro tem.
F. Regular Legislative Session
   1. Convenes: First Monday in December of each even-numbered year.
   2. Length of Session: Session is continuous until November 30 of the following even-numbered year. It may recess from time to time, and may be recalled into regular session.
G. Special Legislative Session
   1. Convenes: When called by the governor.
   2. Length of Session: No limit on length of session.
   3. Subject(s) To Be Considered: May consider only subject(s) specified in the governor's proclamation convening the legislature.
H. Bill Introduction
   1. Time Limitation: No limitation on the introduction of legislation except the legislative schedule established for committee action.
I. Standing Committees
   1. Average Number
      a. Senate: 17.
      b. Assembly: 20.

      2. Committee Hearings Open to the Public
        a. Senate.
        b. Assembly.
J. Bill-to-Law Process
      1. By Whom Referred to Committee
        a. Senate: Rules Committee.
        b. Assembly: Speaker of the assembly.
      2. Required Readings: Three readings of a bill are required before a final vote can take place, and these readings must occur on separate days except by a two-thirds vote.
      3. Formal Floor Debate: Occurs after the third reading, and bills are seldom amended from the floor during this debate.
      4. Recorded Vote on Final Passage
        a. Senate: Votes are recorded manually.
        b. Assembly: Votes are recorded by electronic vote tabulation.
      5. Passage of a Bill: Minimum vote required to pass a bill in each house is a majority of the elected members.
      6. Fate of a Passed Bill Before Adjournment: The governor either signs the bill into law or vetoes it. If governor neither signs nor vetoes the bill within 12 days (Sundays included), it becomes law.
      7. Fate of a Passed Bill After Adjournment
        a. Regular Session: The last day on which either house may pass a bill, except statutes calling elections; statutes providing for tax levies or appropriations of usual current expenses of the state; and urgency statutes, is August 31 of even-numbered years. All other bills given to the governor during the twelve days prior to August 31 of that year become law unless vetoed by September 30.
        b. Special Session: Governor either signs or vetoes the bill. If the governor does neither, the bill becomes law after 12 days.
      8. Passage of a Bill Over the Governor's Veto: Requires a two-thirds vote of the elected members of both houses.

Colorado

A. Official Names
      1. Both Houses: General assembly.
      2. Upper House: Senate.
      3. Lower House: House of representatives.
B. Convening Place: State Capitol Building, 200 E Colfax Avenue, Denver, CO 80203.
C. Number of Legislators
      1. Senators: 35.
      2. Representatives: 65.
D. Terms of Office
      1. Governor: 4 years.
      2. Senators: 4 years.
      3. Representatives: 2 years.

E. Legislative Officers and Leaders: Elected by all members of their respective chambers.
   1. Senate
      a. President of the senate.
      b. President pro tem.
   2. House: Speaker of the house.
F. Regular Legislative Session
   1. Convenes: The first session begins annually on the Wednesday after the first Tuesday in January. The Second session is basically limited to considerations of budget and fiscal matters.
   2. Length of Session: No limit on length of session.
G. Special Legislative Session
   1. Convenes: When called by the governor or by a two-thirds vote of the members of each house.
   2. Length of Session: No limit on length of session.
   3. Subject(s) To Be Considered: May consider subject(s) specified in the governor's proclamation convening the legislature. Only if the legislature convenes itself may it determine subject(s) to be considered.
H. Bill Introduction
   1. Time Limitations
      a. First Session: Legislation must be introduced by the 60th legislative day.
      b. Second Session: Legislation must be introduced by the 30th legislative day.
   2. Exceptions to Time Limitations: Appropriations bills and bills introduced by the Committee on Delayed Bills.
I. Standing Committees
   1. Average Number
      a. Senate: 10.
      b. House: 11.
   2. Committee Hearings Open to the Public
      a. Senate.
      b. House.
J. Bill-to-Law Process
   1. Referred to Committee
      a. Senate: President of the senate.
      b. House: Speaker of the house.
   2. Required Readings: Three readings of a bill are required before a final vote can take place; however, second and third readings must occur on separate days.
   3. Formal Floor Debate: Occurs during the meeting of the Committee of the Whole, and bills are frequently amended from the floor during this debate.
   4. Recorded Vote on Final Passage
      a. Senate: Votes are recorded manually.
      b. House: Votes are recorded by electronic vote tabulation.
   5. Passage of a Bill: Minimum vote required to pass a bill in each house is a majority of the elected members.

6. Fate of a Passed Bill Before Adjournment: The governor either signs the bill into law or vetoes it. If the governor does neither within ten days (Sundays included), the bill becomes law.
7. Fate of a Passed Bill After Adjournment: The governor either signs the bill into law or vetoes it. If the governor does neither, after 30 days (Sundays included), the bill becomes law.
8. Passage of a Bill Over the Governor's Veto: Requires a two-thirds majority vote of the elected members of both houses.

Connecticut

A. Official Names
   1. Both Houses: General assembly.
   2. Upper House: Senate.
   3. Lower House: House of representatives.
B. Convening Place: State Capitol, 210 Capitol Ave, Hartford, CT 06115.
C. Number of Legislators
   1. Senators: 36.
   2. Representatives: 151.
D. Terms of Office
   1. Governor: 4 years.
   2. Senators: 2 years.
   3. Representatives: 2 years.
E. Legislative Officers and Leaders: Elected by all the members of their respective chambers, except the president of the senate, the lieutenant governor, who is appointed by the governor.
   1. Senate
      a. President: The lieutenant governor, who serves ex officio.
      b. President pro tem.
   2. House: Speaker of the house.
F. Regular Legislative Session
   1. Convenes: Annually. On the Wednesday after the first Monday in January in odd-numbered years; on the Wednesday after the first Monday in February in even-numbered years. The second session of the legislature is basically limited to budget and fiscal matters.
   2. Length of Session: Sessions in odd-numbered years cannot continue beyond the first Wednesday after the first Monday in June. Sessions in even-numbered years cannot continue beyond the first Wednesday after the first Monday in May.
G. Special Legislative Session
   1. Convenes: When called by the governor.
   2. Length of Session: No limit on length of session.
   3. Subject(s) To Be Considered: May consider only subject(s) specified in the governor's proclamation convening the legislature.

H. Bill Introduction
  1. Time Limitations: Time limitations on the introduction of legislation is fixed by the legislature when adapting rules for the biennium.
  2. Exceptions to Time Limitations: Bills at the request of the governor for emergency or necessity, emergency legislation designated by presiding officers, legislation revisions, and omnibus validation acts.
I. Standing Committees
  1. Average Number
    a. Joint: 22.
  2. Committee Hearings Open to Public
    a. Usually open, certain matters specified by statute can be discussed in executive session upon a two-thirds vote of committee members present and voting and stating the reason for such executive session.
J. Bill-to-Law Process
  1. By Whom Referred to Committee
    a. Senate: President pro tem.
    b. House: Speaker of the house.
  2. Required Readings: Three readings of a bill are required before a final vote can take place; however, bills or joint resolutions may receive a second reading on the same day.
  3. Formal Floor Debate: Occurs after the second reading, and bills are frequently amended from the floor during this debate.
  4. Recorded Vote on Final Passage
    a. Senate: A record of the votes is not required on bills; however, it can be required upon request of the members.
    b. House: Role call is not required, but is usually taken.
  5. Passage of a Bill: Minimum vote required to pass a bill in each house is a majority of those present and voting.
  6. Fate of a Passed Bill Before Adjournment: The governor either signs or vetoes the bill. If the governor does neither, within five days of receipt of the bill (Sundays and legal holidays excluded), the bill becomes law.
  7. Fate of a Passed Bill After Adjournment: The governor either signs or vetoes the bill. If the governor does neither, in 15 days from its receipt (Sundays and legal holidays excluded), the bill becomes law.
  8. Passage of a Bill Over the Governor's Veto: Requires a two-thirds majority of the elected members of both houses.

Delaware

A. Official Names
  1. Both Houses: General assembly.
  2. Upper House: Senate.
  3. Lower House: House of representatives.
B. Convening Place: Legislative Hall, Dover, DE 19901.

C. Number of Legislators
   1. Senators: 21.
   2. Representatives: 41.
D. Terms of Office
   1. Governor: 4 years.
   2. Senators: 4 years.
   3. Representatives: 2 years.
E. Legislative Officers and Leaders: Elected by the members of their respective chambers, except the president of the senate, the lieutenant governor, who is appointed by the governor.
   1. Senate
      a. President: the lieutenant governor, who serves ex officio.
      b. President pro tem.
   2. House: Speaker of the house.
F. Regular Legislative Session
   1. Convenes: Annually on the second Tuesday in January. The legislature meets in two annual sessions, each adjourning sine die. Bills may carry over from first to second session.
   2. Length of Time: Sessions cannot continue beyond June 30.
G. Special Legislative Session
   1. Convenes: When called by the governor or by a joint call of the presiding officers of both houses.
   2. Length of Session: No limit on length of session.
   3. Subject(s) To Be Considered: Either the governor or the legislature can determine the subject(s) to be considered.
H. Bill Introduction
   1. Time Limitation: Time limitation on the introduction of legislation exists in the house only and is fixed during the month of May by a resolution proposed by the majority leader.
   2. Exceptions to Time Limitation: Exceptions are permitted by a majority vote of the house.
I. Standing Committees
   1. Average Number
      a. Senate: 16.
      b. House: 18.
      c. Joint: 1.
   2. Committee Hearings Open to the Public
      a. Senate.
      b. House.
J. Bill-to-Law Process
   1. By Whom Referred to Committee
      a. Senate: President pro tem.
      b. House: Speaker of the House.
   2. Required Readings: Two readings of a bill are required before a final vote can take place. These readings must occur on separate days.
   3. Formal Floor Debate: Occurs after the second reading, and bills are frequently amended from the floor during this debate.

4. Recorded Vote on Final Passage: Votes are recorded manually.
5. Passage of a Bill: Minimum vote required to pass a bill in each house is a majority of the elected members.
6. Fate of a Passed Bill Before Adjournment: The governor either signs the bill into law or vetoes it. If the governor does neither within five days (Sundays excluded), the bill becomes law.
7. Fate of a Passed Bill After Adjournment: The Governor either signs the bill into law or vetoes it. If the governor does neither within 30 days (Sundays included), the bill dies.
8. Passage of a Bill Over the Governor's Veto: Requires a majority vote of three-fifths of the elected members of both houses.

Florida

A. Official Names
   1. Both Houses: Legislature
   2. Upper House: Senate.
   3. Lower House: House of representatives.
B. Convening Place: State Capitol. Senate: Capitol South Wing; house: Capitol North Wing, Tallahassee, FL 32301.
C. Number of Legislators
   1. Senators: 40.
   2. Representatives: 120.
D. Terms of Office
   1. Governor: 4 years.
   2. Senators: 4 years.
   3. Representatives: 2 years.
E. Legislative Officers and Leaders: Elected by all members of their respective chambers.
   1. Senate
      a. President of the house.
      b. President pro tem.
   2. House
      a. Speaker of the house.
      b. Speaker pro tem.
F. Regular Legislative Session
   1. Convenes: Annually on the Tuesday after the first Monday in April. Legislature meets in an organizational session on the 14th day following each general election.
   2. Length of Session: Session is limited to 60 calendar days; however, session may be extended for an indefinite period of time by a three-fifths vote of members of both houses.
G. Special Legislative Session
   1. Convenes: When called by the governor or by a joint call of the presiding officers of both houses.
   2. Length of Session: Session is limited to 20 calendar days; however, session may be extended for an indefinite period of time by a three-fifths vote of members of both houses.

3. Subject(s) To Be Considered: Either the governor or the legislature determines the subject(s) to be considered.

H. Bill Introduction
1. Time Limitations
   a. Senate: Legislation must be introduced by the 18th legislative day.
   b. House: General bills and joint resolutions must be introduced by the second Friday after the first Tuesday of the session, however, local bills must be introduced by the seventh Friday after the first Tuesday of the session.
2. Exceptions to Time Limitations: Exceptions are permitted by a two-thirds vote or by a recommendation of the Rules Committee.

I. Standing Committees
1. Average Number
   a. Senate: 16.
   b. House: 22.
2. Committee Hearings Open to the Public
   a. Senate.
   b. House.

J. Bill-to-Law Process
1. By Whom Referred to Committee
   a. Senate: President of the senate.
   b. House: Speaker of the house.
2. Required Readings: Three readings of a bill are required before a final vote can take place. These readings must occur on separate days except by a two-thirds vote of the chamber to change the rule.
3. Formal Floor Debate: Occurs after the second reading. Bills are frequently amended from the floor during this debate.
4. Recorded Vote on Final Passage: Votes are recorded by electronic vote tabulation.
5. Passage of a Bill: Minimum vote required in each house is a majority of those present.
6. Fate of a Passed Bill Before Adjournment: The governor either signs the bill into law or vetoes it. If the governor does neither within seven days (Sundays included), the bill becomes law.
7. Fate of a Passed Bill After Adjournment: The governor either signs the bill into law or vetoes it. If the governor does neither within 15 days of receipt (Sundays included), the bill becomes law.
8. Passage of a Bill Over the Governor's Veto: Requires a vote of two-thirds of the elected members in both houses.

Georgia

A. Official Names
1. Both Houses: General assembly.
2. Upper House: Senate.
3. Lower House: House of representatives.
B. Convening Place: State Capitol, Capitol Square SW, Atlanta, GA 30334

C. Number of Legislators
   1. Senators: 56.
   2. Representatives: 180.
D. Terms of Office
   1. Governor: 4 years.
   2. Senators: 2 years.
   3. Representatives: 2 years.
E. Legislative Officers and Leaders: Elected by all members of their respective chambers, except the president of the senate, the lieutenant governor, who is appointed by the governor.
   1. Senate
      a. President: The lieutenant governor, who serves ex officio.
      b. President pro tem.
   2. House
      a. Speaker of the house.
      b. Speaker pro tem.
F. Regular Legislative Session
   1. Convenes: Annually on the second Monday in January. The legislature meets in two annual sessions. There is no set time for adjournment. Bills may carry over from the first to second session.
   2. Length of Session: Session is limited to 40 legislative days.
G. Special Legislative Session
   1. Convenes: When called by the governor or by a petition of three-fifths members of each house.
   2. Length of Session: Session is limited to 70 days if called by the governor, and 30 days if called at petition of legislature, except for impeachment proceedings.
H. Bill Introduction
   1. Time Limitation: Legislation must be introduced by the 33rd legislative day.
   2. Exceptions to Time Limitation: Exceptions are permitted by a three-fifths vote.
I. Standing Committees
   1. Average Number
      a. Senate: 19.
      b. House: 28.
   2. Committee Hearings Open to the Public
      a. Senate.
      b. House.
J. Bill-to-Law Process
   1. By Whom Referred to Committee
      a. Senate: President of the senate.
      b. House: Speaker of the house.
   2. Required Readings: Three readings of a bill are required before a final vote can take place, and these readings must occur on separate days.
   3. Formal Floor Debate: Occurs after the third reading, and bills are frequently amended from the floor during this debate.

4. Recorded Vote on Final Passage
   a. Senate: Votes are recorded by an electronic vote tabulation except on local bills.
   b. House: A record of the votes is not required; however, on bills, can be required upon request of member. Roll call is not required, but is usually taken.
5. Passage of a Bill: Minimum vote required to pass a bill in each house is a majority of the membership.
6. Fate of a Passed Bill Before Adjournment: The governor either signs bill into law or vetoes it. If the governor does neither within five days (Sundays excluded), the bill becomes law. The state constitution prohibits veto of a constitutional amendment.
7. Fate of a Passed Bill After Adjournment: The governor either signs the bill into law or vetoes it. If the governor does neither within 30 days (Sundays excluded), the bill becomes law. If the governor vetoes the bill, it is returned to the presiding officer of the house in which it originated. Such bills may be considered by the house at any time during the first ten days of the next regular session, for purposes of overriding the veto. The state constitution prohibits veto of constitutional amendments.
8. Passage of a Bill Over the Governor's Veto: Requires a two-thirds vote of the members of both houses.

Hawaii

A. Official Names
   1. Both Houses: Legislature.
   2. Upper House: Senate.
   3. Lower House: House of representatives.
B. Convening Place: State Capitol Building, 415 S Beretania, Honolulu, HI 96813.
C. Number of Legislators
   1. Senators: 25.
   2. Representatives: 51.
D. Terms of Office
   1. Governor: 4 years.
   2. Senators: 4 years.
   3. Representatives: 2 years.
E. Legislative Officers and Leaders: Elected by all members of their respective chambers.
   1. Senate
      a. President of the senate.
      b. Vice president of the senate.
   2. House
      a. Speaker of the house.
      b. Vice speaker of the house.

F. Regular Legislative Session
1. Convenes: Annually on the third Wednesday in January. The legislature meets in two annual sessions. There is no set time for adjournment. Bills may carry over from the first to the second session.
2. Length of Session: Session is limited to 60 legislative days; however, session may be extended for not more than 15 days by petition of two-thirds members of each house.
G. Special Legislative Session
1. Convenes: When called by the governor or by a petition of two-thirds members of each house.
2. Length of Session: Session is limited to 30 legislative days but may be extended for not more than 15 days by petition of two-thirds of the members of each house.
3. Subject(s) To Be Considered: Either the governor or the legislature can determine the subject(s) to be considered.
H. Bill Introduction
1. Time Limitations: Time limitations on the introduction of legislation are established during the course of the session.
2. Exceptions to Time Limitations: Exceptions are permitted by a two-thirds vote.
I. Standing Committees
1. Average Number
a. Senate: 17.
b. House: 20.
2. Committee Hearings Open to the Public
a. Senate.
b. House.
J. Bill-to-Law Process
1. By Whom Referred to Committee
a. Senate: President of the senate.
b. House: Speaker of the house.
2. Required Readings: Three readings of a bill are required before a final vote can take place. These readings must occur on separate days.
3. Formal Floor Debate: Occurs after the second reading. Bills can be amended from the floor during this debate; however, no floor amendments can be voted upon until a copy of the amendments has been presented to each member.
4. Recorded Vote on Final Passage: Votes are recorded manually.
5. Passage of a Bill: Minimum vote required to pass a bill is a majority of the membership of each house.
6. Fate of a Passed Bill Before Adjournment: The governor either signs the bill into law or vetoes it. If the governor does neither within ten days (Saturdays, Sundays, holidays, and days on which the legislature is in recess prior to adjournment excluded), the bill becomes law. The constitution prohibits the governor from vetoing a constitutional amendment.
7. Fate of a Passed Bill After Adjournment: Governor either signs the bill into law or vetoes it. If the governor does neither within 45 days (Sat-

urdays, Sundays, and holidays excluded), the bill becomes law. If a bill is given to the governor within ten days of the legislature's adjournment and the governor indicates that he or she will return it with objections, the legislature may convene on the 45th day after its adjournment to consider the governor's objections. If the legislature chooses not to reconvene to consider the governor's objections to the bill, the bill dies on the 45th day. The constitution prohibits the governor from vetoing a constitutional amendment.

8. Passage of a Bill Over the Governor's Veto: Requires a two-thirds vote of the members of both houses.

Idaho

A. Official Names
   1. Both Houses: Legislature.
   2. Upper House: Senate.
   3. Lower House: House of representatives.
B. Convening Place: Idaho State House, Boise, ID 83720.
C. Number of Legislators
   1. Senators: 35.
   2. Representatives: 70.
D. Terms of Office
   1. Governor: 4 years.
   2. Senators: 2 years.
   3. Representatives: 2 years.
E. Legislative Officers and Leaders: Elected by the members of their respective chambers, except the president of the senate, the lieutenant governor, who is appointed to this office by the governor.
   1. Senate
      a. President: The lieutenant governor, who serves ex officio.
      b. President, pro tem.
   2. House: Speaker of the house.
F. Regular Legislative Session
   1. Convenes: Annually on the Monday that falls on or is nearest the ninth day of January.
   2. Length of Session: No limit on length of session.
G. Special Legislative Session
   1. Convenes: When called by the governor.
   2. Length of Session: Session is limited to 20 calendar days.
   3. Subject(s) To Be Considered: May consider only subject(s) specified in the governor's proclamation convening the legislature.
H. Bill Introduction
   1. Time Limitations: House: Individual members of the house must introduce legislation by the 25th day. All committees except the Appropriation, State Affairs, Revenue and Taxation, and Ways and Means committees must introduce legislation by the 45th day. Senate: Individual

members of the senate must introduce legislation by the 20th day. All committees except Finance, State Affairs, Judiciary and Rules must introduce legislation by the 35th day.

  2. Exceptions to Time Limitations: Exceptions are permitted by the speaker, who may designate any committee to serve as a privileged committee, either temporarily or for the remainder of the session.

I. Standing Committees
  1. Average Number
    a. Senate: 9.
    b. House: 13.
  2. Committee Hearings Open to Public
    a. Senate.
    b. House.

J. Bill-to-Law Process
  1. By Whom Referred to Committee
    a. Senate: President of the senate.
    b. House: Speaker of the house.
  2. Readings: Three readings of a bill are required before a final vote can take place. These readings must occur on separate days except by a two-thirds vote.
  3. Formal Floor Debate: Occurs after the third reading. Bills can be amended from the floor during this debate. In order for a bill to be amended; however, it must be transferred from the third reading calendar to another order of business.
  4. Recorded Vote on Final Passage
    a. Senate: Votes are recorded manually.
    b. House: Votes recorded by electronic vote tabulation.
  5. Passage of a Bill: Minimum vote required to pass a bill in each house is a majority of those present.
  6. Fate of a Passed Bill Before Adjournment: The governor either signs the bill into law or vetoes it. If the governor does neither within five days (Sundays excluded), the bill becomes law.
  7. Fate of a Passed Bill After Adjournment: The governor either signs the bill into law or vetoes it. If the governor does neither within ten days (Sundays excluded), the bill becomes law.
  8. Passage of a Bill Over the Governor's Veto: Requires a three-fifths vote of the elected members of both houses.

Illinois

A. Official Names
  1. Both Houses: General assembly.
  2. Upper House: Senate.
  3. Lower House: House of representatives.
B. Convening Place: State House, State Capitol Complex, Springfield, IL 62706.

C. Number of Legislators
   1. Senators: 59.
   2. Representatives: 177.
D. Terms of Office
   1. Governor: Changed from 2 to 4 years with the 1978 election.
   2. Senators: All senators were elected in 1972 for a 10-year term, and elections will be every 10 years thereafter. Senate districts are divided into three groups for the purpose of insuring staggered terms:
      a. One group elects senators for terms of 4 years, 4 years, and 2 years.
      b. A second group elects senators for terms of 4 years, 2 years, and 4 years.
      c. A third group elects senators for terms of 2 years, 4 years, and 4 years.
   3. Representatives: 2 years.
E. Legislative Officers and Leaders: Elected by all members of their respective chambers.
   1. Senate: President of the senate.
   2. House: Speaker of the house.
F. Regular Legislative Session
   1. Convenes: Annually on the second Wednesday in January. The legislature meets in two annual sessions. Bills may carry over from first to second session.
   2. Length of Session: No limit on length of sessions.
G. Special Legislative Session
   1. Convenes: When called by the governor or by a joint call of the presiding officers of both houses.
   2. Length of Session: No limit on length of sessions.
   3. Subject(s) To Be Considered: Either the governor or the legislature can determine the subject(s) to be considered.
H. Bill Introduction
   1. Time Limitations
      a. Odd-Numbered Years: Legislation must be introduced by April 3.
      b. Even-Numbered Years: All bills are referred to the Rules Committee for decision.
   2. Exceptions to Time Limitations: Exceptions are permitted by three-fifths vote; however, in odd-numbered years, bills may be exempted from the April 3 deadline by the Rules Committee. In even-numbered years, committee bills and revenue and appropriation bills are exempt from the limitation.
I. Standing Committees
   1. Average Number
      a. Senate: 15.
      b. House: 20.
   2. Committee Hearings Open to the Public
      a. Senate.
      b. House.
J. Bill-to-Law Process
   1. By Whom Referred to Committee
      a. Senate: Committee on Assignments
      b. House: Committee on Assignments

2. Required Readings: Three readings of a bill are required before a final vote can take place. These readings must occur on separate days.
3. Formal Floor Debate: Occurs after the third reading. Amendments may be submitted at the second reading only, not during final formal floor debate.
4. Recorded Vote on Final Passage: Votes are recorded by electronic vote tabulation.
5. Passage of a Bill: Minimum vote required to pass a bill in each house is a majority of the membership.
6. Fate of a Passed Bill Before Adjournment: The governor either signs the bill into law or vetoes it. If the governor does neither within 60 days after it is received (Sundays excluded), the bill becomes law.
7. Fate of a Passed Bill After Adjournment: The governor either signs the bill into law or vetoes it. If the governor does neither within 90 days (Sundays excluded), the bill becomes law. If the governor is unable to return a bill and his or her objections to the legislature due to adjournment, and the bill and the governor's objections are filed with the secretary of state within 60 days of the governor's receipt of the bill, the secretary of the state then returns the bill and the governor's objections to the originating house promptly upon the next meeting of that house. In the interim, the bill does not become law.
8. Passage of a Bill Over the Governor's Veto: Requires a three-fifths vote of the members of both houses.

Iowa

A. Official Names
   1. Both Houses: General assembly.
   2. Upper House: Senate
   3. Lower House: House of representatives.
B. Convening Place: State Capitol, E Tenth Grand Avenue, Des Moines, IA 50319.
C. Number of Legislators
   1. Senators: 50.
   2. Representatives: 100.
D. Terms of Office
   1. Governor: 4 years.
   2. Senators: 4 years.
   3. Representatives: 2 years.
E. Legislative Officers and Leaders: Elected by all members of their respective chambers, except the president of the senate, the lieutenant governor, who is appointed to that position by the governor.
   1. Senate
      a. President: lieutenant governor, who serves ex officio.
      b. President pro tem.
   2. House
      a. Speaker of the house.
      b. Speaker pro tem.

F. Regular Legislative Session
1. Convenes: Annually on the second Monday in January. The legislature meets in two annual sessions, of no specified length. Bills carry over from first to second session.
2. Length of Session: No limit on length of session
G. Special Legislative Session
1. Convenes: When called by the governor or by a petition of two-thirds of the members of each house.
2. Length of Session: No limit on length of session.
3. Subject(s) To Be Considered: Either the governor or the legislature may determine subject(s) to be considered.
H. Bill Introduction
1. Time Limitations
a. Senate: In odd-numbered years, legislation must be introduced by Friday of the seventh week. In even-numbered years, legislation must be introduced by Friday of the second week.
b. House: In odd-numbered years, legislation must be introduced by the 61st calendar day. In even-numbered years, legislation must be introduced by the 15th calendar day.
2. Exceptions to Time Limitations
a. Senate: Bills cosponsored by the majority and minority floor leaders are exempt from the limitation.
b. House: Exceptions are permitted by a majority vote of the membership unless a written request for drafting the bill was submitted before the deadline. Committee bills are exempt from the limitation.
I. Standing Committees
1. Average Number
a. Senate: 15.
b. House: 15.
2. Committee Hearings Open to the Public
a. Senate.
b. House.
J. Bill-to-Law Process
1. By Whom Referred to Committee
a. Senate: Majority leader, president pro tem, or two assistant majority leaders.
b. House: Speaker of the house.
2. Required Readings: Two readings of a bill are required before a final vote can take place. These readings must occur on separate days.
3. Formal Floor Debate: Occurs after the second reading. Bills are frequently amended from the floor during this debate.
4. Recorded Vote on Final Passage: Votes are recorded by electronic vote tabulation.
5. Passage of a Bill: Minimum vote required to pass a bill in each house is a majority of the membership.
6. Fate of a Passed Bill Before Adjournment: The governor either signs the bill into law or vetoes it. If the governor does neither within three days (Sundays excluded), the bill becomes law.

7. Fate of a Passed Bill After Adjournment: The governor either signs the bill into law or vetoes it. Bills passed within three days of the end of the legislative session must be deposited by the governor with the secretary of state within 30 days following adjournment. The governor must give his or her reasons for disapproving a bill.
8. Passage of a Bill Over the Governor's Veto: Requires a two-thirds vote of the members of both houses.

Indiana

A. Official Names
  1. Both Houses: General assembly.
  2. Upper House: Senate.
  3. Lower House: House of representatives.
B. Convening Place: State House or State Capitol, 200 W Washington, Indianapolis, IN 46204.
C. Number of Legislators
  1. Senators: 50.
  2. Representatives: 100.
D. Terms of Office
  1. Governor: 4 years.
  2. Senators: 4 years.
  3. Representatives: 2 years.
E. Legislative Officers and Leaders: Elected by all members of their respective chambers, except the president of the senate, the lieutenant governor, who is appointed to that position by the governor.
  1. Senate
    a. President: The lieutenant governor, who serves ex officio.
    b. President pro tem.
  2. House: Speaker of the house.
F. Regular Legislative Session
  1. Convenes: Annually on the second Monday in January. The legislature meets in an organizational session on the third Tuesday after the first Monday in November for one day only.
  2. Length of Session:
    a. Odd-Numbered Years: sessions are limited to 61 legislative days or to an April 30 adjournment deadline.
    b. Even-Numbered Years: sessions are limited to 30 legislative days or to a March 15 adjournment deadline.
G. Special Legislative Session
  1. Convenes: When called by the governor.
  2. Length of Session: Session is limited to 30 legislative days within 40 calendar days.
  3. Subject(s) To Be Considered: Either the governor or the legislature may determine the subject(s) to be considered.

H. Bill Introduction
   1. Time Limitations
      a. Senate: In odd-numbered years, legislation must be introduced by the 12th session day. In even-numbered years, legislation must be introduced by the fourth session day.
      b. House: In odd-numbered years, legislation must be introduced by the 16th session day. In even-numbered years, legislation must be introduced by the fourth session day.
   2. Exceptions to Time Limitation: Exceptions are permitted in the senate by consent of the Rules and Legislative Procedure Committee. Exceptions are permitted in house by a two-thirds vote.
I. Standing Committees
   1. Average Number
      a. Senate: 16.
      b. House: 22.
   2. Committee Hearings Open to the Public
      a. Senate.
      b. House.
J. Bill-to-Law Process
   1. By Whom Referred to Committee
      a. Senate: President pro tem.
      b. House: Speaker of the house.
   2. Required Readings: Three readings of a bill are required before a final vote can take place. These readings must occur on separate days except by a two-thirds vote.
   3. Formal Floor Debate: Occurs after the third reading, and bills are seldom amended from the floor during this debate.
   4. Recorded Vote on Final Passage
      a. Senate: Votes are recorded by electronic vote tabulation.
      b. House: Votes are recorded by electronic vote tabulation except concurrence in senate amendments.
   5. Passage of a Bill: Minimum vote required to pass bill in each house is a majority of the membership.
   6. Fate of a Passed Bill Before Adjournment: The governor either signs the bill into law or vetoes it. If the governor does neither within seven days (Sundays excluded), the bill becomes law.
   7. Fate of a Passed Bill After Adjournment: The Governor either signs the bill into law or vetoes it. If the governor does neither within seven days (Sundays excluded), the bill becomes law.
   8. Passage of a Bill Over the Governor's Veto: Requires a majority vote of the members of both houses.

Kansas

A. Official Names
   1. Both Houses: Legislature.
   2. Upper House: Senate.
   3. Lower House: House of representatives.

B. Convening Place: State House, Topeka, KS 66612.
C. Number of Legislators
   1. Senators: 40.
   2. Representatives: 125.
D. Terms of Office
   1. Governor: 4 years.
   2. Senators: 4 years.
   3. Representatives: 2 years.
E. Legislative Officers and Leaders: Elected by all members of their respective chambers.
   1. Senate
      a. President of the senate.
      b. Vice president of the senate.
   2. House
      a. Speaker of the house.
      b. Speaker pro tem.
F. Regular Legislative Session
   1. Convenes: Annually on the second Monday in January. The legislature meets in two annual sessions, of no specified length. Bills may carry over from first to second session.
   2. Length of Session
      a. Odd-Numbered Years: Sessions are not limited in length.
      b. Even-numbered years: Sessions are limited to 90 calendar days; however, both sessions may be extended for an indefinite period of time by a two-thirds vote of elected members of each house.
G. Special Legislative Session
   1. Convenes: When called by the governor or by a petition to the governor of two-thirds of the members of each house.
   2. Length of Session: No limit on length of session.
   3. Subject(s) To Be Considered: Either the governor or the legislature can determine the subject(s) to be considered.
H. Bill Introduction
   1. Time Limitations
      a. Odd-Numbered Years: Individuals must introduce legislation by the 36th calendar day. Committees must introduce legislation by the 45th calendar day.
      b. Even-Numbered Years: Individuals must introduce legislation by the 14th calendar day. Committees must introduce legislation by the 30th calendar day.
   2. Exceptions to Time Limitations: Exceptions are permitted by a majority vote. Other exceptions are bills introduced by the committes on Ways and Means, Senate Committee on Organization, Calendar Committee, Rules Committee, Senate Committee on Federal and State Affairs, House Committee on Calendar and Printing, and authorized select committees.
I. Standing Committees
   1. Average Number
      a. Senate: 16
      b. House: 19.

      2. Committee Hearings Open to the Public
        a. Senate.
        b. House.

J. Bill-to-Law Process
      1. By Whom Referred to Committee
        a. Senate: President of the senate.
        b. House: Speaker of the house.
      2. Required readings: Two readings of a bill are required before a final vote takes place. These readings must occur on separate days except by a two-thirds vote.
      3. Formal Floor Debate: Occurs during the meeting of the Committee of the Whole. Bills are frequently amended from the floor during this debate.
      4. Recorded Vote on Final Passage
        a. Senate: Votes are recorded manually.
        b. House: Votes are recorded by electronic vote tabulation.
      5. Passage of a Bill: Minimum vote required to pass a bill in each house is a majority of the membership.
      6. Fate of a Passed Bill Before Adjournment: The governor either signs the bill into law or vetoes it. If the governor does neither within ten days (Sundays excluded), the bill becomes law.
      7. Fate of a Passed Bill After Adjournment: The governor either signs the bill into law or vetoes it. If the governor does neither within ten days (Sundays excluded), the bill becomes law.
      8. Passage of a Bill Over the Governor's Veto: Requires a two-thirds vote of the members of both houses.

Kentucky

A. Official Names
      1. Both Houses: General assembly.
      2. Upper House: Senate.
      3. Lower House: House of representatives.
B. Convening Place: State Capitol, Frankfort, KY 40601.
C. Number of Legislators
      1. Senators: 38.
      2. Representatives: 100.
D. Terms of Office
      1. Governor: 4 years.
      2. Senators: 4 years.
      3. Representatives: 2 years.
E. Legislative Officers and Leaders: Elected by all members of their respective chambers, except the president of the senate, the lieutenant governor, who is appointed by the governor.
      1. Senate
        a. President: The lieutenant governor, who serves ex officio.
        b. President pro tem.

    2. House
       a. Speaker of the house.
       b. Speaker pro tem.

F. Regular Legislative Session
    1. Convenes: Tuesday after the first Monday in January of even-numbered years.
    2. Length of Session: Session is limited to 60 legislative days.

G. Special Legislative Session
    1. Convenes: When called by the governor.
    2. Length of Session: No limit on length of session.
    3. Subject(s) To Be Considered: May consider only subject(s) specified in the governor's proclamation convening the legislature.

H. Bill Introduction
    1. Time Limitations: All legislation must be introduced before the final ten days.
    2. Exceptions to Time Limitations: Exceptions are permitted by a majority vote of elected members.

I. Standing Committees
    1. Average Number
       a. Senate: 15.
       b. House: 15.
    2. Committee Hearings Open to the Public
       a. Senate.
       b. House.

Bill-to-Law Process
    1. By Whom Referred to Committee
       a. Senate: Committee on Committees.
       b. House: Committee on Committees.
    2. Required Readings: Three readings of a bill are required before a final vote can take place. These readings must occur on separate days except by a majority vote, in which case the second and third readings may be skipped.
    3. Formal Floor Debate: Occurs after the third reading. Bills are frequently amended from the floor during this debate.
    4. Recorded Vote on Final Passage
       a. Senate: Votes are recorded manually.
       b. House: Votes are recorded by electronic vote tabulation.
    5. Passage of a Bill: Minimum vote required to pass a bill in each house is two-fifths of the elected members.
    6. Fate of a Passed Bill Before Adjourment: The governor either signs the bill into law or vetoes it. If the governor does neither within ten days (Sundays excluded), the bill becomes law.
    7. Fate of a Passed Bill After Adjournment: The governor either signs the bill into law or vetoes it. If the governor does neither within ten days (Sundays excluded), the bill becomes law.
    8. Passage of a Bill Over the Governor's Veto: Requires a majority vote of the members of both houses.

Louisiana

A. Official Names
   1. Both Houses: Legislature.
   2. Upper House: Senate.
   3. Lower House: House of representatives.
B. Convening Place: State Capitol, 900 Riverside NW, Baton Rouge, LA 70804.
C. Number of Legislators
   1. Senators: 39.
   2. Representatives: 105.
D. Terms of Office
   1. Governor: 4 years.
   2. Senators: 4 years.
   3. Representatives: 4.
E. Legislative Officers and Leaders: Elected by all members of their respective chambers.
   1. Senate
      a. President of the senate.
      b. President pro tem.
   2. House
      a. Speaker of the house.
      b. Speaker pro tem.
F. Regular Legislative Session
   1. Convenes: Annually on the third Monday in April.
   2. Length of Session: Session is limited to 60 legislative days in 85 calendar days.
G. Special Legislative Session
   1. Convenes: When called by the governor or by a petition of the majority of members of each house.
   2. Length of Session: Session is limited to 30 calendar days.
   3. Subject(s) To Be Considered: May consider subject(s) specified in governor's proclamation convening the legislature; however, if legislature convenes itself, it may determine subject(s) to be considered.
H. Bill Introduction
   1. Time Limitations: All legislation must be introduced by the 15th calendar day.
   2. Exceptions to Time Limitations: Exceptions are permitted by a two-thirds vote of elected members.
I. Standing Committees
   1. Average Number
      a. Senate: 15.
      b. House: 15.
   2. Committee Hearings Open to the Public
      a. Senate.
      b. House.

J. Bill-to-Law Process
   1. By Whom Referred to Committee
       a. Senate: President of the senate.
       b. House: Speaker of the house.
   2. Required Readings: Three readings of a bill are required before a final vote can take place. These readings must occur on separate days.
   3. Formal Floor Debate: Occurs after the third reading. Bills are frequently amended from the floor during this debate.
   4. Recorded Vote on Final Passage: Votes are recorded by electronic vote tabulation.
   5. Passage of a Bill: Minimum vote required to pass a bill in each house is a majority of the members.
   6. Fate of a Passed Bill Before Adjournment: The governor either signs the bill into law or vetoes it. If the governor does neither within ten days (Sundays included) of receiving it, the bill becomes law. The constitution prohibits the governor from vetoing a constitutional amendment.
   7. Fate of a Passed Bill After Adjournment: The governor either signs the bill into law or vetoes it. If the governor does neither within 20 days (Sundays included) of receiving it, the bill becomes law. The constitution prohibits the governor from vetoing a constitutional amendment.
   8. Passage of a Bill Over the Governor's Veto: Requires a two-thirds majority vote of the members of both houses.

Maine

A. Official Names
   1. Both Houses: Legislature.
   2. Upper House: Senate.
   3. Lower House: House of representatives.
B. Convening Place: State House, Augusta, ME 04330.
C. Number of Legislators
   1. Senators: 33.
   2. Representatives: 151.
D. Terms of Office
   1. Governor: 4 years.
   2. Senators: 2 years.
   3. Representatives: 2 years.
E. Legislative Officers and Leaders: Elected by all members of their respective chambers.
   1. Senate: President of the senate.
   2. House: Speaker of the house.
F. Regular Legislative Session
   1. Convenes: Annually on the first Wednesday after the first Tuesday in January. The second session of legislature is basically limited to budget

and fiscal matters, but can include legislation considered in the governor's call, study committee legislation, and initiate measures.

    2. Length of Session: No limit on length of session.

G. Special Legislative Session

    1. Convenes: When called by the governor or by a vote of the majority of each part in each house.

    2. Length of Session: No limit on length of session.

    3. Subject(s) To Be Considered: May consider subject(s) specified in governor's proclamation convening the legislature; however, only if legislature convenes itself may it determine the subject(s) to be considered.

H. Bill Introduction

    1. Time Limitations: Legislation in drafted form must be introduced by the fourth Friday after convening. Legislation in final form must be introduced no later than the sixth Tuesday following the fourth Friday after convening.

    2. Exceptions to Time Limitations: Exceptions are permitted by the approval of a majority of the members of the Legislative Council. Bills to facilitate legislative business are exempt from the limitation.

I. Standing Committees

    1. Average Number: 22 joint committees.

    2. Committee Hearings Open to the Public

      a. Senate.

      b. House.

J. Bill-to-Law Process

    1. By Whom Referred to Committee: In the senate, the secretary of the senate; in the house, the clerk of the house. Should there be disagreements between the clerk and the secretary, the speaker of the house and the president of the senate make the assignment. If they cannot agree, the Legislative Council resolves the issue, subject to approval of disapproval by the membership of either house.

    2. Required Readings: Two readings of a bill are required before a final vote can take place. These readings must occur on separate days except by a three-fourths vote of the members of the chamber.

    3. Formal Floor Debate: Occurs after the second reading. Bills are seldom amended from the floor during this debate.

    4. Recorded Vote on Final Passage:

      a. Senate: A record of the votes is not required on a bill in the senate; however, it can be requested by the members.

      b. House: A record of the votes is not required on a bill in the house; however, it can be requested by the members.

    5. Passage of a Bill: Minimum vote required to pass a bill in each house is a majority of the members present and voting.

    6. Fate of a Passed Bill Before Adjournment: The governor either signs the bill into law or vetoes it. If the governor does neither within ten days (Sundays excluded), the bill becomes law.

    7. Fate of a Passed Bill After Adjournment: The governor either signs the bill into law or vetoes it. If the governor does neither and does not return the

bill to the legislature within the first three days of the next meeting, the bill becomes law.

8. Passage of a Bill Over the Governor's Veto: Requires a two-thirds vote of the members present in both houses.

Maryland

A. Official Names
   1. Both Houses: General assembly.
   2. Upper House: Senate.
   3. Lower House: House of delegates.
B. Convening Place: State House, State Circle, Annapolis, MD 21401.
C. Number of Legislators
   1. Senators: 47.
   2. Delegates: 141.
D. Terms of Office
   1. Governor: 4 years.
   2. Senators: 4 years.
   3. Delegates: 4 years.
E. Legislative Officers and Leaders: Elected by all members of their respective chambers.
   1. Senate
      a. President of the senate.
      b. President pro tem.
   2. House: Speaker of the house.
F. Regular Legislative Session
   1. Convenes: Annually on the second Wednesday in January.
   2. Length of Session: Session is limited to 90 calendar days; however, session may be extended for 30 additional days by a three-fifths vote of the members of each house.
G. Special Legislative Session
   1. Convenes: When called by the governor or by a petition of the majority of members of each house.
   2. Length of Session: Session is limited to 30 calendar days.
   3. Subject(s) To Be Considered: Either the governor or the legislature can determine the subject(s) to be considered.
H. Bill Introduction
   1. Time Limitations: Legislation must be introduced before the last 35 days. Appropriations bills must be introduced by the third Wednesday of January. New governors must introduce legislation in the first ten days after convening of the legislature.
   2. Exceptions to Time Limitations: Exceptions are permitted by a two-thirds vote.
I. Standing Committees
   1. Average Number
      a. Senate: 6.
      b. House: 5.

J. Bill-to-Law Process
1. By Whom Referred to Committee
   a. Senate: President of the Senate.
   b. House: Speaker of the House.
2. Required Readings: Three readings of a bill are required before a final vote can take place. These readings must occur on separate days except by a two-thirds vote.
3. Formal Floor Debate: Occurs after the second readings. Bills are frequently amended from the floor during this debate.
4. Recorded Vote on Final Passage: Votes are recorded by electronic tabulation.
5. Passage of a Bill: Minimum vote required to pass a bill in each house is a majority of the membership.
6. Fate of a Passed Bill Before Adjournment: The governor either signs the bill into law or vetoes it. If the governor does neither within six days (Sundays excluded), the bill becomes law. The constitution prohibits the governor from vetoing a constitutional amendment.
7. Fate of a Passed Bill After Adjournment: The governor either signs the bill into law or vetoes it. If the governor does neither within 30 days (Sundays excluded), the bill becomes law. The constitution prohibits the governor from vetoing a constitutional amendment.
8. Passage of a Bill Over the Governor's Veto: Requires a three-fifths vote of both houses. The governor may veto items in supplementary appropriations and capital construction bills only.

Massachusetts

A. Official Names
1. Both Houses: General court.
2. Upper House: Senate.
3. Lower House: House of representatives.
B. Convening Place: State House, Beacon Hill, Boston, MA 02133.
C. Number of Legislators
1. Senators: 40.
2. Representatives: 240.
D. Terms of Office
1. Governor: 4 years.
2. Senators: 2 years.
3. Representatives: 2 years.
E. Legislative Officers and Leaders: Elected by all members of their respective chambers.
1. Senate: President of the senate.
2. House: Speaker of the house.
F. Regular Legislative Session
1. Convenes: Annually on the first Wednesday in January.
2. Length of Session: No limit on length of session.

G. Special Legislative Session
   1. Convenes: When called by the governor or the legislature.
   2. Length of Session: No limit on length of session.
   3. Subject(s) To Be Considered: Either the governor or the legislature can determine the subject(s) to be considered.

H. Bill Introduction
   1. Time Limitation: Legislation must be introduced by the first Wednesday in December.
   2. Exceptions to Time Limitation: Exceptions are permitted by a four-fifths vote. Other exceptions are requests of the governor, special commissions or committees with specific reporting dates, and home-rule petitions.

I. Standing Committees
   1. Average Number
      a. Senate: 4.
      b. House: 4.
      c. Joint: 21.
   2. Committee Hearings Open to the Public
      a. Senate.
      b. House.

J. Bill-to-Law Process
   1. By Whom Referred to Committee: In both houses the clerk refers the bill to committee, subject to approval or disapproval by the presiding officer of either house.
   2. Required Readings: Three readings of a bill are required before a final vote can take place. These usually occur on separate days; however, if rules are suspended, all readings may be on the same day.
   3. Formal Floor Debate: Occurs after the second reading. Bills are frequently amended from the floor during the floor debate unless engrossed.
   4. Recorded Vote on Final Passage:
      a. Senate: A record of the votes is not required on bills in the senate; however, it can be required upon request of members. This is not based on constitutional requirement.
      b. House: A record of votes is not required on bills in the house; however, it can be required upon request of members. This is not based on constitutional requirement.
   5. Passage of a Bill: Minimum vote required to pass a bill in each house is a majority of those present and voting. This is not a constitutional requirement.
   6. Fate of a Passed Bill Before Adjournment: The governor either signs the bill into law or vetoes it. If the governor does neither within ten days (Sunday and legal holidays excluded), the bill becomes law.
   7. Fate of a Passed Bill After Adjournment: Governor either signs the bill into law or vetoes it. If the Governor does neither within ten days (Sundays and legal holidays excluded) after receipt, the bill dies.
   8. Passage of a Bill Over the Governor's Veto: Requires a two-thirds vote of the members present in each house.

Michigan

A. Official Names
   1. Both Houses: Legislature.
   2. Upper House: Senate.
   3. Lower House: House of representatives.
B. Convening Place: State Capitol, Lansing, MI 48913.
C. Number of Legislators
   1. Senators: 38.
   2. Representatives: 110.
D. Terms of Office
   1. Governor: 4 years.
   2. Senators: 4 years.
   3. Representatives: 2 years.
E. Legislative Officers and Leaders: Elected by the members of their respective chambers, except the president of the senate, the lieutenant governor, who is appointed by the governor.
   1. Senate
      a. President: The lieutenant governor, who serves ex officio.
      b. President pro tem.
      c. Assistant president pro tem.
      d. Associate president pro tem.
   2. House
      a. Speaker of the house.
      b. Speaker pro tem.
      c. Associate speakers pro tem.
F. Regular Legislative Session
   1. Convenes: Annually on the second Wednesday in January. The legislature meets in two annual sessions. Bills may carry over from first to second session.
   2. Length of Session: No limit on length of session.
G. Special Legislative Session
   1. Convenes: When called by the governor.
   2. Length of Session: No limit on length of session.
   3. Subject(s) To Be Considered: May consider only subject(s) specified in governor's proclamation convening the legislature.
H. Bill Introduction
   1. Time Limitations: No time limitation exists on the introduction of legislation.
I. Standing Committees
   1. Average Number
      a. Senate: 17.
      b. House: 33.
      c. Joint: 5.
   2. Committee Hearings Open to the Public
      a. Senate.
      b. House.

J. Bill-to-Law Process
1. By Whom Referred to Committee
    a. Senate: President of the senate (subject to approval or disapproval by the senate membership).
    b. House: Speaker of the house.
2. Required Readings: Three readings of a bill are required before a final vote can take place. The second and third readings must occur on separate days.
3. Formal Floor Debate: In both the senate and the house, bills are frequently amended from the floor during the formal floor debate.
    a. Senate: Occurs during a meeting of the Committee of the Whole.
    b. House: Occurs after the second reading.
4. Recorded Vote on Final Passage
    a. Senate: Votes are recorded manually.
    b. House: Votes are recorded by electronic vote tabulation.
5. Passage of a Bill: Minimum vote required to pass a bill in each house is a majority of the members elected and serving.
6. Fate of a Passed Bill Before Adjournment: The governor either signs the bill into law or vetoes it. If the governor does neither within ten days (Sundays included) after receiving it, the bill becomes law.
7. Fate of a Passed Bill After Adjournment: The governor either signs it into law or vetoes it. If the governor does neither within 14 days (Sundays included) after receiving the bill, it dies.
8. Passage of a Bill Over the Governor's Veto: Requires a two-thirds vote of the members of both houses elected and serving.

Minnesota

A. Official Names
1. Both Houses: Legislature.
2. Upper Houses: Senate.
3. Lower House: House of representatives.
B. Convening Place: State Capitol, Aurora Ave Park, St Paul, MN 55155.
C. Number of Legislators
1. Senators: 67.
2. Representatives: 134.
D. Terms of Office
1. Governor: 4 years.
2. Senators: 4 years.
3. Representatives: 2 years.
E. Legislative Officers and Leaders: Elected by all members of their respective chambers.
1. Senate: President of the senate.
2. House: Speaker of the house.
F. Regular Legislative Session

      1. Convenes: First Monday in January, or the day after if the first Monday falls on a legal holiday in odd-numbered years.

      2. Length of Session: Session is limited to 120 legislative days.

G. Special Legislative Session

      1. Convenes: When called by the governor.

      2. Length of Session: No limit on length of session.

      3. Subject(s) To Be Considered: Either the governor or the legislature may determine the subject(s) to be considered.

H. Bill Introduction

      1. Time Limitation: No limitation of time exists on the introduction of legislation.

I. Standing Committees

      1. Average Number

        a. Senate: 15.

        b. House: 16.

      2. Committee Hearings Open to the Public

        a. Senate.

        b. House.

J. Bill-to-Law Process

      1. By Whom Referred to Committee

        a. Senate: President of the senate.

        b. House: Speaker of the house.

      2. Required Readings: Three readings of a bill are required before a final vote can take place. These readings must occur on separate days except by a two-thirds vote.

      3. Formal Floor Debate: Occurs after the second reading. Bills are frequently amended from the floor during this debate.

      4. Recorded Vote on Final Passage: Votes are recorded by electronic vote tabulation.

      5. Passage of a Bill: Minimum vote required to pass a bill in each house is a majority of the membership.

      6. Fate of a Passed Bill Before Adjournment: The governor either signs the bill into law or vetoes it. If the governor does neither within three days (Sundays excluded), the bill becomes law.

      7. Fate of a Passed Bill After Adjournment: The governor either signs the bill into law or vetoes it. If the governor does neither within 14 days, the bill dies.

      8. Passage of a Bill Over the Governor's Veto: Requires a two-thirds vote of the elected members of both houses.

Mississippi

A. Official Names

      1. Both Houses: Legislature.

      2. Upper House: Senate.

      3. Lower House: House of representatives.

B. Convening Place: New Capitol Senate Chambers or New Capitol House Chambers, 400 High, Jackson, MS 39202.
C. Number of Legislators
  1. Senators: 52.
  2. Representatives: 122.
D. Terms of Office
  1. Governor: 4 years.
  2. Senators: 4 years.
  3. Representatives: 4 years.
E. Legislative Officers and Leaders: Elected by all the members of their respective chambers, except the president of the senate, the lieutenant governor, who is appointed by the governor.
  1. Senate
    a. President of the senate: the lieutenant governor, who serves ex officio.
    b. President pro tem.
  2. House: Speaker of the house.
F. Regular Legislative Session
  1. Convenes: Annually on Tuesday after the first Monday in January.
  2. Length of Session: Session is limited to 90 calendar days. The first session of a new legislature however, is limited to 125 calendar days every other even year at the beginning of the gubernatorial term. Session may be extended for 30 calendar days by a two-thirds vote of those present. There is no limit on extension of the extended session.
G. Special Legislative Session
  1. Convenes: When called by the governor.
  2. Length of Session: No limit on length of session.
  3. Subject(s) To Be Considered: May consider only subject(s) specified in the governor's proclamation convening the legislature.
H. Bill Introducion
  1. Time Limitations: In the 90-day session, legislation must be introduced by the 16th day. In the 125-day session, legislation must be introduced by the 51st day.
  2. Exceptions to Time Limitations: Exceptions are permitted by a two-thirds vote of the membership present. Other exceptions are revenue, local, and private bills.
I. Standing Committees
  1. Average Number
    a. Senate: 31.
    b. House: 25.
    c. Joint: 4.
  2. Committee Hearings Open to the Public
    a. Senate.
    b. House.
J. Bill-to-Law Process
  1. By Whom Referred to Committee
    a. Senate: President of the senate.
    b. House: Speaker of the house.
  2. Required Readings: Three readings of a bill are required before a final

vote can take place. These readings must occur on separate days, except by a two-thirds vote.

3. Formal Floor Debate: Occurs after the third reading. Bills are frequently amended from the floor during this debate.
4. Recorded Vote on Final Passage
   a. Senate: Votes are recorded manually.
   b. House: Votes are recorded by electronic vote tabulation.
5. Passage of a Bill: Minimum vote required to pass a bill in each house is a majority of those present and voting. This is not based on a constitutional requirement.
6. Fate of a Passed Bill Before Adjournment: The governor either signs the bill into law or vetoes it. If the governor does neither within five days (Sundays excluded), the bill becomes law.
7. Fate of a Passed Bill After Adjournment: The governor either signs the bill into law or vetoes it. If the governor does neither within 15 days (Sundays excluded), the bill becomes law. The governor is required to return the bill to the legislature with his or her objections to it within three days after the beginning of the next session.
8. Passage of a Bill Over the Governor's Veto: A two-thirds vote of the members of both houses is required to override a veto of a bill or an item in a bill.

Missouri

A. Official Names
   1. Both Houses: General assembly.
   2. Upper House: Senate.
   3. Lower House: House of representatives.
B. Convening Place: State Capitol, Jefferson City, MO 65101.
C. Number of Legislators
   1. Senators: 34.
   2. Representatives: 163.
D. Terms of Office
   1. Governor: 4 years.
   2. Senators: 4 years.
   3. Representatives: 2 years.
E. Legislative Officers and Leaders: Elected by all the members of their respective chambers, except the president of the senate, the lieutenant governor, who is appointed by the governor.
   1. Senate
      a. President of the senate: The lieutenant governor, who serves ex officio.
      b. President pro tem.
   2. House
      a. Speaker of the house.
      b. Speaker pro tem.
F. Regular Legislative Session
   1. Convenes: Annually on the Wednesday after the first Monday in January.

    2. Length of Session
      a. Odd-Numbered Years: Session may not extend beyond June 30.
      b. Even-Numbered Years: Session may not extend beyond May 15.
G. Special Legislative Session
    1. Convenes: When called by the governor.
    2. Length of Session: Session is limited to 60 calendar days.
    3. Subject(s) To Be Considered: May consider only subject(s) specified in the governor's proclamation convening the legislature.
H. Bill Introduction
    1. Time Limitations
      a. Odd-Numbered Years: Legislation must be introduced by the 16th legislative day.
      b. Even-Numbered Years: Legislation must be introduced by the 13th legislative day.
    2. Exceptions to Time Limitations: Exceptions are permitted by the majority of the elected members or by a request of the governor. Other exceptions are appropriations bills.
I. Standing Committees
    1. Average Number
      a. Senate: 20.
      b. House: 33.
    2. Committee Hearings Open to the Public
      a. Senate.
      b. House.
J. Bill-to-Law Process
    1. By Whom Referred to Committee
      a. Senate: President pro tem.
      b. House: Speaker of the house.
    2. Required Readings: Three readings of a bill are required before a final vote can take place. These readings must occur on separate days.
    3. Formal Floor Debate: Occurs after the committee report and formal printing. Bills are frequently amended during this debate.
    4. Recorded Vote on Final Passage
      a. Senate: Votes are recorded manually.
      b. House: Votes are recorded by electronic vote tabulation.
    5. Passage of a Bill: Minimum vote required to pass a bill is a majority of the elected members of each house.
    6. Fate of a Passed Bill Before Adjournment: The governor either signs the bill into law or vetoes it. If the governor does neither within 15 days and does not return it to the legislature, a joint resolution must be passed by the legislature in order for the bill to become law.
    7. Fate of a Passed Bill After Adjournment: The governor either signs the bill into law or vetoes it. When the legislature is adjourned or recessed for 30 days or more, the governor may return a bill to the secretary of state within 45 days with his or her reasons for disapproval.
    8. Passage of a Bill Over the Governor's Veto: A bill in odd-numbered years is returned to the legislature for consideration when it reconvenes the following year. In even-numbered years the legislature may reconvene on

the first Wednesday following the first Monday in September for not more than ten days to consider vetoed bills. An override requires a two-thirds vote of the elected members of both houses.

Montana

A. Official Names
   1. Both Houses: Legislature.
   2. Upper House: Senate.
   3. Lower House: House of representatives.
B. Convening Place: State Capitol, State Capitol Station, Helena, MT 59601.
C. Number of Legislators
   1. Senators: 50.
   2. Representatives: 106.
D. Terms of Office
   1. Governor: 4 years.
   2. Senators: 4 years. After each decennial reapportionment, lots will be drawn for half of the senators to serve an initial 2-year term; subsequent elections will be for 4-year terms.
   3. Representatives: 2 years.
E. Legislative Officers and Leaders: Elected by all members of their respective chambers.
   1. Senate
      a. President of the senate.
      b. President pro tem.
      c. Majority floor leader.
      d. Minority floor leader.
   2. House
      a. Speaker of the house.
      b. Speaker pro tem.
      c. Majority floor leader.
      d. Minority floor leader.
F. Regular Legislative Session
   1. Convenes: First Monday in January of odd-numbered years.
   2. Length of Session: Session is limited to 90 legislative days.
G. Special Legislative Session
   1. Convenes: When called by the governor or by a petition of a majority of members of each house.
   2. Length of Session: No limit on length of session.
   3. Subject(s) To Be Considered: Either the governor or the legislature may determine subject(s) to be considered.
H. Bill Introduction
   1. Time Limitations: Regular bills must be introduced by the 18th day. Revenue bills must be introduced by the 25th day.
   2. Exceptions to Time Limitations: Exceptions are permitted by a two-thirds vote. Other exceptions are appropriations bills.

I. Standing Committees
    1. Average Number
        a. Senate: 15.
        b. House: 16.
    2. Committee Hearings Open to the Public
        a. Senate.
        b. House.
J. Bill-to-Law Process
    1. By Whom Referred to Committee
        a. Senate: President of the senate.
        b. House: Speaker of the house.
    2. Required Readings: Three readings of a bill are required before a final vote can take place. These readings must occur on separate days.
    3. Formal Floor Debate: Occurs after the second reading. Bills are frequently amended from the floor during this debate.
    4. Recorded Vote on Final Passage: Votes are recorded by electronic vote tabulation.
    5. Passage of a Bill: Minimum vote rquired to pass a bill in each house is a majority of those present and voting.
    6. Fate of a Passed Bill Before Adjournment: The governor either signs the bill into law or vetoes it. If the governor does neither within five days (Sundays included), the bill becomes law.
    7. Fate of a Passed Bill After Adjournment: The governor either signs the bill into law or vetoes it. If the governor does neither within 25 days (Sundays included), the bill becomes law.
    8. Passage of a Bill Over the Governor's Veto: Requires a two-thirds vote of the members present in both houses. Items vetoed in any appropriations bill may be restored by a three-fifths vote of the members of both houses. No appropriations can be made in excess of the recommendations contained in the governor's budget unless three-fifths of the members vote to do so. The excess approved by the three-fifths vote is subject to veto by the governor.

Nebraska

A. Official Names: Legislature. One house only (unicameral); members go by the title of senator.
B. Convening Place: State Capitol, 1445 K, Lincoln, NE 68509.
C. Number of Legislators
    1. Senators: 49.
D. Terms of Office
    1. Governor: 4 years.
    2. Senators: 4 years.
E. Legislative Officers and Leaders: Elected by the members of the legislature, except the president of the senate, the lieutenant governor, who is appointed by the governor.

    1. President of the Senate: the lieutenant governor, who serves ex officio.

    2. Speaker of the Legislature.

F. Regular Legislative Session

    1. Convenes: Annually on the first Wednesday after the first Monday in January. The legislature meets in two annual sessions, each adjourning sine die. Bills may carry over from first to second session.

    2. Length of Session: In odd-numbered years, session is limited to 90 legislative days, in even-numbered years, session is limted to 60 legislative days. Both sessions may be extended for an indefinite period, however, by a four-fifths vote of members.

G. Special Legislative Session

    1. Convenes: When called by the governor or by a petition of two-thirds of the members.

    2. Length of Session: No limit on length of session.

    3. Subject(s) To Be Considered: Either the governor or the legislature may determine the subject(s) to be considered.

H. Bill Introduction

    1. Time Limitation: Legislation must be introduced in the first ten legislative days.

    2. Exceptions to Time Limitation: Exceptions are permitted by a three-fifths vote or by request of the governor. Other exceptions are permitted with the approval of a majority of members of a committee and three-fifths of the elected members of the legislature.

I. Standing Committees

    1. Average Number 13.

    2. Committee hearings are open to the public.

J. Bill-to-Law Process

    1. By Whom Referred to Committee: Senate Referral Committee.

    2. Required Readings: Two readings of a bill are required before a final vote can take place. These readings must occur on separate days.

    3. Formal Floor Debate: Occurs after the first readings. Bills are frequently amended from the floor during this debate.

    4. Recorded Vote on Final Passage: Votes are recorded by electronic vote tabulation.

    5. Passage of a Bill: The minimum vote required to pass a bill in the legislature is a majority of the elected members.

    6. Fate of a Passed Bill Before Adjournment: The governor either signs the bill into law or vetoes it. If the governor does neither within five days (Sundays excluded), the bill becomes law.

    7. Fate of a Passed Bill After Adjournment: The governor either signs the bill into law or vetoes it. If the governor does neither within five days (Sundays excluded), the bill becomes law.

    8. Passage of a Bill Over the Governor's Veto: Requires a three-fifths vote of the elected members of the legislature. Items vetoed in any appropriations bill may be restored by a three-fifths vote of the elected members. Appropriations in excess of those recommended in the governor's budget can be made only by a three-fifths vote of the elected members; these excess appropriations are subject to veto by the governor.

Nevada

A. Official Names
  1. Both Houses: Legislature.
  2. Upper House: Senate.
  3. Lower House: Assembly.
B. Convening Place: State Capitol, Carson City, NV 89701.
C. Number of Legislators
  1. Senators: 20.
  2. Assemblypersons: 40.
D. Terms of Office
  1. Governor: 4 years.
  2. Senators: 4 years.
  3. Assemblypersons: 2 years.
E. Legislative Officers and Leaders: Elected by the members of their respective chambers, except the president of the senate, the lieutenant governor, who is appointed to that post by the governor.
  1. Senate
    a. President: The lieutenant governor, who serves ex officio.
    b. President pro tem.
  2. Assembly
  a. Speaker of the assembly.
    b. Speaker pro tem.
F. Regular Legislative Session
  1. Convenes: Third Monday in January of odd-numbered years.
  2. Length of Session: Session is limited to 60 calendar days. An indirect restriction occurs, since the legislators' pay stops but there is no limit on their daily allowance. Despite this, the session may continue.
G. Special Legislative Session
  1. Convenes: When called by the governor.
  2. Length of Session: Session is limited to 20 calendar days. An indirect restriction occurs, since the legislators' pay stops after 20 calendar days, but there is no time limit on their daily expense allowance.
  3. Subject(s) To Be Considered: May consider only subject(s) specified in governor's proclamation convening the legislature.
H. Bill Introduction
  1. Time Limitation: Bills in draft form must be introduced by the 13th calendar day.
  2. Exceptions to Time Limitation: Exceptions are permitted in the house by a vote of two-thirds present. Other exceptions are committee bills.
I. Standing Committees
  1. Average Number
    a. Senate: 9.
    b. Assembly: 13.
  2. Committee Hearings Open to the Public
    a. Senate.
    b. Assembly.

J. Bill-to-Law Process
1. By Whom Referred to Committee
    a. Senate: Introducer.
    b. Assembly: Introducer.
2. Required Readings: Three readings of a bill are required before a final vote can take place. These readings must occur on separate days except by two-thirds vote.
3. Formal Floor Debate: Occurs after the third reading. Bills are frequently amended from the floor during this debate.
4. Recorded Vote on Final Passage: Votes are recorded by electronic vote tabulation.
5. Passage of a Bill: The minimum vote required to pass a bill in each house is a majority of those elected.
6. Fate of a Passed Bill Before Adjournment: Governor either signs the bill into law or vetoes it. If the governor does neither within five days (Sundays excluded), the bill becomes law.
7. Fate of a Passed Bill After Adjournment: Governor either signs the bill into law or vetoes it. If the Governor does neither within ten days (Sundays excluded), the bill becomes law.
8. Passage of a Bill Over the Governor's Veto: A two-thirds vote of the elected members in both houses is required to override the governor's veto of a bill or an item within a bill.

New Hampshire

A. Official Names
1. Both Houses: General court.
2. Upper House: Senate.
3. Lower House: House of representatives.
B. Convening Place: State House, Concord, NH 03301.
C. Number of Legislators
1. Senators: 24.
2. Representatives: 400.
D. Terms of Office
    1. Governor: 2 years.
    2. Senators: 2 years.
    3. Representatives: 2 years.
E. Legislative Officers and Leaders: Elected by all members of their respective chambers.
1. Senate: President of the senate.
2. House: Speaker of the house.
F. Regular Legislative Session
1. Convenes: First Wednesday after the first Tuesday in January of the odd-numbered years. Legislature meets in organizational session on the first Wednesday of December of even-numbered years.

2. Length of Session: Session is limited, because there is a constitutional limit of 90 days on expenses or the date of July 1, whichever occurs first.
G. Special Legislative Session
   1. Convenes: When called by the governor or the legislature.
   2. Length of Session: Session is limited because there is a constitutional limit of 15 days on salary and expenses.
   3. Subject(s) To Be Considered: Either the governor of the legislature may determine the subject(s) to be considered.
H. Bill Introduction
   1. Time Limitation: Bills must be received for drafting by the fourth Thursday of April.
   2. Exceptions to Time Limitations: Exceptions are permitted by a two-thirds vote of the membership or by the approval of the Joint Rules Committee.
I. Standing Committees
   1. Average Number
      a. Senate: 20.
      b. House: 23.
   2. Committee Hearings Open to the Public
      a. Senate.
      b. House.
J. Bill-to-Law Process
   1. By Whom Referred to Committee
      a. Senate: President of the senate.
      b. House: Speaker of the house.
   2. Required Readings: Three readings of a bill are required before a final vote can take place. The first and second readings are by title upon introduction and before referral to committee. The second and third readings must occur on separate days.
   3. Formal Floor Debate: Occurs after the second reading. Bills are frequently amended from the floor during this debate.
   4. Recorded Vote on Final Passage: A record of the votes is not required on bills; however, it can be required by request of members.
   5. Passage of a Bill
      a. Senate: Thirteen of the 24 Senators must be present for a quorum to be declared and business to proceed. The affirmative vote of at least 10 of the 13 is necessary to render acts and proceedings valid.
      b. House: A majority of the members constitutes a quorum for the conduct of business. When less than two-thirds of the members are present, the assent of two-thirds of those members present is necessary to render acts and proceedings valid.
   6. Fate of a Passed Bill Before Adjournment: The governor either signs the bill into law or vetoes it. If the governor does neither within five days (Sundays excluded), the bill becomes law.
   7. Fate of a Passed Bill After Adjournment: The governor either signs the bill into law or vetoes it. If the governor does neither within five days (Sundays excluded) after receiving it, the bill dies.

8. Passage of a Bill Over the Governor's Veto: Requires a two-thirds vote of members of both houses who are present.

New Jersey

A. Official Names
 1. Both Houses: Legislature.
 2. Upper House: Senate.
 3. Lower House: General Assembly.
B. Convening Place: State House, Trenton, NJ 08625.
C. Number of Legislators
 1. Senators: 40.
 2. Assemblypersons: 80.
D. Terms of Office
 1. Governor: 4 years.
 2. Senators: 4 years, except for senate terms beginning in January of second year following the US decennial census, which are for two years only.
 3. Assemblypersons: 2 years.
E. Legislative Officers and Leaders: Elected by all members of their respective chambers.
 1. Senate
  a. President of the senate.
  b. President pro tem.
 2. General Assembly
  a. Speaker of the general assembly.
  b. Speaker pro tem.
F. Regular Legislative Session
 1. Convenes: Annually on the second Tuesday in January. The legislature meets in two annual sessions. Bills may carry over from first to second session.
 2. Length of Session: No limit on length of the session.
G. Special Legislative Session
 1. Convenes: When called by the governor or by a petition of the majority of members of each house.
 2. Length of Session: No limit on the length of session.
 3. Subject(s) To Be Considered: Either the governor or the legislature may determine the subject(s) to be considered.
H. Bill Introduction
 1. Time Limitation: No limitation of time exists on the introduction of legislation.
I. Standing Committees
 1. Average Number
  a. Senate: 14.
  b. Assembly: 18.
  c. Joint: 2.

    2. Committee Hearings Open to the Public
       a. Senate.
       b. Assembly.

J. Bill-to-Law Process
    1. By Whom Referred to Committee
       a. Senate: President of the senate.
       b. Assembly: Speaker of the general assembly.
    2. Required Readings: Three readings of a bill are required before a final vote can take place. The first and second reading may be on the same day. Upon roll call of three-fourths of the members, the second and third readings may be on the same day.
    3. Formal Floor Debate: Occurs after the third reading. Bills are frequently amended from the floor during this debate.
    4. Recorded Vote on Final Passage: Votes are recorded by electronic vote tabulation.
    5. Passage of a Bill: Minimum vote required to pass a bill in each house is a majority of the members elected.
    6. Fate of a Passed Bill Before Adjournment: The governor either signs the bill into law or vetoes it. If the governor does neither within ten days (Sundays excepted) after receiving it, the bill becomes law. An exception to this rule is: if the house of origin is in temporary adjournment on the tenth day (Sundays excepted) after presentation to the governor, the bill becomes law on the day the house of origin reconvenes unless returned by the governor on that day. The governor may return bills vetoed, suggesting amendments, and bills may be passed in amended form subject to the approval by the governor within ten days after presentation to him or her.
    7. Fate of a Passed Bill After Adjournment: The governor either signs the bill into law or vetoes it. If the governor does neither within 45 days (Sundays excluded) after receiving the bill, it dies.
    8. Passage of a Bill or Item Over the Governor's Veto: Requires a two-thirds vote of the elected members of both houses.

New York

A. Official Names
    1. Both Houses: Legislature.
    2. Upper House: Senate.
    3. Lower House: Assembly.
B. Convening Place: State Capitol, Washington Ave, Albany, NY 12224.
C. Number of Legislators
    1. Senators: 60.
    2. Assemblypersons: 150.
D. Terms of Office
    1. Governor: 4 years.
    2. Senators: 2 years.
    3. Assemblypersons: 2 years.
E. Legislative Officers and Leaders: Elected by all the members of their respec-

tive chambers, except the president of the senate, the lieutenant governor, who is appointed to that post by the governor.

   1. Senate
      a. President: The lieutenant governor, who serves ex officio.
      b. President pro tem.
   2. Assembly: Speaker of the assembly.
F. Regular Legislative Session
   1. Convenes: Annually on the Wednesday after the first Monday in January. The legislature meets in two annual sessions. Bills may carry over from first to second session.
   2. Length of Session: No limit on the length of either session.
G. Special Legislative Session
   1. Convenes: When called by the governor or by a petition of two-thirds members of each house.
   2. Length of Session: No limit on length of session.
   3. Subject(s) To Be Considered: May consider subject(s) specified in governor's proclamation convening the legislature. Only if Legislature convenes itself may it determine the subject(s) to be considered.
H. Bill Introduction
   1. Time Limitations
      a. Senate: The president pro tem may designate a final date for introduction of legislation, but not prior to the first Tuesday of March. Bills recommended by a state department or agency must be submitted to the president pro tem by the third Tuesday of February.
      b. Assembly: Unlimited introduction exists until the first Tuesday in March. Each member may introduce up to ten bills until the last Tuesday in March.
   2. Exceptions to Time Limitations
      a. Senate: Bills by the governor, attorney general, or comptroller must be presented to the president pro tem by the first Tuesday of April to be exempt from the limitations.
      b. Assembly: Exceptions are permitted by a unanimous vote, except on Friday, by the Committee on Rules or by a message from the senate. Exceptions are allowed to members elected in a special election that occurs after the first Tuesday in March. Bills introduced on Friday, and bills from the governor, senate, or Committee on Rules are exempt from these limitations.
I. Standing Committees
   1. Average Number
      a. Senate: 24.
      b. Assembly: 26.
   2. Committee Hearings Open to the Public
      a. Senate.
      b. Assembly.
J. Bill-to-Law Process
   1. By Whom Referred to Committee
      a. Senate: President pro tem.
      b. Assembly: Speaker of the assembly.

2. Required Readings: Three readings of a bill are required before a final vote can take place. In the senate the first and second readings occur upon introduction and before referral to committee. In the assembly the second and third readings can occur on the same day by unanimous consent or special provision of the Rules Committee.

3. Formal Floor Debate: Bills are seldom amended from the floor during the formal floor debate in either chamber.
   a. Senate: Occurs during a meeting of the Committee of the Whole.
   b. Assembly: Occurs after the third reading.

4. Recorded Vote on Final Passage
   a. Senate: A record of votes is not required on bills. It can be required, however, by request of members.
   b. Assembly: Votes are recorded by a "fast" roll call taken by a show of hands. If tabulation of votes is recorded it is done by a "show" roll call taken by individuals' "aye" or "nay."

5. Passage of a Bill: Minimum vote required to pass a bill in each house is a majority of those elected.

6. Fate of a Passed Bill Before Adjournment: The governor either signs the bill into law or vetoes it. If the governor does neither within ten days (Sundays excluded) after receiving it, the bill becomes law.

7. Fate of a Passed After Adjournment: The governor either signs the bill into law or vetoes it. If the governor does neither within 30 days (Sundays included), the bill dies.

8. Passage of a Bill Over the Governor's Veto: Requires a two-thirds vote of those elected in both houses.

New Mexico

A. Official Names
   1. Both Houses: Legislature.
   2. Upper House: Senate.
   3. Lower House: House of representatives.
B. Convening Place: State Capitol, Santa Fe, NM 87501.
C. Number of Legislators
   1. Senators: 42.
   2. Representatives: 70.
D. Terms of Office
   1. Governor: 4 years.
   2. Senators: 4 years.
   3. Representatives: 2 years.
E. Legislative Officers and Leaders: Elected by all members of their respective chambers, except the president of the senate, the lieutenant governor, who is appointed to that post by the governor.
   1. Senate
      a. President of the Senate: The lieutenant governor, who serves ex officio.
      b. President pro tem.
   2. House: Speaker of the house.
F. Regular Legislative Session

1. Convenes: Annually on the third Tuesday in January. The second session of the legislature is basically limited to budget and fiscal matters; however, the legislature may consider bills vetoed by the governor during the preceding session.
2. Length of Session
   a. Odd-Numbered Years: Session is limited to 60 calendar days.
   b. Even-Numbered Years: Session is limited to 30 calendar days.
3. Subject(s) To Be Considered: May consider subject(s) specified in governor's proclamation convening the legislature. Only if the legislature convenes itself may members determine the subject(s) to be considered, which are then unlimited in scope.

G. Special Legislative Session
   1. Convenes: By a petition of three-fifths of the members of both houses.
   2. Length of Session: Thirty calendar days.
   3. Subject(s) To Be Considered: Special sessions are unlimited in scope.

H. Bill Introduction
   1. Time Limitations: Limitations exist only in the first session. Regular bills must be introduced by the 13th legislative day. Appropriations bills must be introduced by the 15th legislative day.
   2. Exceptions to Time Limitations: Exceptions are permitted at the request of the governor.

I. Standing Committees
   1. Average Number
      a. Senate: 7.
      b. House: 12.
   2. Committee Hearings Open to the Public.
      a. Senate.
      b. House.

J. Bill-to-Law Process
   1. By Whom Referred to Committee
      a. Senate: Presiding officer of the senate, at the request of the sponsoring senator.
      b. House: Speaker of the house.
   2. Required Readings: Three readings of a bill are required before a final vote can take place. No more than two readings may take place on the same day.
   3. Formal Floor Debate: Occurs after the third reading. Bills are frequently amended from the floor during the formal floor debate.
   4. Recorded Vote on Final Passage: Votes are recorded by a show of hands.
   5. Passage of a Bill: Minimum vote required to pass a bill in each house is a majority of those present.
   6. Fate of a Passed Bill Before Adjournment: The governor either signs a bill into law or vetoes it. If the governor does neither within three days of receiving it (Sundays excluded), the bill becomes law.
   7. Fate of a Passed Bill After Adjournment: The governor either signs the bill into law or vetoes it. If the governor does neither within 20 days the bill dies.
   8. Passage of a Bill Over the Governor's Veto: Requires a two-thirds vote of those present in both houses.

North Carolina

A. Official Names
   1. Both Houses: General Assembly.
   2. Upper House: Senate.
   3. Lower House: House of representatives.
B. Convening Place: State Legislative Building, Raleigh, NC 27611.
C. Number of Legislators
   1. Senators: 50.
   2. Representatives: 120.
D. Terms of Office
   1. Governor: 4 years.
   2. Senators: 2 years.
   3. Representatives: 2 years.
E. Legislative Officers and Leaders: Elected by all members of their respective chambers, except the president of the senate, the lieutenant governor, who is appointed to that post by the governor.
   1. Senate
      a. President: The lieutenant governor, who serves ex officio.
      b. President pro tem, majority leader.
   2. House
      a. Speaker of the house.
      b. Speaker pro tem, majority leader.
F. Regular Legislative Session
   1. Convenes: First Monday in January, or the day after if the Monday falls on a legal holiday of odd-numbered years.
   2. Length of Session: No limit on length of session.
G. Special Legislative Session
   1. Convenes: When called by the governor or by a petition of three-fifths of the members of each house.
   2. Length of Session: No limit on length of session.
   3. Subject(s) To Be Considered: Either the governor or the legislature may determine the subject(s) to be considered.
H. Bill Introduction
   1. Time Limitations
      a. Senate: In the first annual sessions, state agency bills must be introduced by March 15.
      b. House: No time limit exists on the introduction of legislation.
   2. Exceptions to Time Limitations: Exceptions are permitted by a two-thirds vote in the senate.
I. Standing Committees
   1. Average Number
      a. Senate: 32.
      b. House: 45.
   2. Committee Hearings Open to the Public
      a. Senate.
      b. House.
J. Bill-to-Law Process

1. By Whom Referred to Committee
   a. Senate: President of the senate.
   b. House: Speaker of the house.
2. Required Readings: Three readings of a bill are required before a final vote can take place, and these readings must occur on separate days except by a two-thirds vote.
3. Formal Floor Debate: Occurs after both the second and third readings, and bills are frequently amended from the floor during this debate.
4. Recorded Vote on Final Passage: A record of votes is not required on a bill; however, it can be required by request of the members.
5. Passage of a Bill: Minimum vote required to pass a bill is a majority of those present and voting. This is not based on a constitutional requirement.
6. Fate of a Passed Bill: The governor does not have the power to veto acts of the legislature. This is the only state having such a law. Bills become law 30 days after adjournment of session unless the legislature expressly directs otherwise.
7. Fate of a Passed Bill After Adjournment: Not applicable.
8. Passage of a Bill Over the Governor's Veto: Not applicable.

North Dakota

A. Official Names
   1. Both Houses: Legislative assembly.
   2. Upper House: Senate.
   3. Lower House: House of representatives.
B. Convening Place: State Capitol, Bismarck, ND 58501.
C. Number of Legislators
   1. Senators: 50.
   2. Representatives: 100.
D. Terms of Office
   1. Governor: 4 years.
   2. Senators: 4 years.
   3. Representatives: 2 years.
E. Legislative Officers and Leaders: Elected by all members of their respective chambers, except the president of the senate, the lieutenant governor, who is appointed to that post by the governor.
   1. Senate
      a. President: The lieutenant governor, who serves ex officio.
      b. President pro tem.
   2. House: Speaker of the house.
F. General Legislative Session
   1. Convenes: First Tuesday after the third day in January of odd-numbered years. Legislature meets in an organizational session in December following the general election, to reconvene at a time prescribed by law but no later than January 8.
   2. Length of Session: Session is limited to 80 calendar days.

G. Special Legislative Session
   1. Convenes: When called by the governor.
   2. Length of Session: No limit on length of session.
   3. Subject(s) To Be Considered: Either the governor or the legislature may determine the subject(s) to be considered.
H. Bill Introduction
   1. Time Limitations: Bills must be introduced by the 15th legislative day. Resolutions must be introduced by the 18th legislative day.
   2. Exceptions to Time Limitations: Exceptions are permitted by a two-thirds vote or by the approval of the Committee on Delayed Bills.
I. Standing Committees
   1. Average Number
      a. Senate: 11.
      b. House: 12.
      c. Joint: 1.
   2. Committee Hearings Open to the Public
      a. Senate.
      b. House.
J. Bill-to-Law Process
   1. By Whom Referred to Committee
      a. Senate: President of the senate.
      b. House: Speaker of the house.
   2. Required Readings: Two readings of a bill are required before a final vote can take place. These readings must occur on separate days.
   3. Formal Floor Debate: Occurs after the second reading. In the house bills are seldom amended from the floor during this debate. In the senate, however, bills are frequently amended from the floor during this debate.
   4. Recorded Vote on Final Passage: Votes are recorded by electronic vote tabulation.
   5. Passage of a Bill: Minimum vote required to pass a bill in each house is a majority of those elected.
   6. Fate of a Passed Bill Before Adjournment: The governor either signs the bill into law or vetoes it. If the governor does neither within three days (Sundays included), the bill automatically becomes law.
   7. Fate of a Passed Bill After Adjournment: The governor either signs the bill into law or vetoes it. If the governor does neither within five days (Sundays included), the bill becomes law.
   8. Passage of a Bill Over the Governor's Veto: Requires a two-thirds vote of the members of both chambers.

Ohio

A. Official Names
   1. Both Houses: General assembly.
   2. Upper House: Senate.
   3. Lower House: House of representatives.

B. Convening Place: State House, Broad High St, Columbus, OH 43215.
C. Number of Legislators
   1. Senators: 33.
   2. Representatives: 99.
D. Terms of Office
   1. Governor: 4 years.
   2. Senators: 4 years.
   3. Representatives: 2 years.
E. Legislative Officers and Leaders: Elected by all the members of their respective chambers, except the president of the senate, the lieutenant governor, who is appointed to that post by the governor.
   1. Senate
      a. President: The lieutenant governor, who serves ex officio.
      b. President pro tem—majority leader.
      c. Assistant president pro tem.
      d. Majority whip.
      e. Minority leader.
      f. Assistant minority leader.
      g. Minority whip.
   2. House
      a. Speaker of the house.
      b. Speaker pro tem.
      c. Majority floor leader.
      d. Assistant majority floor leader.
      e. Majority whip.
      f. Minority leader.
      g. Minority whip.
F. Regular Legislative Session
   1. Convenes: Annually on the first Monday in January, or the day after if the first Monday falls on a legal holiday.
   2. Length of Session: No limit on length of session.
G. Special Legislative Session
   1. Convenes: When called by the governor or by a joint call of the presiding officers of both houses.
   2. Length of Session: No limit on length of session.
   3. Subject(s) To Be Considered: Either the governor or the legislature may determine the subject(s) to be considered.
H. Bill Introduction
   1. Time Limitations
      a. Senate: No limitations exist on the introduction of bills.
      b. House: In the regular session, legislation must be introduced by March 15. A resolution to end introduction of bills may be passed by a majority vote.
   2. Exceptions to Time Limitations: House: Exceptions are permitted by a majority vote, on recommendation of a bill by the Reference Committee.
I. Standing Committees
   1. Average Number
      a. Senate: 11.
      b. House: 17.

        2. Committee Hearings Open to the Public
          a. Senate.
          b. House.

J. Bill-to-Law Process
        1. By Whom Referred to Committee
          a. Senate: Rules Committee.
          b. House: Rules Committee.
        2. Required Readings: Three readings of a bill are required before a final vote can take place. These readings must occur on separate days except by two-thirds vote.
        3. Formal Floor Debate: Occurs during a meeting of the Committee of the Whole. Bills are frequently amended from the floor during this debate.
        4. Recorded Vote on Final Passage
          a. Senate: Votes are recorded manually.
          b. House: Votes are recorded by electronic vote tabulation.
        5. Passage of a Bill: Minimum vote required to pass a bill in each house is a majority of the elected members.
        6. Fate of a Passed Bill Before Adjournment: The governor either signs the bill into law or vetoes it. If the governor does neither within ten days (Sundays excluded), the bill becomes law.
        7. Fate of a Passed Bill After Adjournment: The governor either signs the bill into law or vetoes it. If the governor does neither within ten days (Sundays excluded), the bill becomes law.
        8. Passage of a Bill Over the Governor's Veto: Requires a three-fifths vote of the elected members of both houses.

Oklahoma

A. Official Names
        1. Both Houses: Legislature.
        2. Upper House: Senate.
        3. Lower House: House of representatives.

B. Convening Place: State Capitol, 2302 Lincoln Blvd, Oklahoma City, OK 73105.

C. Number of Legislators
        1. Senators: 48.
        2. Representatives: 101.

D. Terms of Office
        1. Governor: 4 years.
        2. Senators: 4 years.
        3. Representatives: 2 years.

E. Legislative Officers and Leaders: Elected by the members of their respective chambers, except the president of the senate, the lieutenant governor, who is appointed to that post by the governor.
        1. Senate
          a. President: The lieutenant governor, who serves ex officio.
          b. President pro tem.

        c. Majority floor leader.

        d. Assistant majority floor leader.

        e. Majority whip.

    2. House

        a. Speaker of the house.

        b. Speaker pro tem.

F. Regular Legislative Session

    1. Convenes: Annually on the Tuesday after the first Monday in January. The legislature meets in two annual sessions. Bills may carry over from the first to the second session.

    2. Length of Session: Session is limited to 90 legislative days.

G. Special Legislative Session

    1. Convenes: When called by the governor.

    2. Length of Session: No limit on length of session.

    3. Subject(s) To Be Considered: May consider only subject(s) specified in the governor's proclamation convening the legislature.

H. Bill Introduction

    1. Time Limitations

        a. Senate: In the first session no limitation on the introduction of legislation exists. In the second session legislation must be introduced by February.

        b. House: In the first session legislation must be introduced by the 19th legislative day. In the second session legislation must be introduced by the tenth legislative day.

    2. Exceptions to Time Limitations: Exceptions are permitted by a two-thirds vote. Other exceptions are revenue and appropriations bills.

I. Standing Committees

    1. Average Number

        a. Senate: 25.

        b. House: 34.

    2. Committee Hearings Open to the Public: Senate and house. Certain matters specified by statute can be discussed in executive session upon a two-thirds vote of committee members present and voting and stating the reason for such executive session.

J. Bill-to-Law Process

    1. By Whom Referred to Committee

        a. Senate: President pro tem.

        b. House: Speaker of the house.

    2. Required Readings: Three readings of a bill are required before a final vote can take place. These readings must occur on separate days.

    3. Formal Floor Debate: Occurs after the third reading. Bills are seldom amended from the floor during this debate.

    4. Recorded Vote on Final Passage: Votes are recorded by electronic vote tabulation.

    5. Passage of a Bill: Minimum vote required to pass a bill in each house is a majority of the elected members.

    6. Fate of a Passed Bill Before Adjournment: The governor either signs the bill into law or vetoes it. If the governor does neither within five days (Sundays excluded), the bill becomes law.

7. Fate of a Passed Bill After Adjournment: The governor either signs the bill into law or vetoes it. If the governor does neither within 15 days (Sundays excluded), the bill dies.
8. Passage of a Bill Over the Governor's Veto: Requires a two-thirds vote of the members of both houses. In the case of a governor's veto of an emergency measure, a three-fourths vote of both houses is required to override the veto.

Oregon

A. Official Names
    1. Both Houses: Legislative assembly.
    2. Upper House: Senate.
    3. Lower House: House of representatives.
B. Convening Place: State Capitol, Salem, OR 97310.
C. Number of Legislators
    1. Senators: 30.
    2. Representatives: 60.
D. Terms of Office
    1. Governor: 4 years.
    2. Senators: 4 years.
    3. Representatives: 2 years.
E. Legislative Officers and Leaders: Elected by all members of their respective chambers.
    1. Senate
        a. President of the senate.
        b. President pro tem.
    2. House
        a. Speaker of the house.
        b. Speaker pro tem.
F. Regular Legislative Session
    1. Convenes: Second Monday in January of odd-numbered years.
    2. Length of Session: No limit on length of session.
G. Special Legislative Session
    1. Convenes: When called by the governor or by a petition of the majority of the members of each house.
    2. Length of Session: No limit on length of session.
    3. Subject(s) To Be Considered: Either the governor or the legislature may determine the subject(s) to be considered.
H. Bill Introduction
    1. Time Limitations:
        a. Senate: Legislation must be introduced by the 36th calendar day.
        b. House: Legislation must be introduced by the 29th calendar day.
    2. Exceptions to Time Limitations: In the house exceptions are permitted with the approval of the House Committee on Legislative Operations and Procedures, or by the speaker of the house. In the senate, exceptions are permitted for priority bills or by the Senate Rules Committee.

I.   Standing Committees
  1. Average Number
    a. Senate: 13.
    b. House: 16.
  2. Committee Hearings Open to the Public
    a. Senate.
    b. House.
J.   Bill-to-Law Process
  1. By Whom Referred to Committee
    a. Senate: President of the senate.
    b. House: Rules Committee.
  2. Required Readings: Three readings of a bill are required before a final vote can take place. These readings must occur on separate days except by a two-thirds vote.
  3. Formal Floor Debate: This occurs after the third reading. Bills are seldom amended from the floor during this debate.
  4. Recorded Vote on Final Passage
    a. Senate: Votes are recorded manually.
    b. House: Votes are recorded by electronic vote tabulation.
  5. Passage of a Bill: Minimum vote required to pass a bill in each house is a majority of the elected membership.
  6. Fate of a Passed Bill Before Adjournment: The governor either signs the bill into law or vetoes it. If the governor does neither within five days (Sundays excluded), the bill becomes law.
  7. Fate of a Passed Bill After Adjournment: The governor either signs the bill into law or vetoes it. If the governor does neither within 20 days (Sundays excluded), the bill becomes law.
  8. Passage of a Bill Over the Governor's Veto: Requires a two-thirds vote of the members of each house present and voting.

Pennsylvania

A.   Official Names
  1. Both Houses: General assembly.
  2. Upper House: Senate.
  3. Lower House: House of representatives.
B.   Convening Place: Main Capitol Building, Harrisburg, PA 17120.
C.   Number of Legislators
  1. Senators: 50.
  2. Representatives: 203.
D.   Terms of Office
  1. Governor: 4 years.
  2. Senators: 4 years.
  3. Representatives: 2 years.
E.   Legislative Officers and Leaders: Elected by the members of their respective chambers, except the president of the senate, the lieutenant governor, who is appointed to that post by the governor.

      1. Senate
        a. President: The lieutenant governor, who serves ex officio.
        b. President pro tem.
      2. House: Speaker of the house.
F. Regular Legislative Session
      1. Convenes: Annually on the first Tuesday in January. The legislature meets in two annual sessions. Bills may carry over from the first to the second session.
      2. Length of Session: No limit on length of session.
G. Special Legislative Session
      1. Convenes: When called by the governor or a petition of a majority of the members of each house.
      2. Length of Session: No limit on length of session.
      3. Subject(s) To Be Considered: May consider only subject(s) specified by the governor.
H. Bill Introduction
      1. Time Limitation: No time limitation exists on the introduction of legislation.
I. Standing Committees
      1. Average number
        a. Senate: 20.
        b. House: 24.
      2. Committee Hearings Open to the Public
        a. Senate.
        b. House.
J. Bill-to-Law Process
      1. By Whom Referred to Committee
        a. Senate: President of the senate.
        b. House: Speaker of the house.
      2. Required Readings: Three readings of a bill are required before a final vote can take place. These readings must occur on separate days.
      3. Formal Floor Debate: Occurs after the second reading. Bills are frequently amended from the floor during this debate.
      4. Recorded Vote on Final Passage
        a. Senate: Votes are recorded manually.
        b. House: Votes are recorded by electronic vote tabulation.
      5. Passage of a Bill: Minimum vote required to pass a bill in each house is a majority of the elected members.
      6. Fate of a Passed Bill Before Adjournment: The governor either signs the bill into law or vetoes it. If the governor does neither within ten days, the bill becomes law. If the tenth day falls on a Sunday, the governor has the following Monday on which to act.
      7. Fate of a Passed Bill After Adjournment: The governor either signs the bill into law or vetoes it. If the governor does neither within 30 days, the bill becomes law. If the 30th day falls on a Sunday, the governor has the following Monday on which to act.
      8. Passage of a Bill Over the Governor's Veto: Requires a two-thirds vote of the elected members of both houses.

Rhode Island

A. Official Names
   1. Both Houses: General assembly.
   2. Upper House: Senate.
   3. Lower House: House of representatives.
B. Convening Place: State House, 82 Smith, Providence, RI 02903.
C. Number of Legislators
   1. Senators: 50.
   2. Representatives: 100.
D. Terms of Office
   1. Governor: 2 years.
   2. Senators: 2 years.
   3. Representatives: 2 years.
E. Legislative Officers and Leaders: Elected by the members of their respective chambers, except the president of the senate, the lieutenant governor, who is appointed to that post by the governor.
   1. Senate
      a. President: The lieutenant governor, who serves ex officio.
      b. President pro tem.
      c. Deputy president pro tem.
   2. House: Speaker of the house.
F. Regular Legislative Session
   1. Convenes: Annually on the first Tuesday of January. The legislature meets in two annual sessions. Bills may carry over from the first to the second session.
   2. Length of Session: Session is limited to 60 legislative days; however, an indirect restriction occurs since the legislators' pay and per diem stops. Despite this, the session may continue until business is concluded.
G. Special Legislative Session
   1. Convenes: When called by the governor.
   2. Length of Session: No limit on length of session.
   3. Subject(s) To Be Considered: May consider only subject(s) specified in the governor's proclamation convening the legislature.
H. Bill Introduction
   1. Time Limitation: Legislation must be introduced by the 42nd legislative day.
   2. Exceptions to Time Limitation
      a. Senate: Exceptions are permitted with the approval of the majority of members present. Exceptions are given to individual local and private bills.
      b. House: Exceptions are permitted with the approval of two-thirds of the members present.
I. Standing Committees
   1. Average Number
      a. Senate: 6.
      b. House: 6.
      c. Joint: 6.

      2. Committee Hearings Open to the Public
         a. Senate.
         b. House.

J. Bill-to-Law Process
    1. By Whom Referred to Committee
       a. Senate: President of senate.
       b. House: Speaker of the house.
    2. Required Readings: Two readings of a bill are required before a final vote can take place. These readings must occur on separate days, except by unanimous consent.
    3. Formal Floor Debate: Occurs after the second reading. Bills are frequently amended from the floor during this debate.
    4. Recorded Vote on Final Passage: A record of votes is not required on bills; however, votes may be recorded upon request of the members.
    5. Passage of a Bill: Minimum vote required to pass a bill in each house is a majority of those members present and voting. This is not a constitutional requirement.
    6. Fate of a Passed Bill Before Adjournment: Governor either signs the bill into law or vetoes it. If the governor does neither within six days (Sundays excluded), the bill becomes law.
    7. Fate of a Passed Bill After Adjournment: Governor either signs the bill into law or vetoes it. If the governor does neither within ten days (Sundays included), the bill becomes law.
    8. Passage of a Bill Over the Governor's Veto: Requires a three-fifths vote of members of both houses present and voting.

South Carolina

A. Official Names
    1. Both Houses: Legislature.
    2. Upper House: Senate.
    3. Lower House: House of representatives.

B. Convening Place: State House, Columbia, SC 29201.

C. Number of Legislators
    1. Senators: 46.
    2. Representatives: 124.

D. Terms of Office
    1. Governor: 4 years.
    2. Senators: 4 years.
    3. Representatives: 2 years.

E. Legislative Officers and Leaders: Elected by the members of their respective chambers except for president of the senate, the lieutenant governor, who is appointed to the post by the governor.
    1. Senate
       a. President: The lieutenant governor, who serves ex officio.
       b. President pro tem.

    2. House
       a. Speaker of the house.
       b. Speaker pro tem.
       c. Speaker emeritus.
F. Regular Legislative Session
    1. Convenes: Annually on the second Tuesday in January. The legislature meets in an organizational session for no more than three days beginning on the first Tuesday after certification of the election of its members. The legislature meets in two annual sessions. Bills may carry over from first to second session.
    2. Length of Session: No limit on length of session.
G. Special Legislative Session
    1. Convenes: When called by the governor.
    2. Length of Session: No limit on length of session.
    3. Subject(s) To Be Considered: Either the governor or the legislature may determine the subject(s) to be considered.
H. Bill Introduction
    1. Time Limitations
       a. Senate: No limitation of time exists on the introduction of legislation.
       b. House: Legislation must be introduced by May 1 and legislation passed by the senate must be introduced in the house prior to May 15.
    2. Exceptions to Time Limitations: Exceptions to time limitations are permitted in the house by a majority vote. Exceptions are given to the General or Deficiency Appropriations acts.
I. Standing Committees
    1. Average Number
       a. Senate: 15.
       b. House: 10.
       c. Joint: 2.
    2. Committee Hearings Open to the Public
       a. Senate.
       b. House.
J. Bill-to-Law Process
    1. By Whom Referred to Committee
       a. Senate: Presiding officer.
       b. House: Speaker of the house.
    2. Required Readings: Three readings of a bill are required before a final vote can take place. These readings must occur on separate days.
    3. Formal Floor Debate: Occurs after the second reading. Bills are frequently amended from the floor during this debate.
    4. Recorded Vote on Final Passage: Votes must be recorded when the legislature is voting to override the governor's veto. In other situations, a record of the final vote is not required, although it can be requested by the members.
    5. Passage of a Bill: Minimum vote required to pass a bill in each chamber is a majority of those present and voting. This is not based on a constitutional requirement.

6. Fate of a Passed Bill Before Adjournment: The governor either signs the bill into law or vetoes it. If the governor does neither within five days (Sundays excluded), the bill becomes law.
7. Fate of a Passed Bill After Adjournment: The governor either signs the bill into law or vetoes it. If the governor does neither and does not return the bill to the legislature within two days after the convening of the next legislative session, the bill becomes law.
8. Passage of a Bill Over the Governor's Veto: Requires a two-thirds vote of the members of each chamber present and voting.

South Dakota

A. Official Names
   1. Both Houses: Legislature.
   2. Upper House: Senate.
   3. Lower House: House of representatives.
B. Convening Place: State Capitol, Pierre, SD 57501.
C. Number of Legislators
   1. Senators: 35.
   2. Representatives: 70.
D. Terms of Office
   1. Governor: 4 years.
   2. Senators: 2 years.
   3. Representatives: 2 years.
E. Legislative Officers and Leaders: Elected by the members of their respective chambers, except the president of the senate, the lieutenant governor, who is appointed to that post by the governor.
   1. Senate
      a. President: The lieutenant governor, who serves ex officio.
      b. President pro tem.
   2. House
      a. Speaker of the house.
      b. Speaker pro tem.
F. Regular Legislative Session
   1. Convenes: Annually in odd-numbered years on the Tuesday after the third Monday in January. In even-numbered years, on the Tuesday after the first Monday in January.
   2. Length of Session: Session is limited to 45 legislative days in odd-numbered years. Sessions are limited to 30 legislative days in even-numbered years.
G. Special Legislative Session
   1. Convenes: When called by the governor.
   2. Length of Session: No limit on the length of session.
   3. Subject(s) To Be Considered: May consider only subject(s) specified in governor's proclamation convening the legislature.
H. Bill Introduction
   1. Time Limitations: In the 45-day session, legislation must be introduced

by the 20th day. In the 30-day session, legislation must be introduced by the eighth day. All committee bills must be introduced by the ninth day.

   2. Exceptions to Time Limitation: The General Appropriations Act is automatically exempt from this limitation. Other exemptions are permitted by a two-thirds vote of the members.

I. Standing Committees

   1. Average Number

     a. Senate: 10.

     b. House: 10.

   2. Committee Hearings Open to the Public

     a. Senate.

     b. House.

J. Bill-to-Law Process

   1. By Whom Referred to Committee

     a. Senate: President of the senate.

     b. House: Speaker of the house.

   2. Required Readings: Two readings of a bill are required before a final vote can take place. These readings must occur on separate days.

   3. Formal Floor Debate: Occurs after the second reading. Bills are frequently amended from the floor during this debate.

   4. Recorded Vote on Final Passage

     a. Senate: Votes are recorded manually.

     b. House: Votes are recorded by electronic vote tabulation.

   5. Passage of a Bill: Minimum vote required to pass a bill in each chamber is a majority of the elected members.

   6. Fate of a Passed Bill Before Adjournment: The governor either signs the bill into law or vetoes it. If the governor does neither within five days (Sundays excluded), the bill becomes law.

   7. Fate of a Passed Bill After Adjournment: The governor either signs the bill into law or vetoes it. If the governor does neither within 15 days (Sundays excluded), the bill becomes law.

   8. Passage of a Bill Over the Governor's Veto: Requires a two-thirds vote of the elected members of both chambers.

Tennessee

A. Official Names

   1. Both Houses: General assembly.

   2. Upper House: Senate.

   3. Lower House: House of representatives.

B. Convening Place: State Capitol, Nashville, TN 37219.

C. Number of Legislators

   1. Senators: 33.

   2. Representatives: 99.

D. Terms of Office
1. Governor: 4 years.
2. Senators: 4 years.
3. Representatives: 2 years.
E. Legislative Officers and Leaders: Elected by all members of their respective chambers.
1. Senate: Speaker of the senate.
2. House
a. Speaker of the house.
b. Speaker pro tem.
F. General Legislative Session
1. Convenes: First Tuesday in January; however, the legislature may and in practice has divided the session to meet in even years also. The legislature meets in an organizational session on the first Tuesday in January, for no more than 15 calendar days, to organize and to introduce bills, then reconvenes on the fourth Tuesday in February.
2. Length of Session: Session is limited to 90 legislative days, including the organizational session. An indirect restriction occurs because of the constitutional limit on legislators' per diem and travel allowance.
G. Special Legislative Session
1. Convenes: When called by the governor or a petition of two-thirds of the members of each house.
2. Length of Session: Session is limited to 30 days. An indirect restriction occurs because of the constitutional limit on legislators' per diem and travel allowance.
3. Subject(s) To Be Considered: Either the governor or the legislature may determine the subject(s) to be considered.
H. Bill Introduction
1. Time Limitations:
a. Senate: General bills must be introduced by the 15th day. Resolutions must be introduced by the 30th legislative day.
b. House: General bills must be introduced by the 20th legislative day.
2. Exceptions to Time Limitations
a. Senate: Exceptions are permitted by the unanimous consent of the Committee on Delayed Bills, or by a two-thirds vote.
b. House: Exceptions are permitted by a two-thirds vote.
I. Standing Committees
1. Average Number
a. Senate: 11.
b. House: 8.
2. Committee Hearings Open to the Public
a. Senate.
b. House.
J. Bill-to-Law Process
1. By Whom Referred to Committee
a. Senate: Speaker of the senate.
b. House: Speaker of the house.

2. Required Readings: Three readings of a bill are required before a final vote can take place. These readings must occur on separate days.
3. Formal Floor Debate: Occurs after the third reading. Bills are frequently amended from the floor during this debate.
4. Recorded Vote on Final Passage: Votes are recorded by electronic vote tabulation.
5. Passage of a Bill: Minimum vote required to pass a bill in each chamber is a majority of the elected membership.
6. Fate of a Passed Bill Before Adjournment: The governor either signs the bill into law or vetoes it. If the governor does neither within five days (Sundays excluded), the bill becomes law.
7. Fate of a Passed Bill After Adjournment: The governor signs the bill into law or vetoes it. If the governor does neither within ten days (Sundays excluded), the bill becomes law.
8. Passage of a Bill Over the Governor's Veto: Requires a majority vote of the elected members of both chambers.

Texas

A. Official Names
   1. Both Houses: Legislature.
   2. Upper House: Senate.
   3. Lower House: House of representatives.
B. Convening Place: Capitol, Austin, TX 78711.
C. Number of Legislators
   1. Senators: 31.
   2. Representatives: 150.
D. Terms of Office
   1. Governor: 4 years.
   2. Senators: 4 years.
   3. Representatives: 2 years.
E. Legislative Officers and Leaders: Elected by the members of their respective chambers, except the president of the senate, the lieutenant governor, who is appointed to that post by the governor.
   1. Senate
      a. President: The lieutenant governor, who serves ex officio.
      b. President pro tem.
   2. House: Speaker of the house.
F. Regular Legislative Session
   1. Convenes: Second Tuesday in January of odd-numbered years.
   2. Length of Session: Session is limited to 140 calendar days.
G. Special Legislative Session
   1. Convenes: When called by the governor.
   2. Length of Session: Session is limited to 30 calendar days.
   3. Subject(s) To Be Considered: May consider only subject(s) specified in the governor's proclamation convening the legislature.

H. Bill Introduction
   1. Time Limitation: All legislation must be introduced within 60 calendar days.
   2. Exceptions to Time Limitations: Exceptions are permitted by a four-fifths vote. Exceptions are automatically given to emergency appropriations or to emergency matters presented by the governor.
I. Standing Committees
   1. Average Number
      a. Senate: 9.
      b. House: 28.
   2. Committee Hearings Open to the Public
      a. Senate.
      b. House.
J. Bill-to-Law Process
   1. By Whom Referred to Committee
      a. Senate: President of the senate.
      b. House: Speaker of the house.
   2. Required Readings: Three readings of a bill are required before a final vote can take place. These readings must take place on separate days except by a four-fifths vote.
   3. Formal Floor Debate: Occurs after the second reading. Bills are frequently amended from the floor during this debate.
   4. Recorded Vote on Final Passage: A record of votes is not required on bills; however, recording may be done upon request of members.
   5. Passage of a Bill: Minimum vote required to pass a bill in each chamber is a majority of the members present and voting. This is not based on a constitutional requirement.
   6. Fate of a Passed Bill Before Adjournment: The governor either signs the bill into law or vetoes it. If the governor does neither within ten days (Sundays excluded), the bill becomes law.
   7. Fate of a Passed Bill After Adjournment: The governor either signs the bill into law or vetoes it. If the governor does neither within 20 days (Sundays excluded), the bill becomes law.
   8. Passage of a Bill Over the Governor's Veto: Requires a two-thirds vote of the members of both chambers present and voting.

Utah

A. Official Names
   1. Both Houses: Legislature.
   2. Upper House: Senate.
   3. Lower House: House of representatives.
B. Convening Place: State Capitol Building, Salt Lake City, UT 84114.
C. Number of Legislators
   1. Senators: 29.
   2. Representatives: 75.

D. Terms of Office
   1. Governor: 4 years.
   2. Senators: 4 years.
   3. Representatives: 2 years.
E. Legislative Officers and Leaders: Elected by all members of their respective chambers.
   1. Senate: President of the senate.
   2. House: Speaker of the house.
F. Regular Legislative Session
   1. Convenes: Annually on the second Monday in January. Second session of the legislature is basically limited to budget and fiscal matters; however, the legislature may consider non-budget matters after a two-thirds vote of the members of each house.
   2. Length of Session
      a. Odd-Numbered Years: Session is limited to 60 calendar days.
      b. Even-Numbered Years: Session is limited to 20 calendar days.
G. Special Legislative Session
   1. Convenes: When called by the governor.
   2. Length of Session: No limit on length of session.
   3. Subject(s) To Be Considered: May only consider subject(s) specified in the governor's proclamation convening the legislature.
H. Bill Introduction
   1. Time Limitation: All legislation must be introduced by the 30th day.
   2. Exceptions to Time Limitation: Exceptions are permitted by a majority vote.
I. Standing Committees
   1. Average Number
      a. Senate: 11.
      b. House: 11.
      c. Joint: 2.
   2. Committee Hearings Open to the Public
      a. Senate.
      b. House.
J. Bill-to-Law Process
   1. By Whom Referred to Committee
      a. Senate: President of the senate.
      b. House: Speaker of the house.
   2. Required Readings: Three readings of a bill are required before a final vote can take place. These readings must occur on separate days, except by a two-thirds vote.
   3. Formal Floor Debate: Bills are frequently amended from the floor during this debate.
      a. Senate: Occurs after the second and third reading.
      b. House: Occurs after the first reading.
   4. Recorded Vote on Final Passage
      a. Senate: Votes are recorded manually.
      b. House: Votes are recorded by electronic vote tabulation.

5. Passage of a Bill: Minimum vote required to pass a bill in each chamber is a majority of the elected members.
6. Fate of a Passed Bill Before Adjournment: The governor either signs the bill into law or vetoes it. If the governor does neither within five days (Sundays excluded), the bill becomes law.
7. Fate of a Passed Bill After Adjournment: The governor either signs the bill into law or vetoes it. If the governor does neither within ten days (Sundays excluded), the bill becomes law.
8. Passage of a Bill Over the Governor's Veto: Requires a two-thirds vote of the members of each chamber.

Vermont

A. Official Names
   1. Both Houses: General assembly.
   2. Upper House: Senate.
   3. Lower House: House of representatives.
B. Convening Place: State House, Montpelier, VT 05602.
C. Number of Legislators
   1. Senators: 30.
   2. Representatives: 150.
D. Terms of Office
   1. Governor: 2 years.
   2. Senators: 2 years.
   3. Representatives: 2 years.
E. Legislative Officers and Leaders: Elected by the members of their respective chambers, except the president of the senate, the lieutenant governor, who is appointed to that post by the governor.
   1. Senate
      a. President: The lieutenant governor, who serves ex officio.
      b. President pro tem.
   2. House: Speaker of the house.
F. Regular Legislative Session
   1. Convenes: Wednesday after the first Monday in January of the odd-numbered years. The legislature may and in practice has divided the session to meet on even years also.
   2. Length of Session: No limit on length of session. An indirect restriction occurs because legislators' pay, per diem, and allowance are limited. The session may continue even after these allowances are exhausted.
G. Special Legislative Session
   1. Convenes: When called by the governor.
   2. Length of Session: No limit on length of session.
   3. Subject(s) To Be Considered: Either the governor or the legislature may determine the subject(s) to be considered.

H. Bill Introduction
  1. Time Limitations
    a. Senate: In odd-numbered years, legislation must be introduced by the 53rd calendar day. In even-numbered years, legislation must be filed with the Legislative Drafting Division 25 days before the session begins.
    b. House: In odd-numbered years, legislation must be introduced within five weeks. Proposals delivered to the Legislative Drafting Division by that time must be introduced within 12 weeks. In even-numbered years, by agreement of the Rules Committee, legislation may be pre-filed by September 1 of the odd year for the next year.
  2. Exceptions to Time Limitations: Exceptions are permitted by a two-thirds vote or by consent of the Rules Committee. Exceptions are made for appropriations and revenue bills. House only: Exceptions are made for committee bills introduced within ten days after the first Tuesday in March.

I. Standing Committees
  1. Average Number
    a. Senate: 12.
    b. House: 14.
    c. Joint: 1.
  2. Committee Hearings Open to the Public
    a. Senate.
    b. House.

J. Bill-to-Law Process
  1. By Whom Referred to Committee
    a. Senate: President of the senate.
    b. House: Speaker of the house.
  2. Required Readings: Three readings of a bill are required before a final vote can take place. Usually these readings occur on separate days; however, if a bill is advanced at the second reading, it may be read for the third time on the same day.
  3. Formal Floor Debate: Occurs after the second reading. Bills are frequently amended during this formal floor debate.
  4. Recorded Vote on Final Passage: A record of votes is not required on bills; however, it can be done upon request of the members. This is not based on constitutional requirement.
  5. Passage of a Bill: Minimum vote required to pass a bill in each chamber is a majority of those members present and voting. This is not based on a constitutional requirement.
  6. Fate of a Passed Bill Before Adjournment: The governor either signs the bill into law or vetoes it. If the governor does neither within five days (Sundays excluded), the bill becomes law.
  7. Fate of a Passed Bill After Adjournment: If adjournment occurs within three days after passage of a bill and the governor refuses to sign it, the bill dies.

8. Passage of a Bill Over the Governor's Veto: A two-thirds vote of the members of both chambers is required to override a veto of a bill or an item of a bill.

Virginia

A. Official Names
  1. Both Houses: General assembly.
  2. Upper House: Senate.
  3. Lower House: House of Delegates.
B. Convening Place: State Capitol, Senate Addition or House Addition, Capitol Square, Richmond, VA 23219.
C. Number of Legislators
  1. Senators: 40.
  2. Delegates: 100.
D. Terms of Office
  1. Governor: 4 years.
  2. Senators: 4 years.
  3. Delegates: 2 years.
E. Legislative Officers and Leaders: Elected by the members of their respective chambers, except the president of the senate, the lieutenant governor, who is appointed to that post by the governor.
  1. Senate
    a. President: The lieutenant governor, who serves ex officio.
    b. President pro tem.
  2. House: Speaker of the house.
F. Regular Legislative Session
  1. Convenes: Annually on the second Wednesday in January. The legislature meets in two annual sessions. Bills may carry from the first to the second session.
  2. Length of Session
    a. Odd-Numbered Years: Session is limited to 30 calendar days.
    b. Even-Numbered Years: Session is limited to 60 calendar days. Session may be extended for 30 more days by a two-thirds vote of the members of each house.
G. Special Legislative Session
  1. Convenes: When called by the governor or a petition of two-thirds of the members of each house.
  2. Length of Session: No limit on length of session.
  3. Subject(s) To Be Considered: Either the governor or the legislature may determine the subject(s) to be considered.
H. Bill Introduction
  1. Time Limitations: Deadlines on the introduction of legislation are set during the session. Municipal charter bills must be introduced on the first day of the session.
  2. Exceptions to Time Limitations: Exceptions are permitted by unanimous vote.

I. Standing Committees
    1. Average Number
        a. Senate: 10.
        b. House: 17.
    2. Committee Hearings Open to the Public
        a. Senate.
        b. House: Committee meetings are open only for the final vote on bills.
J. Bill-to-Law Process
    1. By Whom Referred to Committee
        a. Senate: Clerk of the senate.
        b. House: Speaker of the house.
    2. Required Readings: Three readings of a bill are required before a final vote can take place. These readings must occur on separate days. This is dispensed with for a bill to codify laws or by a four-fifths vote.
    3. Formal Floor Debate: Occurs after the third reading. Bills are frequently amended from the floor during this debate.
    4. Recorded Vote on Final Passage: Votes are recorded by electronic vote tabulation.
    5. Passage of a Bill: Minimum vote required to pass a bill in each chamber is a majority of those present and voting. This majority must be at least two-fifths of the total elected membership.
    6. Fate of a Passed Bill Before Adjournment: The governor either signs the bill into law or vetoes it. If the governor does neither within seven days (Sundays and legal holidays excluded), the bill becomes law.
    7. Fate of a Passed Bill After Adjournment: The governor either signs the bill into law or vetoes it. If the governor does neither within 30 days (Sundays and legal holidays excepted), the bill dies.
    8. Passage of a Bill Over the Governor's Veto: Requires a majority vote of those present and voting in both chambers. This majority must be at least two-fifths of the total elected membership.

Washington

A. Official Names
    1. Both Houses: Legislature.
    2. Upper House: Senate.
    3. Lower House: House of representatives.
B. Convening Place: Legislative Building, Olympia, WA 98504.
C. Number of Legislators
    1. Senators: 49.
    2. Representatives: 98.
D. Terms of Office
    1. Governor: 4 years.
    2. Senators: 4 years.
    3. Representatives: 2 years.
E. Legislative Officers and Leaders: Elected by the members of their respective

chambers, except the president of the senate, the lieutenant governor, who is appointed to that post by the governor.

   1. Senate
      a. President: The lieutenant governor, who serves ex officio.
      b. President pro tem.
      c. Vice president pro tem.
   2. House
      a. Speaker of the house.
      b. Speaker pro tem.

F. Regular Legislative Session
   1. Convenes: Second Monday in January of odd-numbered years.
   2. Length of Session: Session is limited to 60 calendar days.

G. Special Legislative Session
   1. Convenes: When called by the governor.
   2. Length of Session: No limit on length of session.
   3. Subject(s) To Be Considered: Either the governor or the legislature may determine the subject(s) to be considered.

H. Bill Introduction
   1. Time Limitations
      a. Senate: Legislation must be introduced by individual members by the 38th day. No limit of time exists on the introduction of legislation by the committees.
      b. House: Legislation must be introduced by individual members by the 35th day.
   2. Exceptions to Time Limitations: Exceptions are permitted by a two-thirds vote of the elected members.

I. Standing Committees
   1. Average Number
      a. Senate: 17.
      b. House: 22.
   2. Committee Hearings Open to the Public
      a. Senate.
      b. House.

J. Bill-to-Law Process
   1. By Whom Referred to Committee
      a. Senate: President of the senate.
      b. House: Speaker of the house.
   2. Required Readings: Three readings of a bill are required before a final vote can take place. These readings must occur on separate days except by a two-thirds vote.
   3. Formal Floor Debate: Occurs after both the second and third readings. Bills may be amended from the floor after the second reading, only.
   4. Recorded Vote on Final Passage
      a. Senate: Votes are recorded manually.
      b. House: Votes are recorded by electronic vote tabulation.
   5. Passage of a Bill: Minimum vote required to pass a bill in each chamber is a majority of those elected.

6. Fate of a Passed Bill Before Adjournment: The governor either signs the bill into law or vetoes it. If the governor does neither within five days (Sundays excluded), the bill becomes law.
7. Fate of a Passed Bill After Adjournment: The governor either signs the bill into law or vetoes it. If the governor does neither within 20 days (Sundays excluded), the bill becomes law.
8. Passage of a Bill Over the Governor's Veto: A two-thirds vote of the members of both chambers present and voting is required to override a veto.

West Virginia

A. Official Names
   1. Both Houses: Legislature.
   2. Upper House: Senate.
   3. Lower House: House of delegates.
B. Convening Place: State Capitol, 1800 Kanawha Blvd E, Charleston, WV 25305
C. Number of Legislators
   1. Senators: 34.
   2. Delegates: 100.
D. Terms of Office
   1. Governor: 4 years.
   2. Senators: 4 years.
   3. Delegates: 2 years.
E. Legislative Officers and Leaders: Elected by all members of their respective chambers.
   1. Senate: President of the senate.
   2. House: Speaker of the house.
F. Regular Legislative Session
   1. Convenes: Annually on the second Wednesday in January. Following each gubernatorial election, the legislature convenes on the second Wednesday in January to organize, but recesses until the second Wednesday in February for the start of the 60-day session.
   2. Length of Session: Session is limited to 60 calendar days. Session may be extended for an indefinite period of time by a vote of the members of each house. Also, the governor must extend the session until the general appropriations are passed.
G. Special Legislative Session
   1. Convenes: When called by the governor or by a petition of three-fifths of the members of each house.
   2. Length of Session: No limit on length of session.
   3. Subject(s) To Be Considered: May consider subject(s) specified in governor's proclamation convening the legislature. Also, according to a 1955 Attorney General's Opinion, when the legislature has petitioned the governor to be called into session, it may then act on any matter.

H. Bill Introduction
   1. Time Limitations
      a. Senate: Legislation must be introduced by the 41st calendar day.
      b. House: Legislation must be introduced by the 50th calendar day.
   2. Exceptions to Time Limitations: Exceptions are permitted by a two-thirds vote of all members of each house present and voting. Permission of both houses must be granted by a concurrent resolution setting out the title of the bill.
I. Standing Committees
   1. Average Number
      a. Senate: 17.
      b. House: 14.
   2. Committee Hearings Open to the Public
      a. Senate.
      b. House.
J. Bill-to-Law Process
   1. By Whom Referred to Committee
      a. Senate: President of the senate.
      b. House: Speaker of the house.
   2. Required Readings: Three readings of a bill are required before a final vote can take place. These readings must occur on separate days, except by a four-fifths vote.
   3. Formal Floor Debate: Occurs after the three readings. Bills are seldom amended from the floor during the formal floor debate.
   4. Recorded Vote on Final Passage
      a. Senate: Votes are recorded manually.
      b. House: A record of votes is not required; however, the vote can be recorded at the request of members.
   5. Passage of a Bill: The minimum vote to pass a bill in each house is a majority of the members present and voting. A majority of the elected members is needed to repass a bill amended by the other house.
   6. Fate of a Passed Bill Before Adjournment: The governor either signs the bill into law or vetoes it. If the governor does neither within five days (Sundays excluded), the bill becomes law.
   7. Fate of a Passed Bill After Adjournment: The governor either signs the bill into law or vetoes it. If the governor does neither within 15 days (Sundays excluded), the bill becomes law. Appropriations bills become law five days after being received by the governor (Sundays excluded) unless the governor vetoes them.
   8. Passage of a Bill Over the Governor's Veto: A majority vote of the elected members of both houses is required to override the governor's veto. Overrides on supplementary appropriations and budget bills require a two-thirds majority vote of the elected members of both houses.

Wisconsin

A. Official Names
   1. Both Houses: Legislature.

   2. Upper House: Senate.

   3. Lower House: Assembly.

B. Convening Place: State Capitol, Capitol Square, Madison, WI 53702.

C. Number of Legislators
   1. Senators: 33.
   2. Representatives: 99.

D. Terms of Office
   1. Governor: 4 years.
   2. Senators: 4 years.
   3. Representatives: 2 years.

E. Legislative Leaders and Officers: Elected by the members of their respective chambers, except the president of the senate, the lieutenant governor, who is appointed to that post by the governor.
   1. Senate
      a. President: The lieutenant governor, who serves ex officio.
      b. President pro tem.
   2. Assembly
      a. Speaker of the assembly.
      b. Speaker pro tem.

F. Regular Legislative Session
   1. Convenes: Annually on the first Tuesday after January 8. The legislature by joint resolution establishes the calendar dates of session activity for the remainder of the biennium at the beginning of each odd-numbered year. These dates may be subject to change.
   2. Length of Session: No limit on length of session.

G. Special Legislative Session
   1. Convenes: When called by the governor.
   2. Length of Session: No limit on length of session.
   3. Subject(s) To Be Considered: May consider only subject(s) specified in the governor's proclamation convening the legislature.

H. Bill Introduction
   1. Time Limitation: No time limit exists on the introduction of legislation.

I. Standing Committees
   1. Average Number
      a. Senate: 12.
      b. Assembly: 29.
      c. Joint: 6.
   2. Committee Hearings Open to the Public
      a. Senate.
      b. Assembly.

J. Bill-to-Law Process
   1. By Whom Referred to Committee
      a. Senate: Presiding officer.
      b. Assembly: Presiding officer.

2. Required Readings: Three readings of a bill are required before a final vote can take place. In the senate no two readings may occur on the same day. In the assembly the second and third reading must occur on separate days.

3. Formal Floor Debate: Occurs after the second reading. Bills are frequently amended from the floor during this debate.

4. Recorded Vote on Final Passage: A record of votes is not required; however, a record can be made upon request of members. This is not based on constitutional requirement.

5. Passage of a Bill: The minimum vote required to pass a bill in each chamber is a majority of those present and voting. This is not a constitutional requirement.

6. Fate of Passed Bill Before Adjournment: The governor either signs the bill into law or vetoes it. If the governor does neither within six days (Sundays excluded) after receiving it, the bill becomes law.

7. Fate of a Passed Bill After Adjournment: The governor either signs the bill into law or vetoes it. If the governor does neither within six days (Sundays excluded) after receiving it, the bill dies.

8. Passage of a Bill Over the Governor's Veto: Requires a two-thirds vote of the members of both houses present and voting.

Wyoming

A. Official Names
   1. Both Houses: Legislature.
   2. Upper House: Senate.
   3. Lower House: House of representatives.
B. Convening Place: State Capitol, Cheyenne, WY 82001.
C. Number of Legislators
   1. Senators: 30.
   2. Representatives: 62.
D. Terms of Office.
   1. Governor: 4 years.
   2. Senators: 4 years.
   3. Representatives: 2 years.
E. Legislative Officers and Leaders: Elected by all members of their respective chambers.
   1. Senate
      a. President of the senate.
      b. Vice president of the senate.
   2. House
      a. Speaker of the house.
      b. Speaker pro tem.
F. Regular Legislative Session
   1. Convenes: Annually. In odd-numbered years, the session convenes on the second Tuesday in January; In even-numbered years, the session con-

venes on the second Tuesday in February. The second session of the legislature is basically limited to budget and fiscal matters.

   2. Length of Session

      a. Odd-Numbered Years: Session is limited to 40 legislative days.

      b. Even-Numbered Years: Session is limited to 20 legislative days.

G. Special Legislative Session

   1. Convenes: When called by the governor.

   2. Length of Session: No limit on the length of session.

   3. Subject(s) To Be Discussed: Either the governor or the legislature may determine the subject(s) to be considered.

H. Bill Introduction

   1. Time Limitations

      a. In odd-numbered years, legislation must be introduced by the 18th legislative day.

      b. In even-numbered years, legislation must be introduced by the fifth legislative day.

   2. Exceptions to Time Limitations: Exceptions are permitted by a unanimous vote of elected members.

I. Standing Committees

   1. Average Number

      a. Senate: 12.

      b. House: 12.

      c. Joint: 1.

   2. Committee Hearings Open to the Public: Senate and house hearings are not open to the public.

J. Bill-to-Law Process

   1. By Whom Referred to Committee

      a. Senate: President of the senate.

      b. House: Speaker of the house.

   2. Required Readings: Three readings of a bill are required before a final vote can take place. These readings must occur on separate days except by two-thirds vote.

   3. Formal Floor Debate: Occurs during a meeting of the Committee of the Whole. Bills are frequently amended from the floor during this debate.

   4. Recorded Vote on Final Passage: Votes are recorded manually.

   5. Passage of a Bill: The minimum vote required to pass a bill in each house is a majority of the elected members.

   6. Fate of a Passed Bill Before Adjournment: The governor either signs the bill into law or vetoes it. If the governor does neither within three days (Sundays excluded), the bill becomes law.

   7. Fate of a Passed Bill After Adjournment: The governor either signs the bill into law or vetoes it. If the governor does neither and does not file an objection with the secretary of state within 15 days of adjournment (Sundays included), the bill becomes law.

   8. Passage of a Bill Over the Governor's Veto: Requires a two-thirds vote of the elected members of both houses.

American Samoa

A. Official Names
   1. Both Houses: Legislature. (FONO)
   2. Upper House: Senate.
   3. Lower House: House of representatives.
B. Convening Place: Maota Fono, American Samoa 96799.
C. Number of Legislators
   1. Senators: 18.
   2. Representatives: 21.
D. Terms of Office
   1. Governor: 4 years.
   2. Senators: 4 years.
   3. Representatives: 2 years.
E. Legislative Officers and Leaders: Elected by all members of their respective chambers.
   1. Senate:
      a. President of the senate.
      b. President pro tem.
   2. House: Speaker of the house.
F. Regular Legislative Session
   1. Convenes: Annually; odd-numbered years on the second Monday in January and the even-numbered years on the second Monday in July.
   2. Length of Session: Both sessions are limited to 30 legislative days.
G. Special Legislative Session
   1. Convenes: When called by the governor.
   2. Length of Session: No limit on length of session.
   3. Subject(s) To Be Considered: May consider only subject(s) specified in the governor's proclamation convening the legislature.
H. Bill Introduction
   1. Time Limitation: Legislation must be introduced by the tenth legislative day.
   2. Exceptions to Time Limitations: Exceptions are permitted by a two-thirds vote of elected members.
I. Standing Committees
   1. Average Number
      a. Senate: 12.
      b. House: 19.
      c. Joint: 1.
   2. Committee Hearings Open to the Public
      a. Senate.
      b. House.
J. Bill-to-Law Process
   1. By Whom Referred to Committee
      a. Senate: President of the senate.
      b. House: Speaker of the house.
   2. Required Readings: Three readings of a bill are required before a final vote can take place. These readings must occur on separate days.

3. Formal Floor Debate: Occurs after the second reading. Bills are frequently amended from the floor during the formal debate.
4. Recorded Vote on Final Passage: Votes are recorded manually.
5. Passage of a Bill: The minimum vote required to pass a bill in each house is a majority of the membership.
6. Fate of a Passed Bill Before Adjournment: The governor either signs the bill into law or vetoes it. If the governor does neither within ten days (Sundays excluded), the bill becomes law.
7. Fate of a Passed Bill After Adjournment: The governor either signs the bill into law or vetoes it. If the governor does neither within 30 days (Sundays excluded), the bill dies.
8. Passage of a Bill Over the Governor's Veto: A two-thirds vote of the members of both houses is required to override a veto. Override also requires the approval of the secretary of the interior, since American Samoa is a trust territory.

Guam

A. Official Names: One house only. Unicameral Legislature; members go by title of senator.
B. Convening Place: Congress Building, Agana, Guam 96910.
C. Number of Legislators
    1. Senators: 21.
D. Terms of Office
    1. Governor: 4 years.
    2. Senators: 2 years.
E. Legislative Officers and Leaders: Elected by all members of the unicameral legislature.
    1. Speaker of the legislature.
    2. Vice speaker of the legislature.
F. Regular Legislative Session
    1. Convenes: Annually on the second Monday in January. The legislature meets in two annual sessions. Bills may carry over from the first to the second session.
    2. Length of Session: No limit on length of session.
    3. Subject(s) To Be Considered: May consider only subject(s) specified in the governor's proclamation convening the legislature.
H. Bill Introduction
    1. Time Limitation: No time limit on the introduction of legislation.
I. Standing Committees
    1. Average Number: 11
    2. Committee Hearings Are Open to the Public.
J. Bill-to-Law Process
    1. Bills Referred to Committee by: Rules Committee.
    2. Required Readings: Three readings are usually required before a final vote can be taken; however, bills are occasionally passed with two read-

ings and rarely with one. These readings usually occur on separate days.
3. Formal Floor Debate: Occurs after the second reading; however, when budget legislation is considered, it occurs after a meeting of the Committee of the Whole. Bills are frequently amended from the floor during this debate.
4. Recorded Vote on Final Passage: Votes are recorded manually.
5. Passage of a Bill: The minimum vote required to pass a bill is a majority of the senators present and voting.
6. Fate of a Passed Bill Before Adjournment: The governor either signs the bill into law or vetoes it. If the governor does neither within ten days (Sundays excluded), the bill becomes law.
7. Fate of a Passed Bill After Adjournment: The governor either signs the bill into law or vetoes it. If the governor does neither within 30 days (Sundays excluded), the bill dies.
8. Passage of a Bill Over the Governor's Veto: A vote of two-thirds of the members of the senate is required to override a veto.

Puerto Rico

A. Official Names
   1. Both Houses: Legislative assembly.
   2. Upper House: Senate.
   3. Lower House: House of representatives.
B. Convening Place: Capitol, San Juan 00901.
C. Number of Legislators: The constitution provides for selection of additional members from the minority party after a general election in which it elects fewer than nine members in the senate and 17 members in the house. Total senate and house composition can reach 104 members.
   1. Senate: 28.
   2. Representatives: 51.
D. Terms of Office
   1. Governor: 4 years.
   2. Senators: 4 years.
   3. Representatives: 4 years.
E. Legislative Officers and Leaders: Elected by all members of their respective chambers.
   1. Senate: President of the senate.
   2. House: Speaker of the house.
F. Regular Legislative Session
   1. Convenes: Annually on the second Monday in January. The legislature meets in two annual sessions, each adjourning sine die. Bills may carry over from the first to the second session.
G. Special Legislative Session
   1. Convenes: When called by the governor.
   2. Length of Session: Session is limited to 20 days.
   3. Subject(s) To Be Considered: May consider only subject(s) specified in the governor's proclamation convening the legislature.

H. Bill Introduction
   1. Time Limitation: Legislation must be introduced by the 16th day.
   2. Exceptions to Time Limitations: Exceptions are permitted by a majority vote.
I. Standing Committees
   1. Average Number
      a. Senate: 19.
      b. House: 19.
   2. Committee Hearings Open to the Public
      a. Senate: Open.
      b. House: Open.
J. Bill-to-Law Process
   1. By Whom Referred to Committee
      a. Senate: President of the Senate.
      b. House: Speaker of the House.
   2. Required Readings: Three readings of a bill are required before a final vote can take place. These readings can occur on the same day.
   3. Formal Floor Debate: Not applicable; see No. 2 above.
   4. Record Vote on Final Passage: Votes are recorded manually.
   5. Passage of a Bill: The minimum vote required to pass a bill is a majority of the members of both houses.
   6. Fate of a Passed Bill Before Adjournment: The governor either signs the bill into law or vetoes it. If the governor does neither within ten days (Sundays excluded), the bill becomes law.
   7. Fate of a Passed Bill After Adjournment: The governor either signs the bill into law or vetoes it. If the governor does neither within 30 days, (Sundays excluded), the bill dies.
   8. Passage of a Bill Over the Governor's Veto: A two-thirds majority vote of the elected members of both houses is required to override a veto.

Annotated Bibliography

Dona Wilcox Cutting, Patricia A. Goehner,
and Joanne Rabinowe

Andersen K: Working women and political participation, 1952–1972. *American Journal of Political Science* 19:439–453, August 1975. This paper examines the extent to which sex differences in political participation (specifically participation in election campaigns) have narrowed over the last 20 years, and finds that the change is due to a particular group of women: those employed outside the home, who now participate in election campaigns at a rate equal to that of men. The possibility that sociodemographic changes in this group of women account for their increased participation is examined, as is the connection between feminism and participation, and the role of the 1972 election in mobilizing working women.

Anonymous: A consumer speaks out about hospital care. *American Journal of Nursing*, 9:1443–1444, 1976. A postsurgical patient's descriptive account of an "outrageous" two-week hospital stay during which confusion in administering medication, lack of professionalism, mistaken identification of the patient, and other events left the patient with an extremely negative impression of hospital care. The message is clear: the shortcomings of a health care institution are many, and the nurse-manager faces the challenge and responsibility of continually improving the image of nursing, monitoring the practice of nursing, and improving patient care.

Archer H: From bill to law: The legislative process. *Imprint* 23(4):26–29, 1976. A concise article that traces the path of a bill through the legislative processes necessary to become a law. Diagrams are used to outline the steps a bill takes through the House of Representatives and the Senate, with markings to show when input and influence from the public is appropriate.

Archer SE: Politics and economics: How things really work, in Archer SE, Fleshman RP (eds): *Community Health Nursing: Patterns and Practice* 2nd ed. North Scituate, Mass, Duxbury Press, 1979, pp 277–312. A discussion of major political and economic concepts that affect nursing. The uses of decision-making strategies (including the open-system political model), concepts of power, interest groups, and consumer participation in politics are clarified. Economic concepts include the allocation of resources, supply and demand, cost-benefit analysis, marginality, the Consumer Price Index, and opportunity costs. An extensive political and economic bibliography is supplied.

Archer SE, Goehner PA: *Speaking Out: The Views of Nurse Leaders.* New York, National League for Nursing, 1981. Pub. No. 15-1847. The paper reports part of the results of a 1979 nationwide study of nurse administrators from various types of health care agencies and schools of nursing. Respondents indicated that low nurse political involvement is due to lack of preparation for political participation, apathy, and failure to realize the importance of political participation. The overwhelming majority believed that preparation for political participation should be included in all levels of nursing curricula as well as in inservice and continuing education for nurses. Course materials from the graduate course the authors developed at the School of Nursing, University of California at San Francisco, including objectives, content, requirements, and field work, are provided to aid nurse faculty members to develop similar courses.

Ashley JA: *Hospitals, Paternalism, and the Role of the Nurse.* New York, Teachers College Park, 1976. In tracing the social and political history of hospitals and nursing back to the 1800s, discriminatory attitudes toward women and nurses are revealed. This book, an outgrowth of the author's nursing doctoral dissertation, examines: (1) the economic rather than humanistic interests of hospital management (doctors) in the establishment of the first hospital; (2) the practice of medicine as both a business and a profession; (3) the development of the apprentice-subordinate role of the nurse as a saleable commodity and as an ingrained attitude on the part of doctors, the public, and even nurses; (4) the lack of scientific educational programs for nurses; (5) the development of professional organizations: NLN and ANA; and (6) sexual discrimination, economic abuse, lack of political freedom, and poor legal status in nursing. The author states that nursing needs activists and reforms to overcome its passive-submissive public and professional image. Other recommendations include a national health policy that utilizes nurses' abilities and talents, discontinued use of doctors as spokespersons, increased nursing education, and an active consumer advocate for nurses.

Ashley JA: Nurses and the meaning of law and order. *Imprint* 23(4):24–25, 1976. Legislative inequality has impeded nurses' progress since the early 1900s. Courage and active and intelligent participation by all nurses is needed to challenge the powerful medical, hospital, and commercially minded groups that influence the courts and the legislative process to perpetuate this imbalance.

Ashley JA: Power, freedom and professional practice in nursing. *Supervisor Nurse* 6:12–24, 29, 1975. Nurses working in institutions need to develop a strong power base by working collectively. This author feels that in order to change nursing's lack of power, nurses must gain knowledge in politics and work to change their own and the public's attitude toward nursing.

Ashley JA: This I believe about power in nursing. Nursing Outlook 21:637–641, 1973. Nursing has always struggled to recognize and effectively use its actual and potential power. Power for nurses lies in defining nursing to the consumers, the health system, and the educational media, and in differentiating nursing from medicine.

Bandman B, Bandman E: Do nurses have rights? American Journal of Nursing 78:84–86, 1978. B. Bandman states that nurses do not have rights, they have only the privilege of treating patients who consent to a regimen of care. E. Bandman states that nurses, because they have professional responsibilities, must have correlative professional rights. Advocacy calls for intervention in systems on behalf of an individual, and nurses can only accomplish the role of patient advocate if recognition is awarded to their special rights, based on their professional credentials.

Beletz E: The public image: A devoted heart, disciplined hand, not necessarily an inquiring mind. Imprint 23(4):27, 41, 1976. In 1975 students polled citizens to determine the degree to which the public has kept pace with the many changes that have occurred in nursing. Nurses were seen as "sex symbols," "subordinate to physicians," and "lacking intelligence," rather than as "researchers," "innovators," "administrators," and "primary providers of health care versus sick care."

Bernstein MJ, Lesparre M: Washington report: Medigap fraud scored. Hospital, Journal of American Hospital Association 52(12), 1978. Since Medicare coverage is inadequate, the elderly have spent billions of dollars for supplemental health insurance policies that is both duplicative and inadequate. This article has relevance for all nurses working with the aged, and for nurses who have elderly relatives. Nurses must educate the elderly about fraudulent insurance policies.

Bowers HN, Howard GD: Mandates from Washington, DC The Journal of School Health 46:548–551, 1976. The author presents an informative overview of four legislative acts that affect the consumer. The author's key point concerning health prevention education is well supported by his facts and interpretation of the laws.

Bowman RA: The nursing organization as a political pressure group. Nursing Forum 12:72–81, 1973. Because of their large number, nurses have potential for becoming a powerful pressure group. One strong organizational voice that can speak for the entire profession would provide the most desirable representation within the political process. As the visibility of nurses in the political arena increases, the strength of nurses will increase.

Bowman RA, Culpepper RC: Power: Treatment for change. American Journal of Nursing 74:1053–1056, 1974. Nurses' negative self-image has made them powerless, but this powerlessness can be altered through changes in nursing education and group identity. If nurses as a group would mobilize for themselves and also become patient advocates, they could radically change the picture of health care in the United States.

Broder DS: Of presidents and parties. The Wilson Quarterly 11:105–117, 1978. With the election of Dwight D. Eisenhower in 1952, the old pattern of party voting began breaking up. The party system continues to deteriorate.

According to Broder, a split in party politics between President Nixon and Congress and the lack of responsible party system led to Watergate.

Brown B, Gebbie K, Moore JF: Affecting nursing goals in health care. *Nursing Administration Quarterly* 2(3):17–31, 1978. Nursing power is important. The authors define power as the ability and willingness to affect the behavior of others to bring about change. Other important facets of power discussed in this article include sources of power, current approaches to power, and selected strategies to obtain power.

Buell EC, Brigman NE: *The Grass Roots*. Illinois, Scott Foresman & Co, 1968. Readings were selected for this anthology to illustrate and evaluate the present structure and operations of state and local governments and political systems. The authors pose alternatives and highlight some of the problems that must be faced and overcome.

Bullough B: Influences on role expansion. *American Journal of Nursing* 76:1476–1481, 1976. This article emphasizes the fact that nurses should and do have something to say about their own roles. Nurses are instrumental in getting legislation passed to legitimize their practice. The author's review of nursing licensure statutes over the years points out only too clearly what would have happened if nurses had accepted some statutes as final decrees.

Bullough B: Nurse practice acts: How they affect your expanded role. *Nursing* 77:73–81, 1977. This article is an overview of the current status and changing components of nurse practice acts on a national level, with insight into each individual state. The present trend of expanding the scope of practice in some states is significant; however, the nursing section of the state code needs to be revised in every state.

Chamber of Commerce of the United States: *Action Course In Practical Politics*. Washington, Public Affairs Department, 1974. Six pamphlets of practical politics, compiled and designed to be used in conjunction with a 14-hour workshop to guide those who wish to increase their effectiveness in politics. Included are (1) *Political Organization*, (2) *Political Precincts*, (3) *Political Campaigning*, (4) *Political Clubs*, (5) *Political Leaders' Problems*, and (6) *Political Meetings*.

Conway ME: The acquisition and use of power in academia: A dean's perspective. *Nursing Administration Quarterly* 2(3), 1978. The university is attempting to bring about certain behavioral changes and to influence decisions in nursing. Since society needs well-prepared nurses, the university has the obligation to help meet this need by preparing competent resource persons who can use their power to influence decisions and bring about behavioral changes.

Cowart M: *Implementing Health Policy in Baccalaureate Nursing Curricula*. New York, National League for Nursing, 1981. Pub. No. 15-1844. The author emphasizes the importance of public policy, that is, policy adapted by any level of government. Much of health policy falls into the public domain. Teaching about health policy and about the public policy process is essential as a means of incorporating the concept of society into the curriculum as the concepts of man, health, and nursing now are.

Cowart ME: Teaching the legislative process. *Nursing Outlook* 25:777–780, 1977. The evolution and current outline of Flordia State University's undergraduate health-disciplines course in legislation consists of (1) theory and practical experience in the legislative process; (2) change-agent strategies; and (3) an examination of current issues in health care in the state and nation. (4) Practical experience includes orientation to the state capitol and mock committee meetings in class.

Creighton H: Law for the nurse supervisor: Employer's right to temporary reassignment. *Supervisor Nurse* 7:58–60, 1976. Two Pennsylvania nurses were fired on charges of insubordination during a period of political activism. Suit was filed against the hospital for unfair labor practices, and the court ruled for reinstatement. After two appeals, this decision was reversed, based on this argument: Supervisors' orders must be carried out promptly. Failure to do so within a half hour constitutes insubordination. Insubordination is adequate cause for release without warning. Such a release is therefore not an unfair labor practice.

Creighton H: Law for the nurse supervisor: Legality of setting private/special duty fees. *Supervisor Nurse* 1(2):58–62, 1976. This article compares the powerful American Bar Association and American Medical Association to the weak American Nurses' Association, Nurses can only gain power if they unite and work together collectively.

Creighton H: Law for the nurse supervisor: Legal problems in nursing participation in criminal investigations. *Supervisor Nurse* 7(8):44–46, 1976. This article describes recent cases of medical and nursing participation in criminal investigations (usually narcotic enforcement) on state and federal levels that have the potential for medical-nursing malpractice suits. Ethical guidelines for participation by medical personnel in penal, institutional, and police practices are offered.

Creighton H: Law for the nurse supervisor: Right to psychiatric treatment. *Supervisor Nurse* 7(5):70–72, 1976. This article deals with patients' rights in the psychiatric setting and includes legal justification for the civil commitment of the objecting mentally ill person, ramifications of the failure of the staff or the facility to give adequate treatment, and basic necessities that must be provided to the psychiatric patient. A substantial bibliography of articles and court cases is provided.

Delaughery GL, Gebrie KM: *Political Dynamics: Impact on Nurses v. Nursing.* St. Louis, CV Mosby Co, 1975. This book can serve as a reference for historical and current issues of the political and health care systems, the nurses' role in relation to the political arena, and power and change theories. Attention is given to the US Constitution and the Bill of Rights, problems of the city and current issues, social system theory, professionalism, and nurses as political activists and change agents.

Dellefield K: Getting the most from a student bill of rights. *Imprint* 23:40–42, 1976. Nursing education fails to address students' basic rights to give and take responsibility, to be accountable for their actions, and to be assertive decision makers. Nursing students should explore the meaning of rights for themselves and others, the responsibility of obtaining and preserving individual rights, and the significance of contractual agreements (accepting authority and its inherent responsibilities).

Dellefield K: We can make a difference. *Imprint* 23(4):18, 52, 1976. Decisions affecting nursing and health care issues are being made by politicians, not health professionals. Nurses are in a unique position to influence public and political processes because they are the largest profession in the health field, they are respected by the public, and they have knowledge of health care systems. They must unite to identify goals, plan strategies, assume responsibility, and exercise authority in an attempt to influence health care legislation.

Depres LM: A lawyer explains what the National Labor Relations Act really says. *American Journal of Nursing* 76:790–794, 1976. Legal interpretation of Public Law 93-360, which permits collective bargaining in nonprofit hospitals. The law states that (1) supervisory and management personnel cannot interfere in labor organizations, and (2) supervisors may be dues-paying members of professional organizations. The author supports and encourages supervisors to maintain affiliation with professional groups so that such groups can represent all facets of the profession in noneconomic nursing matters.

Diers D: A different kind of energy: Nurse power. *Nursing Outlook* 26:51–55, 1978. Nurses possess power in many areas, including (1) power of numbers: we are large in number; (2) power of position: we are patients' advocates, an alliance with enormous potential; (3) power of politics: the nation's revised health care system under Public Law 93-641 increases and improves the utilization of nurse clinicians; (4) power of knowledge: the proper focus of the development of nursing knowledge is nursing practice; (5) power of pride: we have so much to be proud of in nursing. We stimulated early racial integration in our professional association, we provide economic security for nurses, and we standardized our licensure procedures.

Donaho BA, Parsek JD, Zimmerman A: NAQ forum: Politics and power. *Nursing Administration Quarterly* 2(3):65–70, 1978. A composite of three articles dealing with power as a political force. Nurses have been erroneously viewed by the health care bureaucracy as being without power. Now nursing should take the opportunity to grow, develop, and share its inherent power in order to facilitate care for the individual patient and family, and to influence governmental policy.

Donley R: An inside view of the Washington health scene. *American Journal of Nursing* 79:1946–1949, 1979. Sister Rosemary Donley spent over a year as a Robert Wood Johnson health policy fellow in Washington, DC. In this article she shares her insights into bureaucratic organizations, which will enable the reader to better understand the system and how to use it to his or her advantage.

Dorken H: Avenues to legislative success. *American Psychologist* 32:738–745, 1977. Legislative process is complex. Long-term success is dependent upon a knowledge of the field, organization, delineation of achievable objectives, and a willingness to learn the system and work with it. The establishment of a grassroots legislative network, in which constituents establish a personal relationship with their legislators and alert them to situations in which support is desired, greatly facilitates the legislative process.

Durkin E, Zuckerman S: Legislation affects nursing practice. *Nursing Administration Quarterly* 2(3):39–50, 1978. The authors review current nurse practice acts as they have evolved from the traditional model of nursing to the redefined model of nursing we know today. The expanded role of the nurse is examined, and its impact on recent legislation is discussed. Guidelines for writing to and working with legislators are offered.

Ellis B: Future evolution of nursing role contingent on legislation. *Hospitals, Journal of American Hospital Association* 52(2):81–82, 1978. The evolution of the practice of nursing will depend upon legislation. Control of nursing practice, through revision of the Nurse Practice Act for example, is in the hands of the lawmakers. This article gives suggestions for dealing with lawmakers and uses case studies to point out pitfalls.

Elms RR, Moorhead JM: Will the real nurse please stand up. *Nursing Forum* 16:112–128, 1977. This article is a history of the evolution of the nursing profession. It traces the contributions made by the following nurses: Florence Nightingale, Lillian Wald, Mary Breckenridge, Margaret Sanger, Faye Abdellah, Shirley Chater, Ingeborg Mauksch, and Lydia Hall. A discussion of the three different programs that prepare students to become registered nurses, and their implication on nurses and the profession, is included.

Elsberry ML: Power relations in hospital nursing. *Journal of Nursing Administration* 2(5):75–77, 1972. Sources of power relevant to hospital nursing are legitimate power, referent power, input power, and reward power. Factors that contribute to the lack of power of nurses within the traditional hospital organization are staff line conflict, dual administrative control, inappropriate reward structures, and power and the supervisor's role. Suggested solutions to increase power organizational changes and leadership training.

Fagin C, Maraldo P: *Health Policy in Nursing Curriculum: Why It's Needed.* New York, National League for Nursing, 1981. Pub. No. 15–1845. Nursing as a profession is developing and growing, so it is essential that student nurses understand the political forces that will influence and probably control their practice throughout their careers. Student nurses can be taught that their porfessional responsibilities in health policy need not be an unwelcome burden but rather are an opportunity for professional growth. This understanding can contribute much to nursing being able to exert its political clout.

Fish MS: When does one choose which legal structure in which to practice as a nurse practitioner? *Nurse Practitioner* 1(5):9, 35, 1976. The author suggests types of business relations the nurse practitioner should consider when setting up practice with a physician or a group. Consideration should be given to (1) expenses, (2) taxes, (3) collateral benefits, (4) liability, and (5) continuity (in the event of disability or death of group members). The author believes the corporate structure is the most advantageous for nurse practitioners.

Fleischhaslsei U: Writing your legislator: Some do's and dont's. *Maternal Child Nursing* 3:153–154, 1977. This article tells how to express views to legislators, both verbally and in writing, in an effective manner. Do's and don'ts are presented to facilitate communication.

Gamer M: The ideology of professionalism. *Nursing Outlook* 27(2):108–111, 1979. This article speaks to the issue of education versus experience in preparing nurses for practice. Some historical perspective is given in the comparison of nursing and medical education and the direction each has taken in regard to the goals of prestige, dedication, and money. Academia has stressed education in nursing, while the impetus for an expanded nursing role has come from the practice setting.

Gonzales de Alfaro ME: Legal and civil responsibilities of nurses. *International Nursing Review* 24(6):172–175, 181, 1977. This article focuses on the reluctance of nurses to accept legal and civil responsibility beyond their professional concerns. Because most nurses act at the operational-technical level, it is very important that they contribute information to the political decision-making level of government.

Grimm TJ, Crawford JJ: Viewpoint: Assertiveness training for nurses. *Nursing Administration Quarterly* 2(3):59–63, 1978. The lack of leadership in nursing can be attributed to a lack of self-awareness and a general passivity in interpersonal relations among nurses. Improving nursing services, providing more nursing leaders, and decreasing role conflict could be some of the direct benefits of nurses learning to express their feelings.

Grissum M, Spengler C: *Woman Power and Health Care.* Boston, Little Brown and Co, 1976. This book explores some of the reasons why nurses maintain a relatively powerless role in health care decision making. The authors contend that nursing is greatly influenced by a male-dominated society, and that nurses have generally allowed the men in health care to make the decisions.

Guidelines for Meeting with Legislators, Publication No. 21-1640. New York, National League for Nursing, 1978. Meeting with your legislator should be productive for him or her as well as for you. In this pamphlet, suggestions are given to help ensure a productive session with legislators.

Guidelines for Presenting Testimony on Legislation, Publication No. 21-1624. New York, National League for Nursing, 1978. Some 20,000 bills are introduced during the two-year course of a congressional session. As few as 500 may be signed into law, but many more are the subject of hearings. This pamphlet provides suggestions for preparing testimony for public hearings.

Heide WS: Nursing and women's liberation: A parallel. *American Journal of Nursing* 73:824–826, May 1973. Nursing is characterized as a "feminine" profession, and nurses suffer from the same oppression, prejudices, and limitations as other females in our society. As long as the denial of feminine traits is reviewed as natural and desirable, people will deny part of their humanity, and society will be imbalanced, pathological, and unhealthy. Nurses must undertake consciousness raising, ask questions about professional roles, challenge the status quo, and examine alternatives to the current health care policies.

Herzog TP: The National Labor Relations Act and the ANA: A dilemma of professionalism. *The Journal of Nursing Administration* 6(8):34–36, 1976. The author questions ANA's involvement in collective bargaining. He appears biased in his negative opinion of ANA's future in collective bargaining, and is concerned that it is losing its professional status and is becoming a trade union for nurses.

Hopping B: Step right up and help yourself. *Imprint* 23(4):46, 1976. Nursing

Practice Act. Professional nurses are confronted with the opportunity to grow, to step into new roles that will meet the health care needs of America today with up-to-date interventions.

Hott JP: The struggle inside nursing's body politic. Nursing Forum 15:324–340, 1976. Nursing is being shaped more and more by political decisions. Nurses need to unite and accept responsibility for their profession. Major concerns that need to be addressed include the development of criteria on which to judge competency, establishment of laws that set forth standards for professional capacity, and creation of terminology for specific functions and levels of competency.

Howe F (ed): Women and the Power to Change. New York, McGraw-Hill Book Co, 1975. A collection of essays by women united in their feminist and activist commitment to institutional change on the university campus. Women's education suffers because the university is a male-centered institution with a traditional curriculum, and women employed by the university hold token positions, are awarded less prestige, and are paid less. Alternatives to circumvent the male-centered university are discussed.

Hughes E, Proulx J: Learning about politics. American Journal of Nursing 79:494–495, 1979. Describes a course, called Core III, for graduate-level nurses at the University of Maryland. This course incorporates the socio-economic, cultural, and political aspects of health care.

Jacox A: Address to the next generation. Nursing Outlook 26:38–41, 1978. Consumers are demanding that health professionals be more active in health promotion. Despite internal conflict, nursing needs to define new roles, develop improved knowledge through research, and become constructively and significantly involved in the provision of health care if the profession is to move forward.

Johnson SH: Nursing involvement in national health insurance. Nursing Administration Quarterly 2(3):91–99, 1978. Nurses need to be knowledgeable, involved, and influential in the planning of national health insurance. The positive and negative aspects of the five major proposals (Ullman Plan HR-1, Burleson and McIntyre Plan HR 5200, Kennedy-Griffiths Plan S3, Fulton Plan HR6222, Long-Ribicoff Plan S2470) are discussed and analyzed.

Kalisch BJ: The promise of power. Nursing Outlook 26:42—46, 1978. The critical challenge facing nursing is that of acquiring a solid resource and power base upon which to move the profession forward. The author states that nurses need to form coalitions with health-consumer groups in order to elect public officials who are concerned with the welfare of nurses and health care consumers.

Kalisch BJ, Kalisch PA: A discourse on the politics of nursing. The Journal of Nursing Administration 6:29–33, 1976. Nursing education needs to include the "politics of nursing" in curricula. The future of nursing depends on nurses who can understand, adjust, and take advantage of legislation involving nurses. The authors see nursing administrators as a starting point for the use of democratic principles in institutional politics.

Kelly L: The patient's right to know. Nursing Outlook 24:26–32, 1976. This article focuses on the issues of patients' rights in relation to informed consent, privacy, and medical research. The author elaborates on the requirements for informed consent and discusses the use of consent forms. A comprehensive background of the major legislation affecting patient's rights is also included.

Knowledge of professional nursing legislation. *Nursing Times* 73(18):674–676, 1977. This article discusses the lack of knowledge of nurses in England regarding their "statutory instruments." The author suggests that nurses become knowledgeable about the rules governing definition and classification of terms, approval of training institutions, nursing examinations, qualification of teachers, uniforms and badges, proper use of credential initials, and dismissal of grade classifications for nurses. No information is available on the author, who is referred to as "observer."

Krekeler K: Then education control, now control of practice. *Supervisor Nurse* 5:25–27, 1976. The author states that proposed legislation for institutional licensure and a board of examiners for all types of health personnel education programs is a tactic for maintaining control of nursing education and practice.

Lamb KT: Freedom for our sisters, freedom for ourselves: Nursing confronts social change. *Nursing Forum* 12:329–352, 1973. Nursing's struggle for recognition as a profession is tightly bound to the women's rights movement. Nursing can use the powerful force of sisterhood to increase its professional status by becoming active in the struggle for women's rights.

Lawrence JC: Confronting nurses' political apathy. *Nursing Forum* 15:363–372, 1976. The greatest threat to the nursing profession is nurses' apathy and ignorance of significant health care issues. The author suggests several methods for breaking this present pattern.

Leininger M: Political nursing: Essential for health service and education systems of tomorrow. *Nursing Administration Quarterly* 2(3):1–16, 1978. This article stresses the need for nurses to be knowledgeable about politics and power behavior inside and outside of nursing. Concepts of politics and authority are defined, and are discussed as enabling nurses to make an impact on social and health care systems.

Le Roux, RS: Communication and influence in nursing. *Nursing Administration Quarterly* 2:51–57, 1978. Nurses' inability to influence the health care system in proportion to their strength could be due to their inability to find an audience, to be granted credibility, or to express themselves forcefully. The author, however, contends that the trend toward masters' nursing programs in administration rather than patient-focused clinical practice has brought about an increased emphasis on communication skills.

Levison R: Sexism in medicine. *American Journal of Nursing* 76:426–431, 1976. This article examines and identifies the many areas of medicine in which sexism is supported—from early psychiatry, which considered healthy women to be passive and dependent, to the present-day practice of treating menstruation, pregnancy, and menopause as pathological contributors to female frailty. By identifying the sources of sexism in health care, the nurse may be instrumental in educating ill-informed sources.

Lipset SM: Marx, Engels and American political parties. *The Wilson Quarterly* 2:90–104, 1978. The unique history and culture of America eliminates socialism and class solidarity because of such factors as relatively egalitarian status structure, achievement-oriented value systems, affluence, the absence of an aristocratic or fuedal past, and a history of political democracy prior to industrialization.

Lysaught JP: No carrots, no sticks: Motivation in nursing. *Journal of Nursing Administration* 2(5):43–50, 1972. Focuses on Maslow and Herzberg's respective theories of human motivation and behavior and applies them to nursing.

Matejski MS: Politics, the nurse and the political process. *Nursing Leadership* 2:31–37, 1979. It is imperative that nurses learn about politics if they are going to be heard on matters concerning nursing education, nursing practice, and health care. This article surveys methods of political analysis produced by selected research studies and political scientists.

Merritt S: Winners and losers: Sex difference in municipal elections. *American Journal of Political Science* 21:731–742, 1977. This paper explores the resources and experiences that male and female candidates bring to the local political arena and the characteristics that differentiate winners and losers of both sexes. The comparison of winners and losers suggests that different paths to political success exist for males and females. Success for men is related to social contacts with local politicians, while success for women is related to nonelective political involvement.

Moorhead J: Community health nurses' involvement in legislative activities, in Archer SE, Fleshman RP, (eds): *Community Health Nursing: Patterns and Practice*, ed 2. North Scituate, Mass, Duxbury Press, 1979. The author describes the process she went through in initiating and facilitating the passage of a state law to enable minors to receive treatment for alcohol and other substance abuse without parental consent. Her message is that nurses can and must be more actively involved in legislation. Since nurses and other health providers are increasingly regulated by laws, legislation should not be left to legislators alone.

Mullane MK: Nursing care and the political arena. *Nursing Outlook* 23:699–701, 1975. This article is designed to inspire nurses in areas of political interest. The author predicts "disaster" for the profession if nurses do not become politically involved for their rights as well as for patient rights. Nursing unity is essential for effective influence, and local, state, and national nursing associations are potential sources of collective strength.

Mullane MK: Politics begins at work. *R.N.* 39(7):45–51, 1976. Politics is the act of using influence to bring about change. Yet most nurses associate politics exclusively with government elections and legislation that is determined along party lines. Politics is an essential activity in the nursing profession, because planning plus politics equals change.

Nathanson J: Getting a bill through Congress. *The American Journal of Nursing* 75:1179–1181, 1975. This article outlines the course a bill takes through Congress and the obstacles it may encounter in becoming law. Key legislative terms are defined and explained, such as committee names, bill identification code letters, and terms specific to federal funding legislation.

N-Cap: *Clout*, ed 2, May 1977. American Nurses' Association, Washington, DC. A pamphlet on political action committees (pacs)—what they are and how to get involved in them. Guidelines for forming a state pac are also included. This pamphlet is a useful tool for encouraging and assisting nurses in becoming more politically active.

N-CAP: *Getting Involved in Politics.* Washington, DC, American Nurses' Association. Nurses are the largest group of health care workers in the United States. They have much to gain by becoming politically involved. This pamphlet describes how nurses can do so.

N-CAP: *Know Your Congresspeople.* American Nurses' Association, Washington, DC, 1978. One of the major responsibilities of constituents is to be informed about the people who represent them in the legislature. This pamphlet concisely outlines how to evaluate a legislator's performance.

Novello DJ: The National Health Planning and Resource Development Act. *Nursing Outlook* 24(6):356–358, 1976. The National Health Planning and Resource Development Act of 1974 (Public Law 93–641) has widespread implications for future health care in this country. The purpose of this act was to establish quality health care, at a reasonable cost, to all geographic areas and all groups of citizens. There are many ways in which nurses can become involved in the implementation of this act, such as by becoming members of committees and attending hearings. The author states that it is imperative that nurses become involved.

O'Rourke M: *Health Policy: The Clinical Perspective,* Pub. No. 15-1846. New York, National League for Nursing, 1981. How can nursing realize its hopes for the future through health policy? As experts in nursing, we nurses can and must address the question effectively. We must learn to communicate to legislators and other policy makers about the kinds of professional nursing services that could be provided, how they would differ from present nursing services, and the impact these services would have on the public's health. Nurses can influence health policy if we speak out. Having health legislation and regulations written to include nurses' points of view will, in time, raise the standards of health care provided to the public.

Penniman HP: The state of the two-party system. *The Wilson Quarterly* 11:83–89, 1978. According to the author, the major parties in the United States (Democratic and Republican) are heterogeneous. These parties will continue to dominate congressional, state, and local elections. If direct election of the President should occur, however, the role of major parties in selecting occupants of the White House would be less predictable.

Perry SE: If you are called as an expert witness. *The American Journal of Nursing* 77:458–460, 1977. A short but informative article describing the responsibilities of a legal witness. The author also defines basic trial terminology and includes guidelines for preparation and performance as an expert witness.

The pioneer women in the state legislature. *California Journal* 10:65–66, February 1979. A history of women who served in the 120-member California legislative body from 1918 to 1979. There were four women in the California legislature in 1918 and 11 in 1979 (the highest number ever). An account is given of the California woman legislator's contributions to women's rights and equality. Prior to the 1976 election, California was the third lowest in the nation in the percentage of feminine representation in the state legislature. One possible explanation, recorded in a recent study, is that women have gained more representation in states in which legislators are poorly paid; California has some of the best-paid legislators in the nation.

Powell DJ: Nursing and politics: The struggles outside nursing's body politic. *Nursing Forum* 15:341–362, 1976. Nurses' lack of awareness and involvement in politics have kept their profession under the rule of doctors, health departments, and education departments. The author believes these problems have been with the nursing profession since its inception, and can only be changed if nurses take the initiative to become involved in legislation. The author identifies significant organizations and issues that warrant nursing input now and in the future.

Quinn TA, Salzman E: *California Public Administration: Text and Reading on Decision Making in State Government.* California, California Journal Press, 1978. This book presents an updated, concise review of the inner workings of state government. The book is organized along traditional lines, with sections on each branch of the government; however, the heart of the book is an extensive analysis of the hidden branch of the government, the massive state bureaucracy.

Redman E: *The Dance of Legislation.* New York, Simon & Schuster, 1973. *The Dance of Legislation* follows a bill on National Health Service Corps through the steps to become a law. Eric Redman became actively involved with this bill during the time he worked as a staff member for Senator Warren G. Magnuson. The title is appropriate, for Redman, a novice, learns quickly that he must avoid stepping on too many toes in order to finish the dance victoriously.

Robinson A: Want to get your message across? Write about it. *Imprint* 23(3):45, 1976. One of the effective ways you can provide input and influence your legislators is to write letters to them. The author outlines how to write to legislators, stressing key points. This outline is a very useful tool.

Rogers M: Legislative and licensing problems in health care. *Nursing Administration Quarterly* 2(3):71–78, 1978. This article focuses on problems in the health care system and on specific nursing issues. In the changing health care field there is increased specialization, unionizing of professionals, and lobbying by businesses for control of health. The author contends that nurses must take a strong stand on issues such as expanded role clarification and health care for the people, or the future of the nursing profession is in jeopardy.

Schlatfeldt RM: On the professional status of nursing. *Nursing Forum* 13:16–31, 1974. Nursing is overconcerned with quantity and underconcerned with quality, and this is exemplified by the fact that nursing has yet to delineate a single standard of education. The author states that educators must realistically balance concern for quantity with concern for quality, and that nurses need to become politically astute and seek positions providing opportunities for professional and political influence.

Schorr TM: Nurse power. *American Journal of Nursing* 74:1047, 1974. Nurses' acceptance of powerlessness costs them self-respect. Nurses must be risk takers. They must unite to identify goals, plan strategy, assume responsibility, exercise authority, and be accountable for their actions.

Schroder ES: What goes on in state legislature concerns all nurses. *American Operating Room Nurse* 18:13–14, 1973. The author explains why nurses need to be aware of legislation. Legislation affecting nursing is constantly being passed and if this continues without nurses exercising their influence on legislation, they will lose control over their profession.

Sheahan D: Scanning the seventies. *Nursing Outlook* 26:33–37, 1978. The author describes the need to form a true nursing collective so that nurses can lead, hear, articulate, and advance their hopes and aspirations. The author also describes how a uniform educational system for nursing can be an asset. Rather than having a patchwork system of remedial education programs, nursing needs a single program of professional caliber for all practitioners.

Silverman M, Lee PR: *Pills, Profits and Politics.* California, University of California Press, 1974. Pharmacology is vital to the health and lives of patients. Because pharmacology is such an important field, this book outlines the serious problems that exist within it and the options that are open to the public in regard to drugs and medicine.

Styles MM: Dialogue across the decades. *Nursing Outlook* 26:28–32, 1978. One of the issues discussed in this article is collective bargaining. The author states that collective bargaining does address both personal and professional concerns; however, a large number of nurse-managers feel abandoned by professional organization.

Sullivan RB: Impact of device legislation. *American Operating Room Nurse* 25:658–661, 1977. In 1962 the Kefauver-Harris amendment was added to the Food, Drug, and Cosmetic Act. This amendment has implications for all health care workers involved in the research, production, and use of certain prescription drugs. The law requires all medical devices to be placed in one of three categories. Nurses working in hospitals that test and/or monitor FDA programs need to be aware of this legislation and its impact on nursing care.

Welch S: Women as political animals? A test of some explanations of male-female participation differences. *American Journal of Political Science* 21:711–729, 1977. Based on research, the author gives three major reasons why male and female political participation differs: Women are discouraged from playing an active role in politics, family responsibilities keep women at home and out of political activities, and women as a group have a tendency not to participate in politics. Political socialization theory is discussed in light of these findings.

Werther WB: *Unions: Do They Just Happen or Are They Caused.* New York, National League for Nursing, 1978. A pamphlet addressing (1) what causes unions, (2) why they are needed, (3) why some professionals reject the concept of unions, (4) the conditions for unionizing, (5) the impact of collective action on nursing administrators, and (6) the nurse-executive response to unionizing.

White NS: ERA: The chance for equality. *Nursing Administration Quarterly* 2(3):79–82, 1978. The position of women in society is equated to that of nurses; however, the author views nurses as being in double jeopardy—they are women in a male-dominated society, and they are female professionals in a male-dominated health care provision system. Quoting extensively from Heide, the author discusses the impact ERA will have on nursing. Although the article does not name specific actions to be taken by nurses, it is a "consciousness raiser."

Wood LA: Continuing education: The nurse and the legislative process. *The Journal of Continuing Education* 4(2):19–23, 1973. The author discusses the implementation of a class entitled "The Legislative Process" in a continuing-education program. Besides outlining the curriculum, specific guidelines and recommendations for nurses giving testimony before legislative committees are included.

APPENDIX A

Selected Legislation of Particular Importance to Women:

1919 Through the First Session of the 96th Congress, December 1979

1. Nineteenth Amendment to the Constitution of the United States: "The right of citizens of the United States to vote shall not be denied or abridged by the United States or by any State on account of sex." Passed June 5, 1919; ratified by 36 states; certified August 26, 1920.
2. Women's Bureau, 1920. (Public Law 66-250). The Women's Bureau was created within the Department of Labor to formulate policies and standards to promote the welfare of wage-earning women, to improve working conditions, to increase efficiency, and to advance opportunities for employment.
3. Equal Pay Act of 1963 (PL 88-38) Prohibits discrimination on the basis of sex in the payment of wages for equal work on jobs requiring equal skill, effort, and responsibility and performed under similar working conditions.
4. Title VII of the Civil Rights Act of 1964 (PL 88-352). Prohibits discrimination in employment based on sex as well as upon race, color, religion, and national origin by employers, public and private employment agencies, labor unions, and labor management programs.
5. Comprehensive Health and Manpower Training Act of 1971 (PL 92-157). Prohibits use of federal funds for health professional programs that discriminate on the basis of sex in the admission of persons to their programs.
6. Proposed Equal Rights Amendment. Provides that "equality of rights under the law shall not be denied or abridged by the United States or by any State on account of sex." Passed by the 92nd Congress, March 1972. If ratified by 38 states on or before June

30, 1982, it will become the 27th amendment to the United States Constitution.

7. Equal Employment Opportunity Act of 1972 (PL 92-261). Protects all workers against sex discrimination under Title VII of the Civil Rights Act of 1964.

8. The Higher Education Amendments of 1972 (PL 92-318). Extends coverage of Title VII of the Civil Rights Act to government employees, employees of all educational institutions (except religious schools), and employees of any business or union with 15 or more workers, except religious institutions. Sex discrimination in all federally assisted education programs is prohibited under Title IX.

9. Comprehensive Manpower Act, 1973 (PL 93-203). Extends coverage of Title VI of the Civil Rights Act of 1964 to prohibit sex discrimination in the expenditure of federal manpower funds.

10. Small Business Act of 1974 (PL 93-237). Amends the Small Business Act to prohibit the Small Business Administration from discriminating on the basis of sex or marital status against any person or small business applying for or receiving assistance from the Small Business Administration.

11. Fair Labor Standards Act Amendments of 1974 (PL 93-259). Increases the minimum wage and extends coverage to include state, county, and municipal employees, and domestic workers (the majority of whom are women) who earn more than $50 in a calender quarter or who work for more than eight hours a week for one or more employer.

12. The Education Amendments of 1974 (PL 93-380). Includes the Women's Educational Equity Act, which authorizes the Secretary of Health, Education, and Welfare to make grants to develop special educational programs and activities intended to achieve educational equity for male and female students.

13. The Housing and Community Development Act of 1974 (PL 93-383). Includes provisions that prohibit discrimination on the basis of race, color, national origin, or sex in carrying out community development programs; amends the National Housing Act to prohibit sex discrimination in federally related mortgage loans, insurance guaranties, or related assistance; requires lenders to consider the wife's income as well as the husband's in extending mortgage credit; amends the Civil Rights Act to prohibit sex discrimination in the financing, sale, or rental of housing or in the provision of brokerage services.

14. Equal Credit Opportunity Act of 1974 (PL 93-495). Amends the Consumer Credit Protection Act to prohibit discrimination in credit transactions based on sex or marital status.

15. National Women's Conference Act of 1975 (PL 94-167). Directs

the National Commission on the Observance of International Women's Year, 1975, to organize and convene a national women's conference to evaluate sex discrimination against American women, to recognize the contributions of women to the development of the United States, to assess progress in women's rights, to set goals for the elimination of barriers to full and equal participation by women in all aspects of American life, and to recognize the importance of the contributions of women in developing friendly relations and cooperation among nations and strengthening world peace.

16. International Conventions on the Political Rights of Women (Treaties and Other International Act Series). The Senate, on January 22, 1976, exercised its responsibility to advise and consent, and recommended ratification of the United Nations Convention on Political Rights of Women and the Inter-American Convention on Granting Political Rights to Women. These treaties provide that the contracting parties agree that the right to vote and to be elected to national office shall be neither denied or abridged on account of sex. Both conventions went into force in 1976.

17. Tax Reform Act of 1976 (PL 94-455). Enables some homemakers, under the law on individual retirement accounts, to create tax-deferred retirement accounts; increases the so-called marital deduction enabling an individual to leave $250,000 to a surviving spouse free of estate taxes, a provision of special significance to women, who often outlive their husbands; reduces the gift-tax rate on interspousal gifts up to $200,000, with the first $100,000 being gift-tax free; eliminates the $35,000 income limit on child care deductions, and extends coverage to married couples in which one spouse works part-time or is a student, as well as to separated or divorced parents who have custody of one or more children; and requires that a parent who does not have custody must pay $1,200 at least each per child per year in order to claim any child care deduction.

18. Unemployment Compensation Amendments of 1976 (PL 94-566). Changes benefits of state unemployment compensation laws to include language to the effect that "no person shall be denied compensation under such state laws solely on the basis of pregnancy or termination of pregnancy."

19. Department of Defense Appropriation Authorization Act of 1978 (PL 95-79). Requires the Secretary of Defense to submit a definition of "combat," and to make recommendations on expanding job classifications to which women may be assigned in the military service, as well as on any changes in the law needed to implement these recommendations.

20. Health Planning and Health Services Research and Statistics

Expansion Act of 1977 (PL 94-83). Extends authorizations for family planning services, training programs for family planning clinic staffs, population research and related information, and education programs. Also includes a provision that extends the authorization for rape prevention and control.

21. Departments of State, Justice, and Commerce and the Judiciary and Related Agencies Appropriations Act of 1978 (PL 95-86). Provides additional funding for the Justice Department's Task Force on Sex Discrimination.

22. International Development and Food Assistance Act of 1977 (PL 95-88). Requests that the President determine US contributions to international organizations by at least considering the progress or lack of progress recipient countries have made in promoting the integration of women into their national economies; amends the 1961 Foreign Assistance Act to provide that attention be paid to programs, projects, and activities in developing countries that increase women's integration into their national economies; provides $2 million for the United Nations' Decade for Women, 1976–1985; and prohibits using funds for abortions or involuntary sterilizations.

23. National Science Foundation Authorization Act of 1978 (PL 95-99). Authorizes additional funds for programs designed to assist minorities, women, and the handicapped to obtain education in the sciences.

24. Foreign Assistance and Related Programs Appropriations Act, 1978 (PL 95-148). Authorizes an appropriation not to exceed $3 million for the United Nation's Decade for Women, 1976–1985.

25. Social Security Act Amendments of 1977 (PL 95-171). Increases funding for day care services for the children of welfare recipients and other low-income families.

26. Career Education Incentive Act of 1977 (PL 95-207). Promotes equal opportunity by eliminating bias and stereotyping on the basis of sex, race, or physical handicap; requires all states requesting funds under the act to have a person on their state education agency staff who is experienced in dealing with problems of discrimination and stereotyping in career education on the basis of sex, race, and physical handicap; encourages career development materials that give special emphasis to overcoming sex bias and stereotyping; encourages in-service education to acquaint personnel with changing work patterns of men and women, ways of overcoming sex stereotyping and bias in career education, and ways to help both men and women to broaden their career horizons.

27. Social Security Amendments of 1977 (PL 95-216). Reduces wife's

insurance benefits if she also receives a pension based on her own earnings while a government employee; reduces from twenty to ten years the minimum length of marriage necessary for a surviving spouse or a divorced wife to be eligible for benefits on the basis of her former husband's earnings record; provides for retention of full benefits by widows who remarry after age 60; and authorizes a six-month study of proposals to eliminate dependency and sex discrimination under the Social Security program.

28. Child Abuse Prevention and Treatment and Adoption Reform Act of 1978 (PL 95-266). Establishes a National Center on Child Abuse and Neglect to coordinate research and service activities in the area of child abuse and neglect. Provides for the development of sexual-abuse centers; the development of model adoption legislation and procedures; and the study of unlicensed adoption placements.

29. Federal Employees Part-time Career Employment Act of 1978 (PL 95-437). Provides increased part-time career employment opportunities throughout the federal government. This should benefit the many women who are able or choose to work only part-time.

30. Susan B. Anthony Dollar Coin Act of 1978 (PL 95-447). Authorizes the issuance of a dollar coin commemorating Susan B. Anthony; the coin was issued on January 1, 1979.

31. Comprehensive Employment and Training Act Amendments of 1978 (PL 95-524). Provides for job training and employment opportunities for the economically disadvantaged, unemployed, and underemployed. Special provisions for middle-aged and older workers, Native Americans, migrant or seasonal workers, and youth are included. Discrimination on the basis of race, color, religion, sex, national origin, age, handicap, or political belief is prohibited in all programs funded under this act.

32. Privacy Protection for Rape Victims Act of 1978 (PL 540). Prohibits the admissibility of information or opinion evidence on the past sexual behavior of the alleged victim of rape or assault in a criminal case.

33. Civil Rights Act Amendments of 1978 (PL 95-555). Prohibits discrimination on the basis of sex and pregnancy or pregnancy-related conditions.

34. Educational Amendments of 1978 (PL 95-561). Includes Part C under Title IX, "Women's Educational Equity Act," whose purpose is to provide educational equity for women in the United States, and which establishes the "National Advisory Council on Women's Educational Programs." This is the Title that has generated so much concern over equity in educational opportunities in all areas, including sports.

35. Nurse Training Amendments of 1979 (PL 96-76). Extends through fiscal 1980 the program of assistance for nurse training. Requires the Secretary of Health, Education, and Welfare to study to determine the need to continue federal financial support for nursing education beyond that date. This law required a tremendous amount of effort for passage; the next consideration of these amendments will be even more rigorous.

REFERENCES

Dumas RG: Synopses of selected women's rights legislation and legislation of particular interest to women, in *Nursing's Influence on Health Policy for the Eighties.* Kansas City Mo. American Nurses' Association, American Academy of Nursing, 1979, pp 68–73.

Statutes enacted by the 95th and 96th Congresses.

US Code Congressional and Administrative News. St Paul, Minn, West Publishing Co, 1978 and 1979 eds.

Nurses and the Women's Movement

Sarah Ellen Archer and Ruth P. Fleshman

As PART OF a study of the activities of community nurse-practitioners, in 1975 we conducted a panel of 195 community nurse-
practitioners who volunteered to complete a mailed, anonymous questionnaire. The data reported here were obtained in the second part of a
two-part study. Eighty-eight nurses or 45 percent of those surveyed,
responded (Archer, 1976). I asked the 88 respondents two questions
about the women's movement: "What influence is the women's movement having on nursing?" and "How is the women's movement influencing you?" Their responses have been published previously; we present them here because of their importance to the topic of Chapter 2
and of this book.

Before launching into their responses, we need to know a little about
the nurses who participated in the study. Table B.1 shows their regional
distribution. The largest number, 19 nurses or 22 percent, came from
New England; the Pacific region was second with 16 responses or 18
percent. Only one respondent came from the mountain region. Ony one
of the 88 was male. The largest single age group 25 to 29, contained 23
of the respondents (27 percent). Thirty percent were under 30 years of
age; 36 percent were between 30 and 39 years old; and the remaining
31 percent were 40 or older.

These respondents were a very well prepared group of nurses, much
more so than the nurse population as a whole (See Table B.2). Only three
listed "diploma" as their highest level of preparation. Seventy-two percent (63 nurses) had master's degrees. Five of these community nurse-
pratitioners had completed doctoral degrees, and three others were
enrolled in doctoral programs at the time of their participation in the
study. Table B.3 arrays the type of positions held by these community

nurse-practitioners. Forty-eight percent (41 nurses) were either exclusively involved in direct client service or held joint teaching and service positions. Thirty-eight percent (34 nurses) were nurse-managers and 10 percent (9 nurses) were faculty. Because this is such an atypical group of nurses in terms of their very high level of preparation and the proportion holding managerial or faculty positions, no generalizations regarding the total population of nurses can be made on the basis of the comments of this group of respondents.

WOMEN'S MOVEMENT'S INFLUENCE ON NURSING

Table B.4 contains a listing of the most frequently given responses to the question "What influence do you think the women's movement is having on nursing?" One fourth (22 nurses) indicated that they felt that the women's movement is helping nurses to be more assertive. Other recurrent responses were that the women's movement is increasing the recognition of nurses' skills and value, that it is providing incentives for nurses seeking increased remuneration for nursing services, and that it was increasing opportunities for and pressure to take on more responsible positions. Fifteen said that they felt that nursing had been little affected by the women's movement. Other popular ideas were that the movement had resulted in increasing collaboration and peer relationships between nurses and doctors, and presumably, between women and men; returning control of nursing to nurses; and causing some nurses to resist changes in traditional roles. By and large these responses reflect positive attitudes toward the effect of the women's movement on nursing. At least some think the political involvement of nurses is increasing. Other themes are less positive, such as the belief that the movement is hurting nursing due to backlash. Depending on one's point of view, increasing nurses' aggression and militancy as well as mobility may be either positive or negative changes. There seems to be considerable feeling that the women's movement is having some definite effects on nursing, at least among this group of nurses.

The following are selected verbatim comments respondents made to the question, "What influence do you think the women's movement is having on nursing?"

Creating pressure on top management of the organization to place nurses on decision-making committees of the organization.

Nurses are more aware of inequities in nurse-physician relationships, part of which are sex-related. Nurses are seeking greater responsibility in patient care.

Little overall. I find most nurses and doctors resistant to the changes advocated. Most women I work with continue to be subservient and compliant and unquestioning.

Immense. Recognizing that women are intelligent, responsible, and to be taken seriously has greatly decreased the tension between nurses and doctors (males). However, more women are becoming doctors, considering nursing too "feminine" a role.

At the most radical end of the spectrum, I believe it (the women's movement) attracts attention *from* nursing, e.g., turns focus to lines of work which have rejected women in the past and tends to belittle the so-called "helping professions." But overall, I think it is aiding women to take pride in work well done and to commit themselves to fields of choice, and in the long run I believe it to be a very helpful influence.

Hard to say . . . I think the women's movement points out how RNs have generally been in second-class positions for various reasons. Those RNs who became such because other opportunities were not available are increasingly dissatisfied. Some RNs who are working women, but are basically traditional, may become more defensive. I become more and more pessimistic about nursing every day. It seems the professional elitism is in our way. There are many unmet health needs and we could meet them *if* we wanted to!

1. Younger nurses are not willing to be doctor's handmaidens.
2. Making us fight harder as patient's advocates.
3. Possibly influencing older nurses to resume practice after staying home.
4. Encouraging nurses who seek positions with non-nurse employers to demand higher salaries and benefits.

It is sad, but we seem to need permission to be aggressive and confident. The women's movement is providing this permission. I see it as a human movement since men are breaking stereotypes and entering nursing. I think too that physicians are taking a second look at the potential in nurses.

Very little except with a small number of young nurses. Overall nurses have been programmed to follow orders and to think of themselves as subordinates to almost everyone. They as a group are tremendously defensive, dependent, non-risk takers.

WOMEN'S MOVEMENT'S INFLUENCE ON INDIVIDUAL NURSE

The vast majority of the community nurse-practitioner's responses to the question, "How is the women's movement influencing you?" were positive. Themes such as raising professional role expectations, reinforcing long-held beliefs about personal value, increasing assertiveness, helping others see nurses' contributions to the health team differently, increasing self-confidence, independence, and awareness of inequities are all steps in the right direction. Again, a few indicate political involvement as a result of the influence of the women's movement.

The following are selected verbatim comments respondents made in answer to the question "How is the women's movement influencing you?"

> I do not participate. I am aware of it (women's movement), but have chosen to not get involved other than the business of equal opportunity. No involvement in the emotionalism of women. I know my actions are knowledge based and I don't use the women's movement.
>
> I think they are a little melodramatic. I don't like it. They are disgusting too [sic] many, incuding me. I believe in equal pay for equal work and that's about it. I would still be happy to have the car door opened for me.
>
> Sanctioning my desire to participate actively in a career.
>
> I have become more aware of political issues, ie, the health-care delivery system.
>
> Women's rights are analogous to gay rights, black rights, other civil rights, etc. Let's not take from anyone what he/she is due. However, I don't like to be chastised by feminists who feel I should not be in leadership positions in nursing because I am a man.
>
> Very deeply—being an advocate of equal rights for women and as a dean of a primarily woman's college, I feel responsible to help faculty and students become comfortable with a "new" image of nursing and become comfortable with their female individuality.
>
> I am more assertive with male peers. Pecking order has been revised.
>
> I feel I have a right to guide my own life, I feel some loosening of the restrictions placed on what women were able to do in the past. I feel I could work and have children both.
>
> I belong to a woman's group—am the only nurse in the group. Group has more influence on my role in social situations than in things relating to work. Have better knowledge of myself as a woman, able to share feeling, and get support from other women. (See Table B.5.)

COMMENTARY

The responses of these 88 community nurse-practitioners indicate that the majority feel that the women's movement is having a positive effect on both nursing in general and on them as individuals. Some even see the relationship between the women's movement and politicization. Would that more of us not only saw the relationship but also acted to strengthen it and our political involvement.

Because of the relative invisibility of nurses in the women's movement at the present time, much more work and organizing needs to be done to increase nurses' involvement in all kinds of political activities.

Again, the intent of this book is to help expedite this process. Subsequent studies of nurses and political involvement (Archer & Goehner, forthcoming) and of nurses and the women's movement are much needed.

TABLE B.1
Regional Distribution of Respondents
(N = 88)

Region	Number	Percent
New England (ME, NH, UT, MA, RI, CT)	19	22
Pacific (WA, OR, CA, AK, HI)	16	18
South Atlantic (DE, MD, DC, VA, WV, NC, SC, GA, FL)	11	13
North East Central (OH, IN, IL, MI, WI)	9	10
Middle Atlantic (NY, NJ, PA)	8	9
West North Central (MN, IO, MO, ND, SD, NE, KS)	8	9
West South Central (AR, LA, OK, TX)	8	8
East South Central (KY, TN, AL, MI)	3	4
Mountain (MT, ID, WY, CO, NM, AZ, UT, NV)	1	1
Not Stated	5	6
Total	88	100

TABLE B.2
Highest Level of Preparation Held by Respondents
(N = 86)

Highest Level of Preparation	Number	Percent
Doctorate	5	6
Doctorate in progress	3	4
Master's	63	72
Baccalaureate	12	14
Diploma	3	4
Total	86	100

TABLE B.3
Types of Positions Held by Respondents
(N = 88)

Position	Number	Percent
Direct client services	23	27
Joint service and teaching appointment	18	21
Supervision or department chairperson	17	19
Administration	17	19
Faculty	9	10
Consultation	1	1
Research	1	1
No answer	2	2
Total	88	100

TABLE B.4
Most Frequent Responses to the Question "What Influence Do You Think the Women's Movement Is Having On Nursing?"*
(n = 88)

The Women's Movement Is:	Number
helping us to be more assertive	22
increasing recognition of nurses' skills and value	18
producing incentives for seeking increased remuneration or nursing services	17
increasing opportunities for and pressure to take on more responsible positions	16
having little effect	12
increasing peer relationships and collaboration between nurses and physicians	9
returning control of nursing to nurses	9
causing nursing to resist changes in traditional roles	9
increasing nurses' independent functioning	7
hurting nursing due to antagonism some feel toward women's movement: backlash	6
increasing aggression and militancy	5
increasing nurses' mobility	5
bringing pressure for us to expand nursing roles	4
increasing political involvement regarding Nurse Practice Acts and other issues	4
increasing public awareness of nursing's positive role in health care delivery	4
increasing desire for women's self-help activities	4

*Many respondents gave more than one answer.

TABLE B.5

Most Frequent Responses to the Question "How Is the Women's Movement Influencing You?"*

(N = 88)

The Women's Movement Is:	Number*
raising my professional role expectations and career goals	18
reinforcing long-held beliefs about my own value	14
increasing my assertiveness	11
increasing other's realization of my worth as a member of the health care team	11
making me rethink my relationships with men	11
increasing my self-confidence	11
increasing my independence	9
increasing my awareness of inequities and infringements on my rights	9
increasing my political involvement	8
causing me to take on more responsibility	7
making life more satisfying	5
making life more frustrating; pushing me to do things I don't want to	5
of very little influence	5
of no influence	5
making me less concerned about stereotyped roles of women and nurses	3
opening new career possibilities; providing better benefits at work	3

*Many respondents gave more than one answer.

REFERENCE

Archer, SE and Goehner, PA: Acquiring political clout: guidelines for nurse administrators. *Journal of Nursing Administration*, forthcoming.

A Glossary of Systems Theory Terms

All special fields have their own particular language. This glossary contains some of the most common terms used in systems theory. Knowing them will make reading about the theory easier and help you to be able to enjoy it.

Adaptation. The adjustment that systems make to enable them to survive in their environment and carry out their tasks.

Black box. An operations research term for the system's internal working that transform inputs into outputs and that are concerned with system maintenance. In the poitical systems model, Figure 5.1, the conversion processes' mechanisms for converting inputs to outputs are shown (see throughput).

Boundaries. The parameters or limits of the system that help the system to maintain its integrity and therefore to survive. An open system's boundaries permit exchanges with its environment; a closed system's boundaries do not. A primary management task in open systems is boundary maintenance.

Centralization. Usually one subsystem within a system that plays a dominant part in the operation of the whole system. Changes in the subsystem where this dominant function is centralized are reflected and amplified throughout the system.

Closed system. A system that functions without interacting with its ecosystem and therefore must depend on recycling internal resources to be able to survive. These systems are subject to the second law of thermodynamics, entropy, which predicts an eventual running down as nonrenewable resources are consumed and are therefore no longer available for use.

Consequences. The results of the outputs of the system. Outputs' effects on the environment and on the system via feedback loops are geometric rather than arithmetic—that is, each output has results that in turn have more results or consequences. These consequences go on to infinity. Planners must be concerned with consequences as far as they can be predicted. Computer simulation is a useful aid in considering and planning for the possible long-range consequences of systems' activities.

Control. Constant monitoring (cybernation) of whether and to what extent plans are being carried out and the system is functioning properly. Planning to change plans as feedback indicates change is warranted is a critical aspect of control in systems theory. Control is not a coercive term as applied to systems management.

Cybernation. A term derived from the Greek word for steersman that means guiding or correcting the system's course. Cybernation is a constant monitoring of what is actually going on in the system as a basis for making alterations or adaptations in order to keep the system moving toward its predefined goal.

Differentiation. The effect of the tendency of systems to move toward specializing and dividing the labor among the subsystems—that is, each subsystem's functions become clearly differentiated from those of other subsystems. Bureaucratic systems with their specialized departments and divisions are an example of differentiation.

Environment. The ecosystem in which the system functions. Open systems depend on their environment as a source for their inputs and as a market for their outputs. There are many factors in a system's environment that affect the system, but over which the system has no control; the environment, therefore, imposes a number of givens on the systems.

Equifinality. The sense of purposefulness with which the system adjusts itself in order to achieve its goals and to remain adapted to its environment so that it can survive. A young system may use many paths and means to reach its objectives; its approach may be quite pragmatic. As more regulatory mechanisms, such as rules and policies, are developed, the need for equifinality decreases. Regularized procedures, or hardening of the categories, reduces the need for constant monitoring to be sure that the system is proceeding as planned; there is no other way that the system can operate.

Feedback. The portion of the system's outputs that returns to the system as an input and brings with it information from the environment and other subsystems in the environment about the effects, quality, and consequences of the system's outputs as well as suggestions for changes and new outputs. Feedback may also occur internally as subsystems receive reactions from other subsystems about their work. Feedback occurs naturally in most situations; however, this natural phenomenon can be improved upon by planning feedback loops that constantly supply the system with information about its performance.

Input. Resources that come into the system from its environment and are used to maintain the system and to produce outputs.

Open system. A living system that engages in exchange relationships with its environment. In these exchanges, the system obtains inputs and produces outputs as well as retains some resources to assure its own survival.

Optimization. Modifying and adapting a system to enable it to concentrate its efforts on one particular kind of activity to achieve the best possible outputs. The principle of opportunity costs—that is, resources used for one purpose cannot be used for other purposes also—is operational here and means that optimizing one subsystem can only be done at the expense of other subsystems since some of the resources they would have received went instead to the subsystem being optimized. In systems jargon then, optimizing one subsystem results in suboptimizing all of the rest.

Outputs. The products that an open system releases into its environment.

Progressive segregation. The phenomenon in which subsystems move toward independence and unrelatedness. Progressive segregation takes two forms. The first is decay or degeneration in which the system falls apart. In the second its functions become increasingly differentiated. This second type of progressive segregation occurs in creative and evolutionary processes.

Ripple effect. The continuation of consequences as a result of a system's outputs, as illustrated in Figure 5.1. It derives its name from the effect noted when one drops an object into a calm pool: the ripples go on until the entire pool may be filled. The consequences of outputs from a system can have a ripple effect far beyond and different from those the planners may have intended or envisioned.

Steady state. A dynamic equilibrium rather than a static homeostasis. Through continuous actions and reactions the system maintains a constantly changing but stable relationship with the environment.

Subsystems. The component parts or units of a system that together make up the system. The subsystems are interrelated and interdependent so that a change in one subsystem spills over and affects all of the others.

System maintenance. The system's seeking to survive, when all else fails, by using inputs for this purpose rather than for conversion into outputs. Under normal circumstances as well as those of stress, the system uses some of the resources available to it to maintain operations.

Throughput. The process that takes place inside the system by which inputs are converted into outputs (see Black box).

From Archer SE: Politics and economics: How things really work, in Archer SE, Fleshman RP (eds): *Community Health Nursing: Patterns and Practice,* ed 2. North Scituate, MA, Duxbury Press, 1979.

Index